The Psyc of Pregi and Childbirth

Lorraine Sherr

BA Hons, Dip Clin Psychol, PhD
Senior Lecturer, Department of Public Health,
Royal Free Hospital School of Medicine, University of London

b

**Blackwell
Science**

© 1995 by
Blackwell Science Ltd
Editorial Offices:
Osney Mead, Oxford OX2 0EL
25 John Street, London WC1N 2BL
23 Ainslie Place, Edinburgh EH3 6AJ
238 Main Street, Cambridge
    Massachusetts 02142, USA
54 University Street, Carlton
    Victoria 3053, Australia

Other Editorial Offices:
Arnette Blackwell SA
1, rue de Lille, 75007 Paris
France

Blackwell Wissenschafts-Verlag GmbH
Kurfürstendamm 57
10707 Berlin, Germany

Blackwell MZV
Feldgasse 13, A-1238 Wien
Austria

First published 1995

Set by DP Photosetting, Aylesbury, Bucks
Printed and bound in Great Britain by
Hartnolls Ltd, Bodmin, Cornwall.

DISTRIBUTORS
Marston Book Services Ltd
PO Box 87
Oxford OX2 0DT
(*Orders:* Tel: 01865 791155
        Fax: 01865 791927
        Telex: 837515)

North America
Blackwell Science, Inc.
238 Main Street
Cambridge, MA 02142
(*Orders:* Tel: 800 215-1000
            617 876-7000
        Fax: 617 492-5263)

Australia
Blackwell Science Pty Ltd
54 University Street
Carlton, Victoria 3053
(*Orders:* Tel: 03 347-5552)

A catalogue record for this title is available
from the British Library

ISBN 0–632–03388–6

Library of Congress
Cataloging-in-Publication Data
Sherr, Lorraine.
    The psychology of pregnancy and
    childbirth/Lorraine Sherr.
        p.   cm.
    Includes bibliographical references
    and index.
    ISBN 0–632–03388–6
    1. Pregnancy–Psychological aspects.
    2. Childbirth–Psychological aspects.
    I. Title.
    RG560.S47   1995
    618.2′4′019–dc20   94-48263

To
Liora
Lilian, Lottie
Avrill & Cheryl
Sally, Dolly, Fanyse & Joy
My Female Line

Contents

Acknowledgements

In my opinion personal experience and academic pursuit are closely linked. The birth of my four children Ari, Ilan, Yonatan and Liora, and the baby we lost, prompted my own navigation through the vast literature of childbirth culminating in this book, *The Psychology of Pregnancy and Childbirth*. The writing of this book could be likened to a pregnancy, though no analgesia was offered and no maternity leave earned.

Writing a book provides one with an opportunity to acknowledge people who have contributed, directly or indirectly, intentionally or unintentionally, to the content, direction and illustration of the book. Shula Harris is acknowledged and Janis and Andy Margo should feature. Endless support from Janis Hodges was sustaining. There is the kindly midwife who nursed me through sixteen hours of labour prior to my emergency section, the one who failed to introduce herself when my first baby was delivered, the one who was unable to tell me my blood pressure recording because the information was regarded as confidential (an example of behaviour which has subsequently been used in many lectures); the one who delivered my second baby and showed me the true meaning of a professional. No thanks to the doctors responsible for inserting needles into my veins during my first and last delivery – these are reserved for all those who managed to stay away during my second two!

The care provided by Hugh Begg and John Smith exceeded my expectations. Meg Stacey introduced me to the concept of human relations in obstetrics and Sandra Dicks cared. I have seen those who confirm the need for compulsory training in communication skills and also lectured to many fine doctors and midwives. It is my hope that every woman in labour finds one of the latter at their side. I thank the women who spent hours recording their experiences with me and all those who participated in my research.

Finally I should acknowledge my mother Lilian, who arrived after all my babies and helped us through those early days. I look at my daughter with awe knowing what she has ahead of her – the creation of life.

Lorraine Sherr, January 1995.

Foreword

Yehudi Gordon MB BCh FRCOG FCOGSA MD
Consultant Obstetrician

I am very pleased to write the foreword for Lorraine Sherr's book which explores the psychological events which accompany the primal period – from conception to the end of infancy. Modern obstetrics and paediatrics is compartmentalised and the obstetric model is narrow, focusing to a large extent on the mechanics of labour and the apgar score at birth. As a practising obstetrician I have had an active interest in the psychological and spiritual changes which mothers, fathers and children undergo as they adapt to the transition inherent in the primal period. New parents always experience feelings and emotions related to their own childhood and often issues buried deep in the subconscious emerge and provide an opportunity for self exploration and growth. Healthcare workers are increasingly aware of the importance of the emotions which accompany the birth of a new family; providing information, care and support at this time is exciting and rewarding for the carers, especially if it helps the parents' relationship to develop and mature and helps to create a safe and secure environment for the new baby.

Readers with an interest in the subject will read this book from cover to cover and find a rich assortment of carefully researched information. It is the most complete reference text currently available, a book to be kept and used for reference whenever in-depth knowledge is needed. A significant proportion of the book explores the role of healthcare workers in the psychological adaptation to pregnancy and many aspects of healthcare are analysed including the importance of communication skills between carers and parents. Academic psychological theories, from a range of disciplines are reviewed with a modern balanced, but critical overview. Covering a range of subjects from preconception to late infancy, *The Psychology of Pregnancy and Childbirth* explores a broad spectrum from common daily experiences to rare pathological events.

The Psychology of Pregnancy and Childbirth contains a wealth of information about the needs of new families and will be of interest to psychologists, counsellors, doctors, midwives and nurses. Lorraine Sherr, as a mother of four children, an academic and clinical psychologist, and a lecturer is undoubtedly qualified to write this book.

Introduction

The experience of childbirth is a complex series of events which take place over an extended period of time. It rarely simply spans the nine months of gestation, but is the product of a lifetime of learning, planning and social influence. The nine months may be experienced as an eternity or an instant. The culmination of pregnancy – the birth of a baby – has consequences for the individual for the rest of an individual's life.

Although the academic study of such events is often piecemeal, it is imperative to capture the essence of the experiences in order to understand them, plan and provide good quality care. Psychology, the science of human understanding, is intricately bound up with procreation at many stages, and can aid a better understanding of the core experience of childbirth.

This book sets out to explore these theoretical relationships in depth. A brief understanding of psychology with its different specialities is followed by an overview of some health-related psychological theories, showing how these may be applicable in the field of childbirth. There are some fundamental counselling approaches which will permeate many of the following chapters. These will be set out initially and then enlarged upon within the text.

Psychological applications to childbirth apply not only to the recipient of care, but also have relevance to staff. Chapter 2 sets out major staff issues associated with stress and support. Chapter 3 provides an overview, from a psychological standpoint, of many of the issues which precede pregnancy, such as contraception, pregnancy decisions and fertility issues. This is followed by an exploration of some of the hurdles in staying pregnant (Chapter 4) with a dialogue on termination of pregnancy, pregnancy loss and allied care. Chapter 5 is concerned with communication, a key theme within pregnancy care, and examines the relevant issues, theory and applications in detail. Pregnancy is then examined in Chapter 6 with an in-depth discussion of antenatal care, ante-natal provision and the experiences of pregnant women. Although there are many experiences which are common to all mothers, staff need to be aware of a wide range of unusual or special circumstances which they may well face in their clinical practice. These are outlined in Chapter

7 and include descriptions of abuse in pregnancy, suicide, HIV infection and AIDS, teenage and older pregnancies, women with surgical or medical conditions, rape and many other such situations. Chapter 8 outlines psychological knowledge on the process of birth; Chapter 9 provides an overview of the psychological conditions associated with childbirth. Chapter 10 reviews studies which examine the effect of the baby on the family whilst Chapter 11 looks closely at stillbirth and neo-natal death. The following chapter (Chapter 12) gives an overview of sexual functioning on becoming a parent. Chapter 13 focuses on the development of the young child. Finally, Chapter 14 looks at mental and health problems which children and their families may have to face.

Chapter 1

Psychology and Pregnancy

Psychological insight

Psychological insight can help at many stages in the process of pregnancy and childbirth. Six key stages of such insight have been identified as behaviour change, communication, psychosomatic issues, coping with pregnancy and childbirth, treatment related issues and the whole input of health education.

Behaviour change

The study of human behaviour opens access to a wide area of under-standing concerning behaviour change, triggers, maintainers and relapse. It is important to consider the processes of development over time and how these change as a result of circumstances, social influence, cognitive beliefs, and internal and external triggers. Areas of relevant study for childbirth encompass knowledge of early infant development, transition to parenthood and the impact of pregnancy on behaviour.

Doctor patient communication

Within both clinical and social psychology, a strong tradition of insight has been gathered which explains elements of the doctor patient re-lationship, with a particular focus on communication. This body of knowledge applies to many of the client/professional (and at times professional/professional) interactions which can occur throughout pregnancy, labour, delivery and the post partum period. The theoretical approach which this insight takes to these encounters allows both for an understanding of the underlying processes, and an evaluation of efficacy in terms of outcome satisfaction and behaviour.

Psychosomatic factors

At some level there is an interaction between the psyche and somatic expression of symptoms. In some circumstances the interactions may be trivial, whereas in others they may account for major variation. They therefore need careful attention and integration into the study of pregnancy and childbirth, in order to anticipate the extent to which psychological contributions interact with biological conditions. This extends to cause, expression, experience and subsequent adjustment.

Psychological adjustment

Psychological insight provides access to an understanding of individual coping mechanisms, irrespective of stresses or social circumstances. It can also help to understand the facilitators and hurdles encountered within the process of coping. Coping with childbirth and its related upheaval is a key element in adjustment and also heralds potential avenues for intervention.

Treatment

Psychological science is not restricted to understanding human behaviour, but has evolved a distinct branch for intervention and treatment. Various psychological methods and models of care and treatment can be used to help those encountering challenge, change or trauma. There are many diverse treatment interventions which could be harnessed in the progress of childbirth, including areas such as the management of pain, the organization of wards, the regimens of care, emotional adjustment and the accommodation of the protocols of medical interventions.

Health education

Psychological insight is not only reactive to problems, but may be incorporated into prevention and education initiatives. Health education is a prime example of this and has many applications in the childbirth area. In general, such interventions are associated with the pursuit of good health, utilizing techniques such as information transfer, understanding, compliance and behaviour change.

Areas of psychology explained

Psychology as a discipline has several areas of specialization, many of which can contribute to an understanding of reproduction – some directly, others indirectly. Sadly, much of this knowledge is locked up within the body of psychology and rarely emerges from ivory towers into the labour wards. This chapter will briefly describe the major areas of psychology which may be relevant to childbirth, in direct childbirth-related studies, or in parallel areas where findings may be applicable. The tools of psychology, such as research, observation, understanding human relations and interventions, can also be brought to good use in understanding childbirth. Some of these, especially those associated with counselling, will be elaborated.

Clinical psychology

This refers to the specialized branch of psychology which deals with both normal and abnormal psychological states, including trauma. Treating these conditions involves intervention and support and much of the literature on the subject provides a vast range of research on counselling. These areas are directly relevant to childbirth. This book explores some of the major themes such as anxiety and depression in and around pregnancy and the normal and abnormal states which may be associated with childbirth or child rearing. It also examines clinical understanding of emotional trauma and medical events which may be part of many women's experience of childbirth.

Social psychology

This is the psychology relating to humans within their social environment, with all its accompanying expectations and influences. This type of psychology therefore has direct relevance to childbirth. One of the most important bodies of research in this area concerns the understanding of humans operating within groups. Environmental factors may also influence behaviour and these may range from the simple physical surroundings of a maternity unit, to the complex birth environments with their rules, norms, strictures and impacts on the labouring mother. In addition, social psychology provides much insight into negotiations which may be relevant. Mothers are constantly 'negotiating' health care. Staff may be negotiating work routines, policy and procedures. In particular, much of the literature in this area on communication can be of direct relevance.

Social psychology attempts to provide an understanding of attitudes and attitude formation and this can be directly applied to aid an understanding of reactions to childbirth, health behaviours and medical personnel. Attitude change can only be attempted with a comprehension of attitude formation.

Medical psychology

Medical psychology includes research on the understanding and appraisal of psychosomatic disorders, and the wide impact of medicine and medical care on the psyche. The move of childbirth from home to hospital, mostly as a result of the Peel report, therefore necessitated further direct involvement by medical personnel. Although the rates for simultaneous maternal mortality were affected, such medicalization also presents hazards for both mother and child. These will be explored later in the book with relation to procedures such as induction of childbirth, episiotomy, acceleration of labour and other management techniques. The use of counselling and psychological models will be examined, looking in particular at their efficacy in minimizing the impact of any negative effects of medicalization and enhancing the positive.

Cognitive psychology

This branch of psychology is concerned with the in-depth examination of human thinking, understanding and cognitive processes such as memory, attention, information processing and perception. Many of these are relevant in applied childbirth settings. For example, memory explanations may account for adherence to medical regimens. Motivation and attention may be factors in satisfaction, understanding and compliance in medical settings. Information processing may account for the way women construct their reality during pregnancy and childbirth, how they come to understand aspects of information and how this is integrated. Decision making occurs at multiple stages from the decision to have child, to choices regarding pain management, place of birth, and parenting decisions. Decisions which are made under uncertainty, at times of stress and with varied amounts of information may occur at all stages of pregnancy and childbirth.

Cognitive science has much to contribute at all levels of understanding. For example it may provide interesting explanations of the work of the health care worker, including skilled diagnosis, patient caring and handling explained by cognitive function. Information processing models may reveal explanations for judgement errors, persuasion ramifications and satisfaction/dissatisfaction. It may also provide mental models which can help to explain varied health care behaviour, the adoption of various regimens and the reaction of all individuals within the process.

Health psychology

This area deals with all aspects of human behaviour related to health and its maintenance together with human reactions when health is challenged. Much of the psychology of childbirth literature to date has emerged from this field.

For example, theoretical models of stress and anxiety may be applied to childbirth. Such models do not tend to focus on stress as a negative emotion, but attempt to provide an understanding for stress coping and adaptation. Utilizing such theories therefore preclude blurring between the concepts of stress and strain. A problem with health psychology is that much of it focuses on ill health rather than good health whereas childbirth may be an excellent vehicle to promote the 'normality' of many health issues.

Developmental psychology

This branch of psychology focuses on human development from infant-hood until old age. Traditionally much emphasis has been placed on the developing child, but the notions of life cycles and the emerging adult are now receiving much more attention. These findings are directly applic-able to childbirth and can provide an understanding of the infant, siblings, parenting and grandparenting. Psychologists do not arbitrarily separate the process of pregnancy from development of the infant as medicine does into 'obstetrics' and 'paediatrics'.

A sub-branch of this speciality focuses on disability. This text will attempt to summarize some of the major literature on this subject, with special reference to disabled infants and the subsequent impact on their families.

Applications

The psychology of repetitive behaviour

Much routine care involves repetition of tasks. For example, antenatal care is specifically set up to monitor multiple women and this therefore involves repeated processes on many occasions. The model of repetitive behaviour evolves from construction industry such as a system for car assembly. Here the task of assembly is broken down to minute constituent components. The advantages are the ability to mass produce fairly com-plex products; the disadvantages relate to staff boredom and problems in the lack of a link between the task and the final product. When antenatal care evolves down towards this model, similar problems arise, as perceived not only by the staff but also by the pregnant women.

Repetition always runs the risk of low individualization, forgetting, depersonalization and the uninspired execution of tasks. Subjects blur and individual variation is overlooked. This may lead practitioners to see as trivial and obvious elements which are unique and enormously important to an individual woman. Repetition dulls the ability to pick up variation and nuances – the very reason why such care was set up in the first place.

Social surroundings

Much of psychology is centred around the understanding of people, how they think, behave and evolve. This should never be done in isolation of the environment where they live or work. Environmental psychology attempts to create an understanding of the way in which the environment can shape or change behaviour. Some of the most extreme examples of this school of thought emerge from the famous Zimbardo experiments (Zimbardo 1960; Zimbardo *et al.* 1965). In these studies, everyday volunteers were recruited into a 'prison' study. They were randomly allocated to roles of guards or prisoners. Despite full knowledge of the voluntary nature of the exercise, the slight environmental changes, rules and social norms rapidly affected their behaviour. Guards adopted con-trolling behavioural styles, whilst 'prisoners' become de individuated and subservient. Distress and emotional turmoil were rapidly experienced and the study was abandoned. The lessons from this powerful study must be directly learned within maternity settings. The power of the hospital and of institutionalization and roles can quickly and dramatically affect behaviour of both staff and women.

At a less dramatic level, environmental psychology examines envir-onmental effects. These include the necessity of individual personal space and personalized ownership. In the labour ward, the simple introduction of the mother's own clothing and home-like paraphernalia can ameliorate the often depersonalized atmosphere of a hospital. In special care units, a baby may not feel 'real' or 'as if it belongs' until it is dressed in his or her own clothing, surrounded by toys from the home. Within this context, one can examine the role of home births and understand the positive points of such an experience enabling greater control by the woman or couple, and making it more possible for them to undergo a major life event without completely changing their surroundings.

Environmental considerations regarding interpersonal communi-cations ought to be taken into account when planning interviews, inter-ventions, care and treatment. There is, for example, a fundamental necessity to respect personal space. There is also a need to acknowledge the dramatic influence the environment has on the emotional appraisal of the incident by both the woman and the staff. Factors to be considered include physical environment, emotional factors and cultural influence.

Physical environment
There is no substitute for a quiet and private place where interviews proceed uninterrupted. The environment is filled with technological inventions which interfere with human functioning – some by design, some incidentally. These include telephones ringing, interruptions, noise or distractions. Telephone interruptions usually take precedence over the doctor-patient encounter and the woman invariably waits during such

conversations. Note taking is another example, where pen and paper interfere with the interpersonal processes at work.

Emotional factors
The emotional environment is as important as the physical one. If a woman is to feel at ease and to trust her carers, any efforts to make explicit gestures with regard to emotional care will be positively interpreted. These include social gestures such as the availability of tea and coffee, physiological gestures such as the availability of toilets (and soft toilet paper!); friendship gestures such as photographs, name labels; dialogue gestures such as user friendly information. Prickly emotional guards are raised when nonverbal cues set out to control. These include unpleasant notes pasted on walls and doors (such as 'No Visitors'; 'Please leave the toilets in the same condition as you find them', 'No entry', 'Staff only').

Cultural influence
Cultural factors also contribute to environmental cues. When the care occurs within a single culture, these factors occur naturally. However, in most centres there are cosmopolitan clientele and obstetric departments therefore need to reach out to acknowledge their cultural needs. This can start with simple gestures such as catering for a different language, including appropriate translations of basic information, the availability of translators, or visual aids to assist when language barriers cannot be surmounted. At a more subtle level, cultural effects dictate norms and taboos; when these are not familiar to carers, grave insult and alienation can occur. If the carers have an understanding of the social norms of the society to whom they are delivering care, they may more accurately determine the success of the intervention, understand the pressures and expectations that the client may hold and the support that may be available to them.

Counselling as a model of care

A thread that must run through any psychological analysis of childbirth must be one which elaborates and incorporates counselling as a model in childbirth. Such a model refers to an approach as well as a methodology in care delivery and can be used in support of other models. Counselling skills are complex. Many problems have been encountered when health care workers have presumed that counselling skills are automatic and simply require a desire to counsel or the provision of sufficient time. Unskilled efforts to counsel often end in failure. Fig. 1.1 shows the various levels at which counselling operates.

There are various counselling philosophies and approaches, which provide widely differing theoretical understanding and methodologies. These include psychodynamic, behavioural interventions, cognitive,

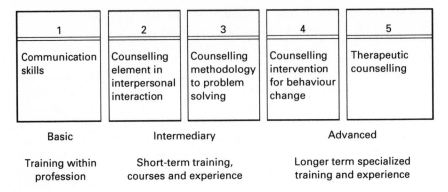

Fig. 1.1   Counselling operates at various levels.

humanistic, transactional analysis, personal construct, gestalt or eclectic approaches which all adapt according to circumstances and the individuals involved. Despite their differences, they all hold in common an understanding of the mental processes intervening between external events and an individual reaction. Counselling is an active and time consuming skill. It requires training, practice and feedback.

Counselling has been formulated for multiple purposes (Sherr, 1991), as shown below.

Support
This is most notable at times of stress, trauma or crisis which typifies many of the events which occur during childbirth.

Provision of factual information
Decision making hinges upon the provision of adequate information. Health care professionals are the guardians of such information and it is to them that women are urged to turn. Counselling may be needed when supplying these details.

Judgements
Judgements are often illogical, made on limited information and not well thought out. Counselling can aid these thought processes, helping re examine courses of action, simplifying the complex or ensuring emotional factors do not cloud the issue at hand.

Decision making
There are mental or cognitive processes which intervene between an event in the world and an individual's reaction to this including the perception of such information, processing, selective attention to components, coding, storage, recall and utilization. Counselling input

into this process can allow for a reinterpretation of the environmental event, and, thereby affect the individual's reaction.

Recovery

Cognitive factors can interact with recovery, to affect the speed of recovery, the impact on the individual, medication and/or support required to facilitate recovery.

Crisis intervention

The need for counselling may be triggered by sudden, unexpected situations or crises. The quality of care given in these circumstances can depend on accessibility, prompt reaction (as crises are often of limited duration), appropriate action and direction. The aim of such counselling is to mobilize the individual as soon as possible. There is wide individual variation in response and in perception of a situation as a crisis.

Easing distress

Counselling can facilitate psychological expression at times of emotional distress and subsequently help with adjustment in the presence of such distress.

Emotional expression

There is a basic human need to talk. Emotions can be submerged or bottled up in traumatic or disturbing situations and counselling allows a safe and helpful occasion for expression of these feelings.

Problem resolution

Counselling may assist in allowing the individual to examine problems, to appraise solutions and to try these out by examining possible outcomes and reactions. This process may enhance problem resolution and promote a problem solving approach to crises in the future.

Skill acquisition

Counselling of individual members of staff may be a process during which professional skills are attended to, adjusted, created or refined.

Advice giving

This may be the form of counselling that health care workers are most familiar with. It may take the form of direct advice, e.g. take iron tablets in pregnancy. Such advice runs the risk of becoming a directive rather a suggestion.

Anticipation

Another type of counselling may take place in the form of warning or alerting interventions. This may relate to, for example, the ways in which labour can commence: a midwife may instruct a woman on the different ways in which labour can commence and how she may react. The diffi-culties with such transfers of information often arise from the fact that the health care practitioner, who is in possession of the information base, may wish to completely take over control of the situation in hand.

Facing the unfaceable
Often the fear of something is greater than the problem itself. When people are able to face up to issues much relief can be generated. Coun-selling helps clients verbalize their fears, examine possible outcomes and plan reaction strategies. This frees the client into action rather than trapping them in avoidance or denial.

Addressing behaviour
Individual expression is a complex mixture of behavioural repertoires. Some behaviours may be confrontational or maladaptive. They may have been previously effective in certain situations but are now useless or even a hindrance. The client, however, may still revert to them. Essentially people possess some behaviours which may render them vulnerable and others which are particular strengths. Counselling can highlight such strengths and draw attention to individual limitations.

Structuring self-perceptions
Thought processes can bring about emotional pain as a result of demanding (even unreasonable) internal standards, negative self per-ceptions, self criticism or denigration. If these can be identified and adjusted, much relief can be generated.

Problems arising from the counselling approach

Counselling as a tool and as a philosophy is not immune from problems. The problems are related to the theory underpinning the approach, the efficiency with which the counselling interventions occur, the available training and the client's readiness and choice to avail themselves of the facilities offered by this approach. Some problems occur when:

- Counsellors take things personally.
- Counsellors are unable to disentangle the client's problems from their own point of view.
- Counsellors attempt to take control.
- Counsellors become overwhelmed by the nature or scale of the problem.
- Counsellors attempt to dispense copious advice. There are many other places for clients to go for this.
- Counsellors ignore their gut intuitions.
- Counsellors are dishonest or false.

- Counsellors suffer from time restrictions or are unavailable when needed.
- Counsellors attempt to solve all the client's problems, thereby promoting dependency, which may be counter productive in the long-term.
- Counselling environments are not private or confidential.
- Counselling is imposed on an unwilling client.
- No limits and boundaries are set for the task of counselling.
- Training is inadequate.
- Brief exposure to basic skills is mistaken for comprehensive training.
- Staff experience burnout.
- Ethnic or cultural barriers are not recognized or respected.

As with all approaches, the counselling and psychological approach has a limited scope and is most effective when used in conjunction with other approaches.

Psychology and feminism

There is an emerging literature on feminism in psychology, much of which is focused on women and reproduction. Oakley (1980) reports that childbirth stands 'uncomfortably at the junction of the worlds of nature and culture'. Ussher (1989) goes further examining how the capacity of women to reproduce has been used to 'subjugate' women in situations where biology has been the excuse for a variety of social acts, such as exclusion from education, employment and positions of power, responsibility and trust.

From this perspective it is important to understand that the role of medicalization of childbirth may also serve to depersonalize women and goes further to pathologize what is a normal female function. Indeed, Ussher (1989) cautions that the psychological attempts to explain deviant motherhood only serve to endorse the notion of pregnancy as an illness. There is an uncanny acceptance throughout the literature that motherhood is a natural state, despite the fact that many women find it challenging, difficult or even unfulfilling (Oakley, 1986). There is a predisposition in the literature to examine social experience through biological criteria.

The last ten years have been marked by an evolving change in the medical profession, in how it approaches pregnancy and childbirth and how this affects women. The natural childbirth movement has been seen as the major trigger for this change. Yet Ussher (1989) argues that the situation is not a simple dichotomy with 'natural' and 'medical' on opposing sides. She argues convincingly that the removal of technology will not remove negative experiences (even if it affects the personal alienation encountered by the women) and that true progress can only be achieved if the whole approach to pregnant women is altered, where pregnancy is placed in context within the female life cycle as a whole. Yet even she falls into the trap of removing choice and control from women. She states that we must 'see childbirth in context, as part of the woman's whole life cycle, giving choice to the individual woman, treating her as a person and not removing control and power from her'. These are passive sentiments and do not give voice to the abilities of women to define their own roles, take their own choices, determine their own levels of control and not to articulate their existence in terms of male concepts, such as power.

These issues can be extended to the very gender specific professional distribution. Most midwives are female, and most obstetricians are male. As women permeate medicine (and this is only a development of the latter half of this century), the balance may alter. Yet women are still not in the positions of power within obstetrics to the same extent as men. At a more subtle level, those who are at a position of power may have adopted 'male' approaches to make it in a male dominated field. Thus many women cite a preference for the gender of their carer. Some prefer midwives, to ensure a female carer. Alternatively, some avoid female doctors as they feel they will not get true care or sympathy. Others avoid male doctors, as they find it difficult to relate to males on such female related issues. Some have no preference either way.

Therapeutic tools used by psychologists

Most occupations invoke the skilled use of tools or instruments. There are no microscopes or stethoscopes in psychology. Instead many of the 'tools' which are used are based on inherent human capacities, applied in a structured way. These may involve such skills as listening, talking or even silence. Some of these tools are seen as fundamental to psychological interventions and specifically so to counselling. By way of example, the next section will highlight a diverse range of tools which psychological science can invoke. Although it is not comprehensive, it will provide a vehicle to understand the diverse ways in which psychological tools can be applied to the process of pregnancy and childbirth. Many of the subjects described will emerge in different forms throughout the chapters of the book. The areas explained will include:

(1) Observation.
(2) Empirical research, with a comprehensive discussion of a variety of relevant theoretical models.
(3) Placebo effects.
(4) Decision making.
(5) Listening.
(6) Questioning.

(7) Crisis intervention.
(8) Pain understanding.
(9) Anxiety understanding.
(10) Problem solving.
(11) Lateral thinking.
(12) Emotion insight and explanation.
(13) Breaking bad news.

Observation

Observational skills reveal much of human interaction patterns which can be recorded and understood.

Nonverbal communication

Nonverbal aspects of communication include body position, facial expression, eye contact and gestures. If listening facilitates the client's expression and ease, the counsellor should face the client with good eye contact in a relaxed and comfortable manner. A counsellor will find difficulty listening to their client if they are suffering from anxiety themselves, which intrudes into the session. They will also find it hard to listen well if they are seated badly (especially behind barriers such as desks or high chairs), if they are eager to interrupt, if they have limited time, or if they are impatient.

Social structures

Uniforms are another nonverbal aspect to communication. They provide trust and symmetry in the eyes of some, yet show a barrier and control for others. Many units abandon uniforms in an attempt to make a statement about friendliness and care. Yet they may abandon some of the positive aspects of this communication inadvertently. A uniform suffices as part of an introduction. In the absence of a uniform staff must, of necessity, fully introduce themselves and explain to women their role and their status. Other apparatus may serve similar purposes. Stethoscopes around a neck indicate a doctor, length of white gowns indicate status, colour and design of head gear, sleeves and aprons all have meaning.

Empirical research

Psychology provides the social science knowledge for using empirical research to examine hypotheses, test these out and understand human behaviour, motivation and actions. Such methodology allows researchers to test out ideas, to operate at a level beyond common sense or intuition, and to explain unexpected, curious or unanticipated events.

Theoretical models

Theory is the ability to move beyond intuition. It allows for models of understanding so that generalizations can be applied to other situations and reactions can be anticipated and even predicted. Such models allow for broader understanding. As psychology is the science of human behaviour, there are numerous theoretical models proposing frameworks for processes and understanding which could be applied to the childbirth experience. A few are set out and explained here.

Theory of satisfaction

This theory (Ley, 1988) predicts a relationship between understanding and memory, which interact with the level of satisfaction. Interrelationships between these variables also show a prediction and understanding of compliance in medical behaviour. The model can be seen in Fig. 1.2. This model is discussed at length in Chapter 4, its applicability could permeate much antenatal and labour/delivery care.

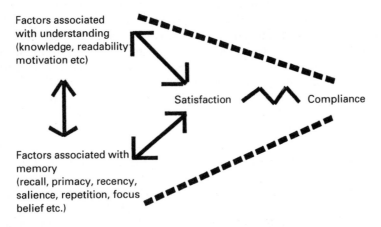

Fig. 1.2　Ley's Model of Communication.

Cognitive explanations of health beliefs and attributions (Marteau, 1989)

Marteau explains how beliefs and attributions influence the health and behaviour of the individual and can interact in health care. As such beliefs and attributions are held by both the recipient of care and the provider, a complex interaction can result. These factors can then affect care in various ways. They may affect staff decisions about treatment strategy and choice, just as they may affect patients' cognitions. a synthesis of the model is set out in Fig. 1.3.

There are numerous critiques of cognitive theories, essentially pointing out that the limitations which underpin such studies are situation or illness specific. Others have cautioned that cognitive explanations are too narrow, without sufficient regard for wider social, economic and envir-

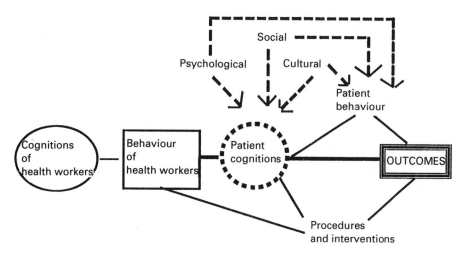

Fig. 1.3   Marteau's model of health beliefs and attributions.

onmental factors, which may have dramatic effects on illness and health behaviours (Winett, 1985).

Theories of sick roles and illness behaviour

Theories differentiate between sick roles and illness behaviour. Willmott (1989) points out the wide range of disagreement about what constitutes illness and how modern technology has been invoked to clarify some disease states. Parsons (1951) described sick roles in detail. This theory provides for social roles where sickness confers a series of expectations and obligations. These are summarized in Fig. 1.4.

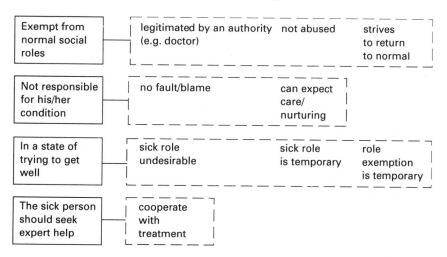

Fig. 1.4   Parson's theory of sick roles.

Limitations have been proposed (Cockerham, 1978) as the concept does not allow for the extensive observed variation and seems to be focused on acute, rather than chronic long-term illness. Parson's model also presumes a one-to-one relationship between carer and patient (often this is inappropriate – especially in childbirth where they may be multiple carers, ranging from doctor, midwife and nurse, to health visitor, anaesthetist and so on). The theory also does not take into account people who are not motivated to get well – a basic presumption of Parsons. Some theories expand on the secondary gains from illness and how individuals can adopt illness behaviour as a way of life to gain attention they require, control, sympathy, care or self satisfaction, or to avoid other painful aspects of their life that good health would necessitate them facing up to. Illness behaviour is the theoretical model which attempts to describe the behaviour that people have or adopt in direct response to illness or disease (Mechanic, 1962). A visual model is shown in Fig. 1.5.

This model allows for behaviour, observation, measurement and change. These can all usefully be incorporated into an understanding of

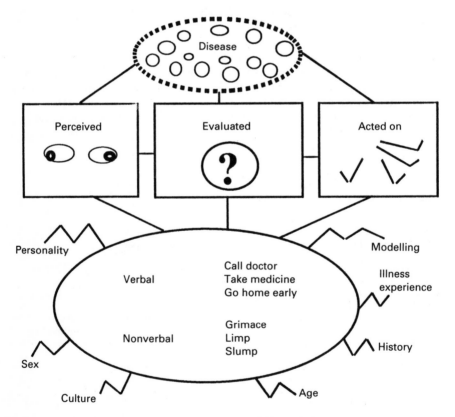

Fig. 1.5   Mechanic's model of illness behaviour.

illness behaviour and much intervention has utilized either this model or derivatives thereof. Normative studies also allow the concept of 'abnormal illness behaviour' to emerge.

Pilowsky (1984) notes the need to accommodate excessive reactions or behaviours which may be disabling, require intervention or simply accommodate individuals who deviate noticeably from the norm. Some of these states may well be observed during a variety of childbirth processes. The model is described in Fig. 1.6.

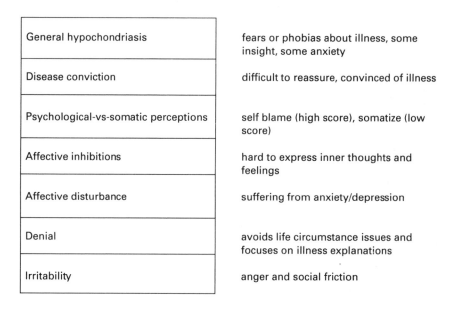

Fig. 1.6 Pilowsky's model of psychological states and illness.

Theories on centredness of care

These theories address the whole person model of care which can either be client, doctor or institution centred. Nichols (1984) has used such a model to provide critique and explanation of a variety of factors in patient handling, adjustment and reaction. For example he emphasizes the doctor-nurse centredness bias in current care and how this may prevent a comprehensive understanding of the emotional needs of seriously ill patients. It can account for problems in giving diagnoses (Ellian & Dean 1985), or in detecting the high level of emotional disturbance which is commonly found in medical care (Mayou & Hawton 1986). Maguire (1985) noted how much psychological morbidity was created by medical conditions and how infrequently staff picked this up. This may well apply to maternity care, where the focus is on the physical well-being of the mother and baby. Nichols (1984) explains how institution centred approaches make such a quest for understanding difficult to contemplate.

Factors connected with the specific institution in question can lead to many difficulties, which could go some way to explaining not only the emotional trauma and pain, but the unexpected behaviour of those caught up in the system (such as passivity, reluctance to ask questions, confusion and anger). Kornfield (1972) has explained the impact of high technology modern hospitals on an individual, as shown in Fig. 1.7.

Geographic confusion
   Where can I go?
   Where should I go?

Subcultural confusion
   Who is who?
   Who does what?
   When do they do it?
   What is good?
   What is bad?

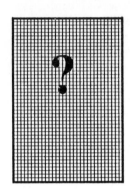

Role confusion
   How do I relate?
   How do I behave?
   How do I communicate?
   How will my needs be met?

Fig. 1.7   Kornfield's concepts on the impact of high technology on the individual.

Theories of control

Theories of control incorporate a variety of notions and have potential wide application in health care generally and childbirth specifically. Thompson (1981) has described a theory of control contributions as shown in Fig. 1.8.

Other theories related to control include: locus of control (Rotter, 1966). This is a theory which attempts to quantify the extent to which individuals perceive themselves or others (or even chance) to be in control of important events. There are some problems with this theory when it tries to predict outcome based purely on the locus of control levels. In doing so,

Type of control	Activity	Situations
Information control	Learning, gather knowledge	Preparation
Behavioural control	Acting on a situation	Preparation
Cognitive control	Altering thinking about a situation	Preparation Accidents Disability
Retrospective control	Making a decision after the event about possible control	Accidents Emergencies Disabilities

Fig. 1.8   Thompson's model of control.

it may fail to differentiate between outcomes (good or bad) when individuals may vary their attributions of control differently. It may also fail to allow for a continuum of experience, where not all individuals feel in personal control (internal), or abdicate control control to others (external). Some oscillate, depending on mood, situation or time, whilst others feel a mixture of the two.

Health related situations have a variety of control problems. These may be associated with the following (Brewin, 1988):

- The degree of control any person has. The level of this control may be unclear. If there is no clarifying information, there will be a great reliance on their self-generated notion of control.
- Control may reside partly in the hands of others.
- Control may not be a unitary concept (either present or absent). Instead, it may fluctuate in degree and have several different ways for exertion. Individuals may show preferences for one way or another without necessarily abdicating control.
- Control in childbirth has been operationalized in terms of antenatal classes, choice in pain management, and coping styles.

Theory of learned helplessness
Seligman (1975) has put forward a theory which takes the notion of control much further and attempts to understand fully and explain psychological states. The experience of uncontrollability can lead to a generalized view that outcomes are inevitable, despite their efforts. This in turn can lead to a learned helplessness in the individual, who perceives that whatever their actions, reactions which are out of their control will still occur. This is different from hopelessness (Alloy *et al*, 1988) which attributes feelings of foreboding and negative outcome to the affected individuals.

Placebo effects
Placebo effects are interesting phenomena which occur when patient reaction is noted, in the absence of true intervention. Rather, the strength of their belief and/or expectations is so strong that they form the presumed trigger for outcome observations. These have been described by Ross & Olson (1982) and Richardson (1989) and are formulated in Fig. 1.9.

Theory of reasoned action
This theory (Fishbein & Ajzen, 1975; Ajzen 1988; Ajzen & Fishbein, 1980) sets out to describe the intervening variables between knowledge, attitudes and behaviour and to explain some of the disparate findings in the literature. Earlier studies showed systematically that knowledge and attitudes contributed to behaviour but did not account for it in totality.

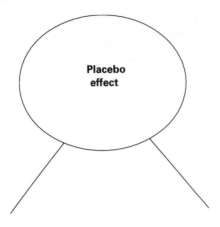

How

Patient factors
but inconsistent research findings
patients vary with occasion

Treatment factors
More serious interventions greater effects
Physical characteristics of placebo
(dose, regimen, size and colour have
effects)

Therapist
Status
Style
Impact

Why
Reassure and relax patient
Encourage positive viewing
of symptoms
Responding to attention
Conditioned responses from
previous treatments
Outcome expectations
Reporting biases/errors

Fig. 1.9   Placebo effects.

Shifting either knowledge or attitudes was often necessary for behaviour change, but in many studies it was not sufficient. The theory attempted to provide a wider base of ingredients, notably social and subjective norms, the influence of others and the mediating effects of intentions, to account for behaviour and behaviour change. The theory is based on the underlying assumptions of rational thinking and perceives behaviour as emanating solely from cognitive processes.

In field work, the model has proved more helpful than earlier linear models, but it still cannot be used to predict behaviour change with certainty.

Health belief model
This model examines the underlying triggers associated with health beliefs and their relative strengths. Such beliefs allow an individual to evaluate

personal perceived susceptibility to negative health threats, to evaluate the seriousness of the health threat, to appraise the efficacy of protection strategies and to assess the obstacles to action. Behaviour change must therefore be aimed at these fundamental belief systems and can only occur when one or more have been addressed. The methodology for addressing these may vary, but often utilizes information input. Personality theory has been grafted into this explanation to account for perceptions about efficacy for change and to adjust the barriers and facilitators of change inherent in the individual's belief in their own ability to bring about change, foster or harness the requisite skills and gain support.

An individual's readiness to carry out health related behaviour is related to three elements:

Motivations which interact with their initial willingness to seek out help and their fundamental intention to adhere to the action plan suggested.

Perceptions of threat, which are related to their beliefs about the severity and importance to them personally of the medical threat or hazard before them.

Efficacy of the remedial action, which is their personal endorsement that the intervention or adjustment will remedy or adjust the undesirable outcome.

Again, this theory is reliant on conscious decision making and takes no account of behaviour which may not be available or accessible to conscious planning. Problems with the theory arise when detailed examinations of information levels, adjustments and beliefs are made. For example, it may be more difficult to shift a strong health belief than to adjust behaviours based on a previous knowledge gap.

Attributional theories
Attributional theories encompass the various attempts by researchers to explain observed events and examine how such explanations may modify or adjust future behaviour. In health care studies, many people have come to causal conclusions about a variety of aspects of these conditions. Change can come about when these attributes are challenged, addressed or adjusted.

Attributional processes may commence early on in any condition. Initially, people will need to attribute cause and explanation to their feelings and experience. There is a wide body of psychological research attempting to explain and understand causal attributions and the role they play in subsequent experience and behaviour within health care settings. As attributions can have far reaching consequences, they may play a key role in understanding health related behaviour, behaviour change and emotional reactions to health threats.

Attributional explanation is seen as a necessity in cognitive coping, rationalizing of threatening health events and reactions to adversity. For some, explanation may be a luxury item, but such attributional theories would see them as a necessity rather than a luxury.

Decision making

There are numerous theories on decision making that are of growing importance in medicine generally, and obstetric care specifically. The changing models of care actively foster decision input from women. Decision making has a role at multiple points within the process of care, commencing from the choice to seek care, the degree of compliance, life style changes and options of choice (Redelmeier, 1993).

It is rare for people to make decisions based on a complete rational examination of all options and pathways available to them. A number of factors intervene and in reality, decisions are usually based on heuristics and simplified processes, limited by available information and mediated by situational factors, biases, stresses and social norms/pressure. Bell *et al.* (1988) conclude that there are multiple errors in the decision making pathways in applied medical settings. Such errors can be time limitations which limit rational processes, misinformation, distrust, certainty (or uncertainty), confusion or fear. Redelmeier (1993) outlines a number of factors which interact with nonoptimal decision making. These include:

Safety and danger perceptions
Decisions are sometimes affected, when they rely on a total understanding of danger and safety levels. People tend to categorize these levels at the extremes with little focus on compromise or intensity.

All or nothing options
There is a disproportionate appeal of options which offer total risk elimination, compared to a partial elimination or reduction.

Framing
It has been clearly articulated that decision making can be dramatically affected by how information is framed. Framing effects can be a function of presentation or interpretation. The only way around such a framing bias is to ensure that those who have to make a decision are given access to all aspects of the situation in hand.

Presentation
The way in which information or a set of facts is presented may dramatically alter the perceptions and understanding of a recipient. These may in turn influence behaviour.

Retrospective bias
Studies which employ retrospective evaluations suffer from bias, as the final outcome may affect what they seek out and report. Often such outcome studies are used to simply provide a summary of the facts, instead of more sound prospective investigations into why the facts happened.

Predicting emotional reactions to the unknown
It is difficult for an individual to fully conceptualize or appreciate the meaning and impact of emotions, especially if the decision is made prior to any experience with the emotion it is anticipated they will feel.

Learning
Past experience can provide a model for learning. However, memory for sensations is often inaccurate. The intensity of concerns can also put disproportionate emphasis on one aspect of a course of action, which will affect the outcome more than another aspect.

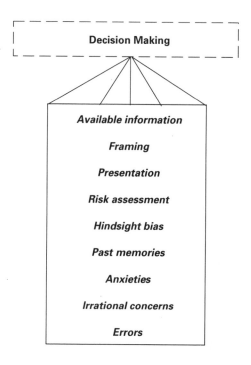

Fig. 1.10   Factors influencing decision making.

Listening

Listening is a difficult skill. Social dialogue teaches turn taking, interruptions and self assertion. Counselling runs contrary to these instincts. Listening includes the words and content of the dialogue and other factors such as pitch, volume, timing, hesitations and flow. At the same time, there may be a host of non-verbal aspects to the communication process which may punctuate the dialogue and at times run counter to it.

Questioning

Questions form a major theme in all dialogue. Counsellors need to be aware of the number of questions they use and the type of questioning style they adopt. These often may determine how the interviewee will answer the questions and may dictate the course of the conversation. Generally questions fall into open and closed categories.

Closed questions

These are questions which limit the scope and extent of the reply – often when the answer is a factual one such as: *'What is the date of your last period?' 'How old are you?'*

These usually prompt reduced or monosyllabic replies. They have a specific role, but when used out of context they may have unfortunate limitations. They serve the function of providing clarification, pacing a wary or shy client, building up confidence or opening up slowly at times of stress or trauma, but their effect is usually to attribute power to the questioner and lower status to the respondent. Short answers from a series of closed questions may hide detail, may dictate the response or may give out messages about acceptable and desirable replies.

Open questions

Open questions allow for freedom of expression and may therefore be time consuming, but achieve high levels of success at eliciting detail and complete histories. Open questions allow the individual to talk freely and to recount their situation in their own way. They remove bias and value judgements, encouraging the client to talk whilst validating notions of an interested, caring listener. They may, however, be perceived as threatening and individual reactions are unpredictable.

Funnelling

Funnelling is an intriguing procedure which may be utilized as a questioning strategy to produce a variety of outcomes. Sherr (1986) explains funnelling as a process where each open question marks the commencement of a new funnel in a diverse subject topic. Questions then progress to become closed, pointed and precise, thereby narrowing and constricting the area of enquiry and the range of possible responses. An untrained or unskilled questioner may rapidly progress down the funnel without the skill to expand the topic or embark on a new funnel if required. Furthermore, such narrowing may engender a 'subservient' client who may tailor responses so as to avoid transgression of the funnel boundaries (Sherr, 1986). Questions which funnel are often helpful in sifting through large chunks of information and in focusing a client towards a specific end. They run the risk of directing answers towards the bias of the questioner.

Judgemental questions

Although psychological interventions aim at achieving non-judgemental status, other models of care do not set out to achieve this. It can thus be difficult to remain non-judgemental, and questioning can make the process and the nature of the judgements obvious, together with the accompanying implied censure, disdain or appraisal. When judgemental questions are perceived, usually clients respond to their need to be appreciated or to meet with approval, rather than supplying accurate responses. This may therefore set up a barrier or resistance which impedes trust and may well hinder the helping process.

This may account for many findings in the literature. For example, most abuse during pregnancy goes unreported. Risk factors for sexually transmitted diseases are often not disclosed and drug use or similar problems may only come to light months after initial meetings.

Silence

Silence is usually uncomfortable and in social dialogue it is quickly filled. In counselling it is used with care. Silence usually has a purpose. It presents a message of its own and may often speak louder than words. It may simply provide time and courage for a client to divulge their story, or it can challenge and prompt the client to think deeper, to examine the content of the conversation or even to move to a deeper plane of disclosure and dialogue. Silence in excess is threatening and should be used with care.

Intervention

A crisis arises when an individual is exposed to an unanticipated circumstance. Crisis situations can occur at many points during childbirth. Crisis reactions include:

Anxiety – This may be expressed as psychological disarray or physical symptoms such as heart palpitations, dry mouth, sweating, stomach churning, shaking knees (or body), increase in body heat.
Panic/terror –This results when the situation is overwhelming and the person feels immobilized, unable to act or react and frozen into their panic without recourse to any form of action or relief.
Uncomfortable feelings – The individual is torn between their feelings of helplessness and their desire to overcome these uncomfortable feelings and relieve their acute anxiety.
Fixation – At this point, the situation is all consuming and may impede other areas of the individual's existence.

Crisis interventions are often determined (or limited) by the amount of access the counsellor has at key timing points. Crisis intervention should aim to:

(1) Directly address the problem.
(2) Break the crisis down into manageable segments when the enormity of the problem leads to the client's mental paralysis.
(3) Be honest. The counsellor needs to be the person who acknowledges the crisis and the full extent of its impact on the individual, rather than deny or provide meaningless platitudes.
(4) Give attention to the individual. The client may need to talk the crisis through. They may have a full and long story which needs to be heard. The counsellor ought to listen to the story as told by the affected person (rather than the counsellor's imagined or personal reaction to a similar situation) which will determine how they cope.
(5) Facilitate decision making. Crisis help comes in the form of facilitating decision making rather than imposing personal solutions.
(6) Ensure that the client is moved to action. This can be done by agreement, contracts or pacing, showing the client one of the pathways out of their paralysis.
(7) Follow up the situation. Survival of a crisis does not imply that an individual has handled the situation to the end. Ideally, it should provide them with insight into the processes they adopted, so that in a subsequent similar situation they can cope with more ease.
(8) Aid prevention. Crisis intervention may be appropriate as an access point to counselling, but often a situation could have been avoided or handled better in the first place if counselling strategies had previously been adopted.

Pain understanding

Pain phenomena are not fully understood. Wherever pain comes from (and this is often a useless question when there is no relief for the pain, despite its origins) the experience of pain is essentially a psychological event. Clients can be helped by minimizing pain, by dulling pain experience, or by being distracted from pain, perhaps incorporating some physical measures (such as posture, stance or muscle tone) both to lessen pain and prevent the development of secondary pain. Relaxation techniques can facilitate pain relief.

Much of the pain literature from psychology has not been fully integrated into the major areas of pain relief and pain management in labour, or even for minor procedures such as amniocentesis or blood specimens, although slowly some ideas are permeating. These ideas should facilitate the following:

● Lead to an understanding of the underlying mechanisms which account for pain experience (such as the Gate theory by Melzack 1973, 1983).

- Appreciate the psychological and social/cultural influences on the perception of pain.
- Evaluate the effects of the context in which pain occurs on the subjective experience.
- Explore the interventions which may affect pain experience, pain fear, thresholds and management. These generally include preparation, emotional and personality factors, cultural and situational factors, biofeedback, variations in pain behaviour, cognitive treatments to challenge and modification of pain related thoughts and cognitions.

These can affect the amount of pain experienced, the action taken in the presence of pain, the level of surrounding stress, and anguish in the anticipation and experience of pain.

Anxiety understanding

Anxiety can be experienced as an unpleasant emotion. Women need to be aware of the link between their mind and their bodies and to understand the flight/fright reaction. They may benefit from anxiety reduction, amelioration or simply understanding their bodily reactions and gathering reassurance from the fact that it is 'normal'. There is a presumption that anxiety is a negative emotion. This is not necessarily accurate. Any intense emotion can be experienced as negative. Yet there may be a purpose for emotion and the removal of the emotion may conceal the purpose it is serving. Theories certainly point to the function of anxiety and how some levels of anxiety are facilitative in coping strategies.

Brewin (1988) has described some theoretical approaches to anxiety (and depression) in some detail and these may help understand the experience. He concludes that generalized anxiety is often characterized by various attentional biases which focus on the negative, particularly threat or danger. In depression, positive material is often less readily introduced to consciousness than negative material. Differential accessibility may play a role in increased negative expectations and provide input where this can be changed. For some individuals, anxiety and depression may then pre-set which pieces of new information are selectively attended, processed, recalled and integrated. Such styles may then perpetuate or feed anxiety and depression levels unless checked. Brewin notes that, despite some limitations of an information processing approach, there has been much support for this theory, which allows for possible pathways to affect thought processes and schemas and to improve mood.

Problem solving

Emotional trauma often renders decision making difficult, impossible or non-fruitful. Computers make logical decisions – people do not. The process of decision making is fascinating. It is often situation and personality dependent. It may rely on simple availability of information without much contemplation of the consequences and implications of the decision. Social norms, expectations, views of self, and non-relevant information may all cloud decision making. In everyday life, this often does not matter. However, in crisis times problem solving and decision making may be key elements in adjustment. Helping to think through options, imagine positive and negative outcomes and plan strategies to deal with these may allow clients to mobilize their decision making abilities and ensure that optimum decisions are made, even in difficult or limited situations.

Lateral thinking

Alternative framing is a technique which may help move a problem forward which cannot be simply resolved. When problems are faced they may be overwhelming or be viewed in a way which renders them difficult to counter. One method of helping is for the counsellor to assess the problems objectively and to help the patient see other sides, or different sides, to the problem.

Emotion insight and explanations

Emotional reactions can be experienced with such intensity that they can overwhelm people. Heron (1977) differentiates anger, fear, grief and embarrassment. When overwhelmed by emotions, understanding is necessary to eliminate fear and allow for unrestricted choices. Extreme emotional experiences can affect a woman's self-image, can engender feelings of helplessness and hopelessness, can lead to constant failure when unattainable (or unrealistic) goals are set or can impede full functioning by misattributions of causality. In such circumstances, people may constantly attribute events to internal causes and therefore feel helpless about control over their life. Help can be given by allowing people to express their emotions, by working on their self-image and by altering attributions.

Breaking bad news

In obstetrics there may, sadly, be occasions of bad news. These may be associated with grief and bereavement and are expounded in the relevant chapters in this book. Bad news training has become more widely accepted after the widespread acknowledgement of the pain and suffering experienced by unskilled handling of bad news. Such untrained attempts often compounded the experience for people at the very time when they were needy or vulnerable. Psychological understanding of emotions has allowed some insight into the experience of giving and receiving bad news. Based on this understanding, intervention can provide an optimum reaction to bad news situations.

Themes of the book

Within this broad context, the chapters of this book will explore a variety of themes, all focusing on the psychological literature. There are vast bodies of supplementary literature available for some areas of study; others there is none. Some topics are briefly covered and readers will be referred to good source text books to follow up these topics. The major themes which will be described are:

- The impact of childbirth on the mother and father.
- The psychological cost of the medicalization of childbirth.
- The psychological understanding of processes and procedures during pregnancy, childbirth and the early neonatal period.
- The jump between empirical and research findings and practical applications.

Throughout this text, quotations from women themselves will be used, as their words often speak louder than many columns of data or tables of empirical studies. These quotations were drawn from interviews in the course of a study on communications in obstetrics (Sherr, 1989).

References

Ajzen, I. (1988) *Attitudes, Personality and Behaviour.* Open University Press, Milton Keynes.

Ajzen, I. & Fishbein, M. (1980) *Understanding Attitudes and Predicting Social Behavior.* Prentice Hall, New Jersey.

Alloy, L., Abramson, L., Metalsky, G. & Hartlage, S. (1988) The hopelessness theory of depression: attributional aspects. *B. Jnl. of Clin. Psych.*, 27, 3–18.

Bell, D., Raiffa, H. & Tuersley, A. (1988) *Decision Making.* Cambridge University Press, New York.

Brewin, C. (1988) *Cognitive Foundations of Clinical Psychology.* Lawrence Erlbaum, Hove.

Cockerham, W. (1978) *Medical Sociology.* Prentice Hall, Englewood Cliffs.

Ellian, M. & Dean, G. (1985) To tell or not to tell the diagnosis of multiple sclerosis. *Lancet*, ii, 27–8.

Fishbein, M. & Ajzen, I. (1975) *Beliefs Attitude Intention and Behavior: an Introduction to Theory and Research.* Addison Wesley, Reading, Massachusetts.

Heron, J. (1977) *Behaviour Analysis in Education and Training Human Potential.* Research Project, University of Surrey, Guildford, Surrey.

Kornfield, D. (1972) The hospital environment: its impact on the patient. *Advances in Psychosomatic Medicine*, 8, 252–70.

Ley, P. (1988) *Communicating with Patients: Improving Communication Satisfaction and Compliance*, Croom Helm, London.

Maguire, P. (1984) Communication skills and patient care. In *Health Care and Human Behaviour* (eds. A. Steptoe and A. Mathews), Academic Press, London.

Maguire, P. (1985) Improving the detection of psychiatric problems in cancer patients. *Soc. Sci. and Medicine*, 20, 819–823.

Marteau, T. (1989) Health beliefs and attributions. In *Health Psychology* (ed. A. Broome) Chapman and Hall, London.

Mayou, R. & Hawton, K. (1986) Psychiatric disorder in the general hospital. *B. Jnl. of Psych.*, 149, 172–90.

Mechanic, D. (1962) *Students under Stress: a Study in the Social Psychology of Adaptation.* Free Press, New York.

Mechanic, D. (1986) The concept of illness behaviour: culture situation and personal predisposition. *Psychological Medicine*, 16, 1–7.

Melzack, R. (1973) *The Puzzle of Pain.* Basic Books, New York.

Melzack, R. (1983) *The Challenge of Pain.* Penguin Books, Harmondsworth.

Nichols, K. (1984) *Psychological Care in Physical Illness.* Croom Helm, Beckenham.

Nichols, K. (1989) Institutional versus client centred care in general hospitals. In: *Psychology and Health* (ed. A. Broome) Chapman and Hall, London.

Oakley, A. (1980) *Women Confined.* Martin Robertson, Oxford.

Oakley, A. (1986) Feminism, motherhood and medicine: who cares: In *What is Feminism?* (Ed. J. Mitchell and A. Oakley). Basil Blackwell, Oxford.

Parsons, T. (1951) *The Social System*, Free Press, New York.

Pilowsky, I. (1984) Pain and illness behaviour assessment and management. In *Textbook of Pain* (eds Wall and Melzack) Churchill Livingstone, London.

Redelmeier, D., Rozin, P. & Kahneman, D. (1993) Understanding patient's decisions – cognitive and emotional perspectives. *Jnl. of the American Medical Association*, July 7, **270**(1) 72–6.

Richardson, P. (1989) Placebos: their effectiveness and modes of action. In *Health Psychology* (Ed. A. Broome) Chapman and Hall London.

Ross, M. & Olson, J. (1982) Placebo effects in medical research and practice. In *Social Psychology and Behavioural Medicine* (Ed. J. Eiser) John Wiley, Chichester.

Rotter, J. (1966) Generalised expectancies for internal versus external control of reinforcement. *Psychological Monographs*, 80, 1, 609, 1– 28.

Seligman, M.E.P. (1975) *Helplessness On Depression Development and Death.* Freeman, San Francisco.

Sherr, L. (1986) *Client interviewing for Lawyers.* Sweet and Maxwell, London.

Sherr, L. (1989) *Communication and Anxiety in Obstetric Care.* Unpublished PhD Thesis, Warwick University.

Sherr, L. (1991) *HIV and AIDS in Mothers and Babies.* Blackwell Scientific Publications, Oxford.

Thompson, S. (1981) Will it hurt less if I can control it? A complex answer to a simple question. *Psychological Bulletin*, 910, 89–101.

Ussher, J. (1989) *The Psychology of the Female Body.* Routledge, London.

Willmott, M. (1989) The sick role and related concepts. In *Psychology and Health.* (Ed. A. Broome) Chapman and Hall, London.

Winett, R. (1985) Ecobehaviour assessment in life styles concepts and methods. In *Measurement strategies in health psychology* (Ed. P. Karoly), John Wiley and Sons, New York.

Zimbardo, P. (1960) Involvement and communication: discrepancy as determinants of opinion conformity, *Jnl. of Abnormal and Social Psychology*, 60, 86–94.

Zimbardo, C., Weisenberg, I., Firestone, I. & Levy, B. (1965) Communicator effectiveness in producing public conformity and private attitude change. *Jnl. of Personality*, 33, 233–55.

Chapter 2

Staff Stress and Support Groups

In order to provide quality care, staff must not limit their understanding of the psychological experience of childbirth solely to the recipient of care. The complexity of the process demands a clear understanding of the emotional factors for care providers as well as for women and their families. Obstetric work is a speciality which may generate much staff stress and anxiety. Provision of care must therefore include an analysis of this stress together with an evaluation of support and its efficacy.

Staff support

Staff support is an insurance policy for continued high level input. Unsupported staff soon reach breaking point and cannot be expected to provide high level input over extended periods of time. Some staff feel no need for support. However, this does not mean they do not have needs. A good staff training system will ensure that input can be tailored to these needs. For example, Sherr & George (1988) found that staff in the UK preferred educational meetings to support groups. It was possible that such staff gained beneficial input from the content of such meetings, as well as deriving benefit from the informal contacts made around such meetings. Thus the provision of educational updates and seminars may play a vital role in informing staff and in supporting them.

The literature on staff needs and staff support spans a wide range of specialist areas. Some general lessons can be learned from these for reference to obstetric situations. Within obstetrics, the majority of literature is focused on special care units, but these may share many aspects with the labour ward, ante-and post-natal care, and allied clinics.

The provision of staff support groups has often been put forward as one solution to staff difficulties in a number of settings. Staff needs vary widely and an understanding of staff coping, frustration, hurdles and the demands of optimal care form an essential part of understanding the ideal staff protocols in order to maximize staff satisfaction, efficiency and productivity.

Stress and health care

Health care in general and intensive care in particular provide demanding and often stressful occupational needs (Parkes, 1985). Stresses emanate from a variety of sources, many of which have been documented (Menzies, 1960). These range from stresses associated with caring for very ill or dying patients to more mundane sources. Furthermore, the structures of nursing and medical hierarchies often in themselves create defences or barriers to coping and caring tasks.

As medical care evolves to a more patient-centred approach, particularly an approach aimed at the whole person rather than discrete tasks, the experience of care may be more fulfilling but the emotional involvement may also be heightened.

Inadequate staffing and demanding work schedules also contribute to work related stress (Caldwell & Weiner, 1981). Work environments can trigger many of the annoyances and difficulties faced by staff. These may create different, and at times greater, stressors. They can involve hurdles faced via interpersonal relationships, role and status factors (Cook & Mandrillow, 1982), discipline issues, autonomy and authority divisions (Birch, 1979), the doctor/nurse divide, work structures, work schedules and decision making.

'Burn out' is the term, originally described by Maslach (1978) which marks the culmination of stress factors within working situations. This widely debated term is supposed to describe a state of emotional exhaustion which renders staff unable to continue in their previously demanding task with efficacy and may ultimately result in resignation. The effects have been expressed in a variety of ways in the literature. These include:

- Increased absenteeism
- Minor ailments
- Lack of enthusiasm
- Overwhelmed reactions to new demands
- Inability to be motivated
- Problems in initiating new plans of action
- Hurdles undertaking new or existing work with enthusiasm and commitment

Maslach elaborates on the concept via a stage theory. Staff in the presence of unabated stressors initially show high enthusiasm, but this is impossible to sustain over prolonged periods of time. They then move to an experience of minor physical complaints or somatic symptoms, which include headaches, non-specific infections, colds, virus infections, flu and so on. Thereupon they proceed to lose enthusiasm, become cut off from the task in hand and finally insensitive and emotionally blunted to patient needs and colleague problems. Their insensitivity progresses to intolerance. They progress through periods of low mood. The entire scenario culminates in an eventual withdrawal (Bennett, *et al.* 1991). In summary, Maslach & Jackson (1981) define burn out as a combination of:

(1) Emotional exhaustion – feelings of being emotionally overextended and exhausted by one's work.
(2) Depersonalization – an unfeeling and impersonal response to clients.
(3) Lack of personal accomplishment – a tendency to evaluate oneself negatively, particularly in relation to work and dissatisfaction with personal accomplishment at work.

This type of pattern has been described in the literature within many settings and has been held responsible for effects such as rapid staff turnover, frequent job changes, losses to the professions and dissatisfaction within wards by other staff and patients alike. Withdrawal and turnover then feed into the system in turn. This overburdens the current enthusiastic staff and aggravates the situation of staff shortages.

A variety of theoretical models have been proposed to account for burn out (Bennett, *et al.*, 1991). Freudenberger (1977) proposes a 'depletion model' which highlights organizational conditions such as ambiguous roles, staff shortages and over demanding work. All of these conditions can result in a slow depletion of individual resourcefulness and energy as time passes. Pines, *et al.*, (1981) highlight the problems of tedium and diminished personal growth. Cherniss (1980) and Meier (1983) describe a model of 'competence in crisis'. Here staff generate a set of high expectations for themselves, often coupled with low coping ability. Such situations can result from inexperience but will culminate in crisis and ultimately in burn out. The positive aspects of this model are that it allows for improvement over time, as experience and expertise are gathered – most other models present a downward linear prognosis, whereas this one allows for learning and rejuvenation. Other studies have shown a deterioration of commitment and resolve over time and with excessive exposure to the stressors of work (Karger, 1981). Maslach (1982) provides a comprehensive theoretical model to account for burn out where she combines multiple factors contributing to staff reaction, including situational triggers, social context and the demands and nature of the job, as well as the behaviour of the individual within the work situation.

Factors which may be involved in burn out include:

- *Age* – This is a negative factor where increased age is associated with decreased burn out.
- *Experience* – Length of experience also correlates negatively with burn out.
- *Relationships* – People who are single or alone are more likely to experience burn out than those within a relationship or family.

- *Family* – People with children are less likely to experience burn out than childless carers.
- *Exposure* – The amount of time spent actively working may relate to burn out, but findings are inconclusive (some studies report length of exposure as a protection whereas others report it as a predictor). It may be that the nature of exposure rather than the pure length of time is the key variable here.
- *Variation* – Variation is reported as a form of protection against burn out, where the cumulative effects of experience can be used to their full, whilst the factor of change can protect against the severity of relentless exposure to specific types and patterns of stress.
- *Gender* – Maslach found roughly equal distribution of burn out between the sexes. Any gender effects that are reported may reflect overriding gender distributions within professions, rather than direct gender effects (for example, there are generally more female nursing staff than males, yet more males are in a position of authority within nursing).
- *Intensity* – The intensity of exposure is cited as more likely to trigger burn out than the chronicity of exposure.

Special care baby units, labour wards, pre-and post-natal wards and antenatal clinics bring with them their own unique concerns. When compared with other units, neonatal work is seen to be more stressful with higher work loads, lower autonomy, job satisfaction and peer support (Spinks & Michaelson, 1989). Particular stressors include the following factors.

Organization

Issues of death, handicap and ethics will be described later in this book (see Chapter 11). However, it is often the daily routines of caring, the ward and work organization and the work environment which directly contribute to staff emotions. For example, death and handicap are not the major factors in special care baby units. Daily routines surrounding intensive medical nursing and caring skills are often boring and repetitive. Within such an environment, organizational factors become key elements to staff well being. Seemingly small issues such as duty rotas, task delegation, time keeping, responsibility, team membership, work allocation and tea breaks can take on quite dramatic proportions. Menzies (1960) outlined organizational obstacles, identifying elaborate medical systems and routines as defences against the emotional burden of caring. Frith & Morrison (1986) noted that reductions of resources, management approaches, technology and focus on community care all contributed to organizational difficulties, both by the implementation of change and by the uncertainties experienced during the transition and change to the newer systems.

Personality dynamics

On paper, good working environments and atmospheres have often been described, but in reality they are extremely difficult to create, let alone maintain over time. In most wards, interpersonal factors contribute dramatically to the smooth running of the ward. Interpersonal relationships within the hospital system are often dramatically affected by factors of role and status. Pecking orders exist throughout the health care system, dictating responsibility. These can be the source of much friction. In maternity and special care units there are many professionals working together, including medics, nurses, midwives, technicians, psychologists, social workers, auxiliaries, paediatricians, students, physiotherapists and anaesthetists. Some units with a teaching affiliation may compound the situation by imposing an additional hierarchy of students and teachers within the setting. These are not only potentially stressful, but are often typified by rapid turnover, so the situation will continually repeat itself.

Different ranks of staff may experience difficulties when dealing with each other (Jacobsen, 1983). Cook & Mandrillow, (1982) noted the role of situational support. Parkes (1985) recorded problems arising from failure to carry out precise instructions, and dissatisfaction expressed by students who were chastized, especially if this was in front of other staff or patients. Menzies (1960) enlarged upon this by describing how nurses had neither autonomy nor the recourse to initiative. Nichols *et al.* (1981) also identified inappropriate reactions to errors by superior staff as a source of stress. Parkes (1985) described great discomfort for students who were reprimanded in the presence of others – particularly patients and visitors – which could result in detachment.

Wilson & Underwood (1980) described a phenomen of learned helplessness which was visible in hospital staff. Young doctors described their relationships with consultants as stressors (Frith & Morrison, 1986). Indeed, practices by those in charge correlated highly with performance and motivation measures in studies by Parkes (1981). Parkes (1981) also pointed out that strain and stress were experienced differently by male and female respondents. Folkman & Lazarus (1980) resolved the various findings by differentiating between sex and gender issues. Differences could be explained in terms of gender roles. This was endorsed by findings reported by Parkes (1981) who noted that male student nurses were seen as receiving more favourable treatment than females.

There are many complex factors relating to personality dynamics and characteristics which may impede or facilitate coping. The dynamics of a ward can be complex and if these break down, stress levels may increase.

Even within a well functioning ward, personality factors may result in undue stress on certain individuals or in certain situations.

Skills

Reproductive technology may require specific expertise and experience with unique technology. Such technology, even when mastered, is threatening because it is in a constant state of change and education. Work in labour wards with tiny babies may require a confidence and deftness which does not come easily nor immediately to all. Both these skills require a quality level and a speed of acquisition which are challenges to any staff member. Such skill acquisition and transfer imposes a learning and teaching environment at a practical level on the wards. Learning skills often rely heavily on observation ability, past experience and personal learning ease. The myriad of teaching approaches which were known to be effective are rarely employed when on-the-job training is utilized. There is a wide teaching remit inherent in many levels of staff behaviour, yet teaching skills are rarely part of the curriculum.

Communication

Dissatisfaction with communication is the most consistent complaint put forward by patients (Ley, 1982). Communication difficulties cover a host of interactions. Of foremost importance is the communication between parents and staff. This can relate to communication of information, whether factual or reassuring, or more generally, to communications aimed at easing distress and promoting coping or well being. There is certainly an overlap between communication issues and other areas of stress.

Certain members of staff may have sole responsibility for information provision. Parents may often turn to one member of staff to consolidate information, double check facts or explore the implications of messages received, even though that person neither provided the information in the first place, nor is empowered to elaborate on it. Resultant anxiety can be monitored in both those seeking information (the parents) and those unable to provide adequate responses (the staff). Ley (1982) examined the role of misunderstanding and how it contributed to dissatisfaction and reduced compliance. Inadequate communications can lead to ambiguous messages to parents or result in misinformation, misunderstanding and erroneous conclusions. These factors can often be the trigger which severs relations between staff and parents or cause problems between staff members.

It is a skilful task to be able to provide adequate relevant information in a clear and systematic way. McGuire & Rutter (1976, 1977) showed how

poor medical students were at gathering information during first interviews. The process is hindered by many factors such as:

- Fact overloading
- Use of jargon
- Lack of clarity and blurring
- Problems with full understanding
- Difficulties in recall
- Stress level in the recipient

Even when information has been provided, patient recall is often low.
This can be increased by techniques such as:

Data clustering
For example, providing information which is organized into meaningful
sections, numbering items or linking items.

Subject priming
For example, alerting the recipient to the impending information ('the
most important thing I need to know is ...')

Specific information
This has better recall value than vague information. Thus if a woman is
told 'come to hospital when your contractions are frequent' she may
prefer advice which states 'come to hospital when your contractions are
five minutes apart'.

Avoidance of generalized statements
Such statements such as 'cut down your alcohol', 'exercise regularly' have
less recall than a focused statement on the specific situation.

Improved recall is a realistic goal, given that it has correlated with
improved satisfaction, reduced anxiety and increased compliance (Ley,
1977, Sherr, 1989).

Staff/patient communication

Staff/patient communication is often fraught and open to misunderstandings. Johnson (1982) found that although staff could identify
the general worries that beset patients, they found it difficult to identify
which particular patients experienced specific worries. Indeed, patients,
rather than staff, were better able to understand worries. Staff groups
have been used to facilitate communication between staff and patients on
special care baby units (Mertin & Watson, 1984). These workers described
how staff mistook parental stress reactions and labelled such parents as

'difficult patients'. Groups which succeeded in sensitizing staff to pick up emotional responses had the effect of mobilizing the provision of support for such parents.

Bender & Swan Parente (1983) noted issues between staff and parents which needed resolving. They described rivalry which may emanate from staff taking over the care of the baby. In the absence of good communication, parents may judge staff as capable and potent, irrespective of whether the staff member feels able or helpless. Staff also often judge parents in a similar way. At times of crisis, which difficult labour or admission of a baby to a special unit may represent, parents may need parenting themselves. Issues of separation and attachment may need resolving as well. Dammer & Harpin (1982) described a system where parents and all levels of staff met regularly. They found that parents gained confidence in their ability to look after their baby and that staff reported increased insight into parental anxiety and problems, leading to changes in organization.

In some circumstances, the 'patient' will include the woman and her partner and the baby. Babies may have limited avenues for communication but they do have communication needs which may be demanding and stressful to meet. They need a variety of inputs, such as close, warm handling, and they respond to many environmental stimuli such as light, sound and temperature. Many babies have widely differing cries – some of which can engender disparate emotions such as love, irritation, annoyance, desire to comfort. Babies who are born to drug-addicted mothers are often typified by such 'difficult' levels of arousal and demanding cries.

Staffing

The level of staffing on a unit can be a key ingredient to smooth running and stress abatement. Understaffing places a heavy burden on staff and limits their ability to carry out comprehensive, let alone satisfactory, care. When there are staff shortages, elements of care regimes are, of necessity, sacrificed. Often it is the immediate issue which is responded to, at the expense of the important. Short-term needs usually take precedence and this may set the scene for longer term problems. Understaffing places a double pressure on staff members. Firstly, there is the sheer volume of work which may be impossible to achieve. Secondly, there are the frustrations caused to the sensitive worker who, of necessity, has to deliver a personally unacceptable level of care, but is 'helpless' to do otherwise.

Staffing problems have been noted as severe and constant stressors (Nichols, *et al.* 1981, Leatt Schreck, 1980). Parkes noted that such stress was exacerbated by exhaustion and pressure. Dunn (1985) noted that there is a constant and acute shortage of midwives on intensive neonatal units and quoted the 1984 House of Commons Social Services Committee Report as giving an urgent priority which called for a 28 per cent increase.

Environment

The working environment can have a dramatic effect on staff functioning and stress levels. This includes factors such as:

- Ward size
- Ward layout
- Ward design
- Decoration
- Off ward facilities such as changing and rest/eating facilities
- Lighting
- Daylight access
- Temperature
- Distraction
- Noise
- Overcrowding

Staff interactions

Good communication is not simply contained in the provision of information. Staff need to communicate with each other effectively. Information flow is a key element, as there is constant staff turnover, shift changes and multiple involvement with any patient. This requires meticulous attention to detail if information is to be passed on effectively.

Death of a baby

The arrival of a baby is usually meant to signify a beginning with new birth and life. Death poses a contradiction. Staff may have to face this death, which in itself can be traumatic. In addition, they have to support the parents who are going through the experience of bereavement. Reaction can be intensified if a staff member has built up a relationship with the baby or the parents. This is particularly true if there has been a history of problems where there has been prolonged antenatal admission. Staff may be ill-equipped to deal with their own emotions and reactions, but during this traumatic time they will be the front line workers who are called upon to provide support for parents and relatives.

Parkes (1981) noted that caring for patients who were terminally ill was a particular stressor. This stems not only from the problems raised by the actual death, but as a result of surrounding stressors such as communication regarding the terminal nature of an illness, informational demands, ward protocols about information handling and conflicting needs. Stress can also arise when patients question a staff member who does not have the authority or knowledge to respond adequately (Hackett & Weisman, 1977). In such instances, Parkes (1985) noted that many students used avoidance as a coping mechanism. Patients can keenly sense when they are being fobbed off or avoided, and students were often troubled by their inability to respond adequately. Parkes further noted that senior staff were insensitive to such anxieties experienced by their students. Although she did not measure whether they are insensitive to such anxieties generated in the patients as well, it is not unreasonable to assume that this may follow on. When emotional involvement is present (Parkes, 1985; Field, 1984), the situation can become exceedingly difficult.

When a life is lost, the emotion of guilt is common. Staff may question care, they may experience personal guilt and criticize their own input and competence, or they may feel anger and guilt towards the system in which they find themselves. Some of the practical protocols associated with dying can be particularly distressing, such as laying out a body (Parkes, 1985), visits to the mortuary or funeral attendance. Frith and Morrison (1986) noted that dealing with death was a major stressor for young doctors.

Hay & Oken (1972) further note that repeated exposure to death and dying can erode the ability of staff to cope. This may manifest in staff distancing themselves as a form of self protection. Patients may thus find staff very removed and this may alienate them, hindering their trust and emotional expression.

If a parent has lost a new born baby, communication can be very difficult. When families are questioned (White *et al.* 1984) despite adequate (and appreciated) communications prior to the death, much criticism is levelled at interactions after the event. Families in this study were particularly concerned about the lack of feedback from post mortem examinations, the lack of information about the cause of death, the effects on the mother and, especially, the possibility of recurrence with a future birth.

Handicap

All parents have an immediate and ongoing concern about whether their baby is 'normal'. In special care baby units, this is a particular problem as staff may have a limited capacity to follow up queries and have no idea of the longer term implications of a handicapped or compromised baby in terms of developmental goals, milestones, expectations, achievements and needs. This may be hindered by the staff's own personal notions and prejudices about handicap.

The presence of a physical handicap, which is visible on observation of the baby, can trigger immediate difficulties. Staff need to handle the baby and teach parents, often by way of example, how to act and interact with the baby. This could involve modelling, where parents may overcome difficulties in approaching or touching the baby by observing staff and taking a lead from their example.

The staff to whom parents turn first for advice on prognosis, long-term expectations, provisions, services, demands and the future of their baby may themselves have low experience or exposure to handicaps. Such limitations at source may have long term consequences, as often early adjustment by parents can ease the progression of coping. Kaplan & Mason (1960) described emotional reactions to pre-term babies as intense. Mertin & Watson (1984) emphasized the importance of helping parents to cope with emotional reactions on such occasions.

Handicaps may also raise questions about immediate management, and life and death decision making. This is made all the more difficult in the case of very premature babies, where diagnosis and prognosis may be difficult or speculative. The very nature and degree of uncertainty will load the emotional situation.

Moral and ethical problems

Staff often have to face many moral and ethical dilemmas in reproductive care. Hierarchies within medicine may make this more difficult. It is often unclear which individual or group of individuals in a unit holds responsibility for decision making and how decisions are carried through. Conflict and stress may occur when policy is not adhered to, when policy is at odds with personal conviction, or when disagreement surrounds any factor of the management. A staff member who is called on to provide care which directly conflicts with their own personal beliefs may have considerable difficulty in doing so.

Sims Jones (1986) noted that ethical dilemmas were widespread, especially in special care baby units and described the differing standpoints which may conflict. At one extreme, there are those who believe in a right to life for everyone, whatever the standard of that life. Another school of thought is primarily concerned with the quality of life and endorses the notion that infants who had no meaningful life have the right to die. Another school of thought (utilitarianism) advises an overall policy of 'greatest good for greatest number' which promotes an economic or resource-based approach. Within such a range of possible ethical standpoints, staff need to face their own perceptions honestly. Sims Jones felt that staff who were comfortable with their own views could deliver more effective care. This notion has much appeal, but has not been tested empirically.

Breaking bad news

Facing patients with bad or difficult news can be particularly stressful and can be aggravated by additional hurdles. For example, there are often rules laid down about who can provide such news and a staff member who is prevented from telling news honestly and quickly can experience much stress. There is generally little training for breaking bad news and staff often learn by uncomfortable and even disastrous experience. When there is no debriefing and postvention, such negative experiences can either reinforce bad practices or alienate the staff member from their own emotions, which may further decrease their performance in the future.

Stress reduction

It is usually presumed that wherever there is stress, there is a need to reduce it. Yet this is not necessarily so. Some individuals report that their best work is carried out under some sort of stress or pressure. A level of stress and anxiety provoked by a situation may alarm or warn the individual about possible consequences and help them adopt adequate preparation and coping styles. For every situation, there needs to be an initial examination of the nature of the stress, the effects that it may have and the possible benefits. It is also important to remember that stress can never be entirely removed.

From a psychological stand point, interventions should aim be to:

● Understand the nature, causes and effects of stress.
● Predict stressful situations.
● Anticipate stress.
● Prepare for stress and enhance coping.
● Acknowledge stress and stress inducing situations to allow for adjustment and reaction.
● Provide input where needed to avoid, prevent, reduce or understand stress.

Some intervention techniques are listed below.

Introduction of a counselling model to care
Davis & Fallowfield (1991) note that the adoption of a counselling approach to health care has multiple benefits, which may be interlinked. In the sample of oncology staff they studied who had adopted such an approach professional satisfaction was increased and burn out was decreased. The study reports that few oncology staff had formal counselling training, but a large proportion had attended brief training courses. Those with exposure to such training derived more personal benefit from their work. Similar results were found with medical students who

delivered higher levels of empathy in their care as a result of training, and also reported decreased levels of personal stress when confronted with emotional patients. Davis & Rushton (1989) enhanced self efficacy and helpfulness by training experienced health care professionals in basic counselling skills.

Organizational change
This involves a constant examination and adjustment of ward structures, protocols and policy, allowing for change, re-examination and evaluation.

Staff support groups
These vary greatly in content, aims and objectives. Staff groups are often not validated or evaluated in a systematic way. Research studies reveal a variety of possible outcomes, including successes (Weiner & Caldwell, 1981) and failures (Weiner *et al.*, 1983).

Setting up staff support groups

When setting up any staff support group, planning and understanding should be an integral part of the process. The first priority should be to decide on the purpose of the group. Will it react to problems, will it anticipate problems, or is it there to provide a forum which extends beyond problem-based thinking?

Only when these issues have been considered can some of the practical factors be addressed. These include the question of who, if anyone, should lead the group (an insider or an outsider). Groups can benefit from input from a trained psychologist, social worker or counsellor (Mertin & Watson 1984, Bender & Swan Parente 1983). Practical considerations such as where the meetings should be held, timing, frequency, attendance and even payment, must be resolved. Some units decide that staff support should be held in work time; others decide it should be held out of work time. All of these practical issues occur in the context of staff rota issues, staff shortages, and ward or clinic demands and the subsequent decisions have clear messages about the importance the unit places on the support of its staff.

Support can be emotional, practical, individual or group-based; it can be formal or informal. However, some groups which were established as informal support networks have broken down. Informal support can collapse when there are too many people involved in a situation, when there is no time available to allow support to occur, when no effort is put into such activities, or when the situation gives rise to isolated workers. Support, in whatever form, needs to be part of the ward routine and therefore integrated as such.

However, groups and staff support may initially be seen as highly threatening. Individuals, especially if they were not involved in the decision to set up a group, may perceive the need for the group as a statement of failure or an inability to cope. Prior to any group launch, adequate and sufficient ground work is essential to ensure that the group has a chance of success.

Practical considerations

The way in which a staff group is established may directly determine its success. The group can either be an expression of a caring environment, or an attempt to substitute for one. If a group is treated as a crisis intervention tool, it can only provide limited help – usually linked to a particular crisis. It is preferable to set up a group before problems get so entrenched that they need immediate intervention.

A key factor in any group work is an understanding that participation is voluntary. Groups cannot be imposed on unwilling participants with any success. This is especially noticeable if it is created by senior staff and intended for uptake by junior staff.

Groups must meet regularly. This may help the process and ensure that the group time is not simply seen as a respite from a busy or demanding ward. It needs to provide an active vehicle to address potential or current crises. Participation within a group ought to be voluntary. Issues discussed within the group should be acknowledged as confidential and should not be taken outside of the group. For example, decisions on staff promotion should never include information which has been expressed during group meetings.

Groups are also not exclusively for those who are not coping. Indeed, the examination of coping styles and sharing coping doubts can help members to build up personal coping skills before a crisis occurs. They may find it easier to tolerate uncertainty when they realize that it is an emotion they share with their colleagues.

Aims of staff support groups

Support can have a range of goals. It is helpful to articulate these prior to the start of group meetings, as they may form the basis against which group efficacy and continuation can be measured. At the same time, groups may evolve and the goals which prompt initial group creation may thus give way to higher order needs. This dynamic process should feed into group evaluation.

Groups can fill various roles, some of which have been described by Mertin & Watson (1984). These are as follows:

(1) The group should help staff to understand the implications.
(2) It should allow staff insight to their own and their patients' reactions.

(3) Groups should facilitate communication and allow a forum for information exchange.
(4) A group should provide support at times of crisis.
(5) Groups should use crisis situations to ensure preparedness and appropriate reactions to similar situations in the future.

Groups in other areas of obstetrics can follow similar formats. Although the same crisis issues surrounding an ill baby may not be present, the model still stands. Such groups can then provide skills and reassurance for staff, as well as permission to understand, acknowledge and react to emotional aspects of their work. They can also provide an occasion to relax traditional barriers to allow for free expression and communication.

Composition of groups

Group compositions vary. Some are aimed at a specific professional group, whereas others are interdisciplinary. Some involve staff only, whereas others create a forum for staff/patient dialogue. Group membership is rarely stable. Ward and clinic demands, staff shifts, off duty time and rotation all contribute to variation and turnover of attenders. This can prove frustrating if such variance is not anticipated. Rigid demands can prejudice the successful continuation of a group.

Issues

Groups can provide a forum to address unlimited issues. It is important that they examine process as well as outcomes, problem solving strategies, personality conflicts, and serve as a learning vehicle for the future. Some groups simply voice problems and others discuss issues more generally, whereas others are primarily concerned with the identification and adoption of coping mechanisms. Bender & Swan Parente (1983) reported that groups alleviated stress by allowing for reflection, a forum for expression and an occasion for interpretation.

Evaluation

Group evaluation is essential. This can be informal or formal. It can be done with simple regular assessments or within a more formalized research or empirical paradigm. Rigorous evaluation should involve prior hypotheses about the aims and desired outcomes of the group, meaningful indices about how to measure these and useful tools to provide outcome measures.

There is often a wide variation between practice and ideal. Some workers have shown positive outcomes of groups and others have reported failures. The initial goals of a group would determine the outcome criteria for success. Such criteria may change or evolve and the evaluation may need to be adjusted accordingly. A group may fail on initial criteria but still provide a useful forum for staff. It is unclear how to judge such outcomes. In the long term, studies have examined measures such as staff turnover, staff satisfaction and burn out related factors. Few studies have directly examined enhanced patient handling or crisis resolution. Given that staff who burn out invariably depart, groups may never contain burnt out staff and thus group factors which rely solely on measures allied to burn out may be misdirected. Critical evaluation should involve competence, quality of care, prevention and coping skills.

Pasacreta & Jacobsen (1989) identify the problems that nursing staff may face in an AIDS ward and emphasize the need to contrast this with the challenges and rewards which are also part of the care package. These involve the ability to make a meaningful contribution to a new frontier, of providing care for a needy group of patients who may suffer from discrimination, and the ability to become involved in research and clinical care. They identify differences between nurses who have limited or no previous exposure to patients and those who, on the other hand, specialize in AIDS care. The former group may have concerns about contagion which can manifest in behaviours to remove them from the wards. They may have rational or irrational fears which need accurate, up to date information in order to be managed effectively. The latter group have often come to terms with fears of contagion but these can often be reawakened. Yet their main suffering is with burn out type symptoms (overwork, stress, feeling undervalued and becoming distanced from the emotional pain of the work (Pines & Maslach, 1978). These workers set up a staff support group. Although they claim benefit, no empirical data was gathered.

Implications for practice

Any unit that purports to care for those who pass through it should start the process by caring for the caregivers. Support often comes via informal channels. Formal support, which can come in many forms, should be an extension of this and not a substitute. Statements of caring can be made at the one extreme by inviting a psychologist onto the ward or, at the other, by ensuring staff have adequate changing, relaxation and toilet facilities. If staff are to respond to the emotional burden of their work, they need to feel secure in their ability to navigate their own personal emotions, to reflect on their feelings, to gain support and to learn positively from their experiences. They need to be shielded from unremitting stressors, high intensity exposure and unreasonable burdens. It is rare for staff to feel totally negative or positive. Rather, there is a fluctuating course of emotions which need understanding, support and acknowledgement.

References

Bender, H. & Swan Parente, A. (1983) Psychological and psychotherapeutic support of staff and parents in an intensive care baby unit. In: *Parent Baby attachment in premature infants* (Eds J.A. Davis, M.P.M. Richards & N.R.C. Roberton), Croom Helm, London.

Bennett, L., Michie, P. & Kippax, S. (1991) Quantitative analysis of burnout and its associated factors in AIDS nursing. *AIDS Care,* **3** (2), 181–92.

Birch, J. (1979) The anxious learners. *Nurs. Mirror,* 8 February, 17.

Caldwell, T. & Weiner, M. (1981) Stresses and coping in ICU nursing: a review. *Gen. Hosp. Psychiatry.* 13, 119.

Cherniss, C. (1980) *Professional burnout in human service organizations.* Praeger, New York.

Cook, C. & Mandrillow, M. (1982) Perceived stress and situational supports. *Nursing Management,* 13, 31–42.

Dammer, J. & Harpin, V. (1982) Parents' meetings in 2 neonatal units: a way of increasing support for parents. *BMJ,* Sept. 25, 285.

Davis, H. & Rushton, R. (1989) An evaluation of basic counselling training. *Counselling,* 68, 1–8.

Davis, H. & Fallowfield, L. (1991) *Counselling and Communication in Health Care,* Wiley, Chichester.

Field, D. (1984) We didn't want him to die on his own: nurses' accounts of nursing dying patients. *Journal of Advanced Nursing* 9, 59–68.

Folkman, S. & Lazarus, R. (1980) An analysis of coping in a middle-aged community sample. *Jnl. Hlth. & Social Behaviour,* 21, 219–39.

Freudenberger, H. (1977) Burn out: occupational hazard of the child care worker. *Child Care Quarterly,* 56, 90–99.

Frith, J. & Morrison, L. (1986) What stresses health professionals? A coding system for their answers. *B. Jnl. of Clin. Psych.* 25, 309–10.

Hackett, T. & Weisman, A. (1977) Reactions to the imminence of death. In *Stress and Coping: an Anthology* (Eds A. Monat & R. Lazarus) Columbia Univ. Press, New York.

Hay, D. & Oken D. (1972) The psychological stresses of intensive care. *Psychosomatic Medicine,* 34, 109–114.

Jacobsen, J. (1983) Stress and coping strategies of neonatal intensive care unit nurses. *Research in Nursing and Health,* **6,** (1) 33–40.

Johnson, M. (1982) Recognition of patients' worries by nurses and by other patients. *B. Jnl of Clini. Psych.,* 21, 255–61.

Kaplan, D. & Mason, E. (1960) Maternal reactions to premature birth viewed as an acute emotional disorder. *Am. Jnl. of Orthopsychiatry,* **30**.

Karger, H. (1981) Burnout as alienation. *Social Service Review,* 55, 270–83.

Leatt Schreck, R. (1980) Differences in stress perceived by head nurses across nursing specialities in hospitals. *Jnl. of Advanced Nursing* 5, 31.

Ley, P. (1977) Psychological studies of doctor patient communication. In *Contributions to Medical Psychology Vol 1,* Pergamon Press, Oxford.

Ley, P. (1982) Satisfaction, compliance and communication. *British Jnl. of Clinical Psychology*, 31, 241–54.

Maguire, P. & Rutter, D. (1976) Training medical students to communicate. In: *Communication Between Doctors and Patients* (Ed. A.E. Bennett) Oxford University Press for Nuffield Prov. Hospitals Trust, London.

Maslach, C. (1978) Job burnout: how people cope. *Public Welfare* 36, 56–8.

Maslach, C. (1982) Burnout: a social psychological analysis. In *The Burnout Syndrome: Current Research Theory Interventions* (Ed. J. Jones) London House Press, Park Ridge, Illinois.

Maslach, C. & Jackson, S. (1981) The measurement of experienced burnout. *Jnl. of Occupational Behaviour*, 2, 99–113.

Meier, S. (1983) Towards a theory of burnout. *Human Relations*, 36, 899–910.

Menzies, I. (1960) A case study on the functioning of social systems as a defence against anxiety. *Human Relations*, 13, 95.

Mertin, P. & Watson, J. (1984) Stress in a NICU. *Education*, **13**, (10), 43.

Nichols, K., Springford, V. & Searle, J. (1981) An investigation of distress and discontent in various types of nursing. *Jnl. of Advanced Nursing*, 6, 311.

Parkes, K. (1981) Occupational stress among student nurses: a comparison of medical and surgical wards. *Nursing Times-occasional papers*, 76, 113.

Parkes, K. (1985) Stressful episodes reported by first year student nurses: a descriptive account. *Soc. Sci. Med.*, **20**, (9) 945–53.

Pasacreta, J.V. & Jacobsen, P.B. (1989) Addressing the need for staff support among nurses caring for the AIDS Population. *ONF*, **16**, (5), 659–63.

Pines, A. & Maslach, C. (1978) Characteristics of staff burnout. *Community Psychiatry*, **29**, (4) 233–37.

Pines, A.M., Aronson, E. & Kafry, D. (1981) *Burnout From Tedium to Personal Growth*. The Free Press, New York.

Rutter, D.R. & Maguire, P. (1977) History taking for medical students. *The Lancet*, 558–60.

Sherr, L. (1989) *Anxiety and Communication in Obstetrics*. PhD Thesis, Warwick University.

Sherr, L. & George, H. (1988) *AIDS and Staff Stress*. Abstracts, Psychology and Health International, British Psychological Society.

Sims Jones, N. (1986) Ethical dilemmas in the neonatal intensive care unit. *The Canadian Nurse*, April 24–6.

Spinks, P. & Michaelson, J. (1989) A comparison of the ward environment in a special care baby unit and a children's orthopaedic ward. *Jnl. Reproductive and Infant Psychology*, 7, 47–50.

Weiner, M. & Caldwell, J. (1981) Stressors and coping in ICU nursing: nurse support groups on ICU. *Gen. Hosp. Psychiatry*, 3, 129.

Weiner, M., Caldwell, T. & Tyson, J. (1983) Stress and coping in ICU nursing: why support groups fail. *Gen. Hosp. Psychiatry*, 5, 176–8.

White, M., Reynolds, B. & Evans, T.L. (1984) Handling of death in special care nurseries and parental grief. *BMJ*, 289, 167.

Wilson, D. & Underwood, P. (1980) Learned helplessness at city hospitals. *Persp. Psycho. Care*, 18, 256.

Chapter 3

Getting Pregnant

Pregnancy occurs by design by some and by accident for others. Some couples choose not to have children, and are sometimes referred to as the 'voluntary childless', whereas others have difficulty in conceiving over extended periods of time. Although such difficulties are widespread, actual prevalence is unknown as many do not seek out help. Cartwright (1979), Oakley (1980) and Bourne (1975) conclude that in any given sample some women can take up to six months to conceive and one in ten can take over a year. A small proportion of women have extended problems and therefore choose to undergo fertility treatments.

Counselling for pregnancy decisions

Unplanned pregnancy

Ryan & Dunn, (1988) studied how to deal with unplanned pregnancy. They summarize five methods for dialogue and measure preferences in a sample of college students. The five methods include: marriage, abortion, adoption, becoming a single parent or allowing the grandparents to raise the child.

Marriage was the most preferred option, followed by abortion. Subjects also noted that they would prefer to live as a single parent, rather than have a third party look after their baby (such as with adoption or other family members raising the child).

The mental health implications of giving birth to an unwanted baby were studied by Najman, *et al.*, (1991), who found higher post partum anxiety and depression levels compared to controls. The magnitude of the mental health differences, however, diminished over a six month period. It is of note that in the study population (n = 8556) there were relatively few overall mental health problems.

Family spacing

Some women have subsequent children soon after the first child, whilst others delay for varying periods of time (Dunn, 1988). The reasons for this can be social, economic or family. The effects of family spacing can be measured from the point of view of the mother, the father or the resulting children. Studies have catalogued a variety of advantages and dis-advantages of both short and long gaps between children.

Family planning

Family planning is usually a euphemism for contraception. Contraception has a specific role in the understanding of procreation, as the decision not to procreate is as important as the decision to do so.

Contraception is not a new concept, but the availability of chemical means of reproductive control this century has revolutionized the whole area of birth planning, control and choice. This has had specific effects on women. It is seen as a very modern innovation, yet early literature does exist on a variety of ways in which women in various cultures avoided unwanted pregnancies. These ranged from abstinence and intercourse timing, to older style barrier methods.

Modern fertility control still evokes much political and social debate. The availability of contraception has wide ramifications on sexual beha-viour, freedom and decision making. This in turn may affect traditional female roles, which can suddenly be freed, or place a heavier burden on childbearing decisions which nowadays have to be much more of an active choice for many couples.

First intercourse is rarely protected and young people may only seek advice after exposure. Contraception comes in varying forms, and there are many psychological barriers and facilitators which encourage or discourage their initiation, their continuity, their efficacy or their aban-donment.

Contraception behaviours and practice are intricately bound up with pregnancy and family planning, as well as other issues such as sexually transmitted diseases. Contraception cannot now be divorced from the control of sexually transmitted disease (specifically HIV) which has revolutionized studies in sexuality and the promotion of contraception.

The majority of contraception initiatives are under the control of the female and invariably are initiated outside of the sexual situation (such as the pill, diaphragm, coil). Barrier contraception differs in that it has to be initiated during or immediately preceding sex and may interrupt the pattern of the encounter.

Contraceptive choice and decision making is an interesting area of study. There are those who make active choices and those who, despite knowledge, do not utilize contraception. There are those who use it regularly and those who only use it sporadically.

Methods of contraception can be divided in various ways. Firstly there are those under the control of the male (such as the condom) and those under control of the female (such as the IUD, pill or cap). Secondly, there are those which are utilized prior to the sexual encounter (such as the pill, IUD), those utilized during the sexual encounter (condom, cap) and those utilized after the sexual encounter (morning after pill or even the termination of a pregnancy). Another distinction can be made between the different modes of contraception. These include barrier methods (such as condoms and caps), chemical measures (such as the pill), surgical measures (such as sterilization techniques for both male or female), or behavioural methods (such as the rhythm method or withdrawal).

The understanding of contraceptive behaviour has become the focus of many studies emanating from the literature on sexually transmitted diseases (notably HIV prevention) and from pregnancy avoidance, control or planning. An alarming finding (Boyle, 1991) is that the rate of legal termination of pregnancy in the UK has risen despite the legal, cheap and effective means of contraception. Bracken, *et al.* (1978) and Allen (1981) note the consistent trend that women seeking termination had not utilized, or considered utilizing, contraception when they had conceived.

Contraceptive studies are fraught with problems. Most use self report outcome measures which do not allow for a variety of 'slips twixt cup and lip', such as forgetting, occasional lapses, improper use, or contraceptive failures (such as burst condoms). More sophisticated studies do examine regularity of use and some examine partner corroboration in an attempt to control for this.

Numerous barriers to contraception exist which ought to be fully understood. Studies of pregnant teenagers (Ryan & Sweeney, 1980) showed almost two thirds had made active decisions not to utilize contraception. This was not because they intended to become pregnant (although a third said they did). Ante- and post-natal care afford ideal opportunities to discuss contraception but this is often skated over. This may be as a result of conflicting priorities, poor training, embarrassment, or simply a lack of time.

Boyle (1991) notes the oddity that the majority of studies examining contraception and conception are purely female based, as if males are entirely unconnected with contraception and conception. This extends in the female–male emphasis in education, prevention and intervention efforts. As most of these are geared towards women, endorsing the perpetuating cycle of female responsibility, burden and censure.

A variety of theoretical models which can be used to explain, understand and predict health behaviour (see Chapter 1) are of potential significance in understanding contraceptive behaviour. These models attempt to understand the predictors of contraceptive behaviour, the evaluation of the costs and benefits of the behaviour and the influence of personal, situational and normative factors on beliefs, intentions and behaviour and hurdles experienced during the process. These need to be taken into account for a fuller understanding of contraceptive behaviour.

Side-effects

There are numerous side effects which result from contraceptive use. Boyle (1991) reports that women endure more side effects than men and are expected to do so. Side effects include potential future health hazards, unwanted pregnancy in the event of failure, and interference with the experience of sex.

Availability

The availability of contraceptives varies enormously from country to country. Such availability may be limited by financial constraint, religious doctrine, normative issues or national policy. However, there are also the emotional barriers to access. Allen (1981) recounts the acute fear, anxiety and embarrassment experienced by women and men seeking out contraception.

Normative influences

There are often subtle metamessages associated with contraception which may widen the gap between the intention to consider contraception and the actual act of seeking it out. These encompass the secret, personal nature of sexual relations and worries which surround consultations and disclosure. There are often social, religious or parental sanctions about sex and these may be transferred directly to contraception. Such barriers may hinder dialogue about contraception, the formation of accurately informed opinions, the willingness to seek out advice and/or contraception and finally the intention to use it.

Negotiation

Behaviour which is not discussed nor negotiated is more open to problems than planned behaviour. However, sexual dialogue and discussion is often limited or missing. Any form of dialogue and planning surrounding sexual activity may interfere with spontaneity and remove the excitement or pleasure from the act. Zelnick & Shah (1983) report the increased likelihood of contraceptive use for planned intercourse. Schinke (1984) reports that forward strides can be made when young people are given training on interpersonal negotiation skills. These serve to counteract anxiety and embarrassment and may be useful in promoting contraceptive decision making.

Advantages and disadvantages

There are numerous costs and benefits to contraceptive use. These range from inhibiting factors for the sexual encounter itself, to health and disease prevention and pregnancy prevention.

There has been a great deal of focus on prophylactic contraception in the light of sexually transmitted diseases, notably HIV infection. The past decade has seen concerted health educational efforts to promote condom use. The whole area of AIDS and HIV infection has resulted in attention to sexual encounters, negotiation, partner selection and sexual behaviour. Early in the campaign, few turned to the body of existing knowledge whilst many efforts which utilized fear campaigns were of limited success (Sherr, 1987).

Contraceptive negotiation is not a simple event, and the complexities, especially where women are concerned, must be acknowledged (Sherr, *et al.* 1991). There are many barriers to condom use, even for individuals at high risk of STD or HIV exposure (Sherr, *et al.* 1990). The barriers are often both physical (disliking the smell or feel of condoms) to psychological (interfering with pleasure or possible inferred meaning if condoms are used). There is also the perception that whilst the barriers are within the immediate sexual encounter, the hazards are somewhere in the future. Some aspects of sexual behaviour may not be under simple control and few studies tend to focus on individuals rather than couples.

Previous pregnancy termination has been examined in the light of subsequent contraception. Many studies report a link between abortion and sterilization, although the trend is diminishing with time (Boyle, 1991). Other workers have noted reliable contraceptive practices after termination which either reflect the altering beliefs about pregnancy or result from enhanced professional advice (or a mixture of both).

Ley's theory (1988) about the role of knowledge in behaviour certainly applies here. Adequate and accurate knowledge seems to be a necessary (but not sufficient) component in contraceptive decision making. Many teenagers have erroneous beliefs about the risks of pregnancy at first intercourse. This is compounded by inaccurate ideas about safe and risky periods for conception (Morrison, 1985). Some grossly overestimate the chances of pregnancy from a single encounter, whereas others under-estimate (or even negate) the possibility. The availability of termination may affect such notions as well.

Few studies take on board the fact that contraceptive decisions and attitudes are not static and fluctuate over time, as conditions, perceptions, prompts, plans and desires change.

Infertility

It is ironic that so many people spend so much time avoiding pregnancy when there is another group who expend great energy and suffering seeking out pregnancy.

The true rate of infertility problems is difficult to determine. Infertility statistics are misleading in that they invariably underestimate the number of couples experiencing transient or short-term infertility. Those who seek medical assistance often do so after much heartache and suffering. Hull, *et al.* (1985) estimates that the rate was as high as one in six couples. Failure to conceive, especially if the difficulties are long-term, can bring with it stresses and disappointments for couples.

Fertility options include a series of investigations, the use of fertility drugs, various forms of surgery, laparoscopy, in vitro fertilization (IVF), and GIFT. There are also alternatives such as adoption or fostering, which result in a child but not a pregnancy. The whole process of fertility treatments causes enormous strain, affecting the nature and emotional meaning of sexual behaviour, social reaction and norms, personality variables and self esteem.

Early infertility studies focused on personality correlates of infertile women. They attempted to explain infertility in terms of personality characteristics (usually negative ones). Such psychogenic infertility has little background and more recent investigations tend to examine the emotional costs of infertility and fertility treatments, which may also have been reflected in the earlier study outcomes. Indeed O'Moore & Harrison (1991) examined the link between anxiety and 'reproductive failure'. Such anxiety may be caused by the failure, rather than the other way round.

Psychological consequences for couples who are involuntarily childless can extend from divorce (Coughlan, 1965) to suicide (Schellon, 1957), and a wide range of emotional ramifications (Shaw, 1991). Most studies concentrate on the female partner and there is now a small but growing literature on both male infertility and the effects on couples (Glover, *et al.*, 1992). Callan & Hennessey, (1989) compared involuntary and voluntary childless groups (n = 167) and found that the infertile group had higher expectations of love and a sense of femininity, better quality marriages, but that there were no differences in self esteem ratings and psychological or marital adjustment.

Edelman & Connolly (1986) found a relationship between stress levels and individuals with unexplained infertility. Yet the very presence of infertility, especially if it is unexplained, may be the source of stress and no studies have adequately controlled for this.

Downey & McKinney (1992) described some of the emotional states experienced by infertility clinic attendees (n = 118 women). They noted emotional distress, but this did not equate with psychological impairment. When compared to controls, there were no greater incidence of psychiatric histories, past depressive episodes, current self-esteem or sexual function differences. Indeed, infertile couples reported being happier with their partners than did the controls. On the negative side, self worth and mood changes were more common in the infertile group.

Fertility treatments are emotionally harrowing (Seibel & Taymor 1982). The nature of treatments are such that they entail prolonged stress and tension, exposure to unpleasant and embarrassing investigations. They constantly raise hope, but may deliver disappointment. Their long-term nature also presents a chronic situation for such couples who face endless months of investigation, treatment, monitoring and disappointment tinged with the hopes of success. Relationship strain is commonly documented. This is a result of multiple factors. The pressures for procreation, family life and parenting are intense and there is much sense

of failure for some couples. This is intensified by the burden such interventions place on sex which is monitored, measured, timed and anxiety
laden. Couples undergoing infertility treatments have to adjust simultaneously to the possibility of failure while accommodating the multiple
aspects of intervention and sustaining the motivation to maintain attendance and treatment.

Some people go through extensive procedures, such as tubal surgery,
laparoscopy or in vitro fertilization. There are often emotional, economic
and social costs associated with these.

Although there is widespread acknowledgement of a need for counselling and support for individuals undergoing infertility investigations
(Fouad & Fahje, 1989), there is little comprehensive evaluation of the
efficacy of such support which can point the way forward to effective
care. Individual, couple and group counselling are commonly employed.
The aims of intervention would be:

(1) Provision of information.
(2) Expression of emotions.
(3) Examination of coping skills and styles.
(4) Promotion of communication.
(5) Facilitation with relationship strain, trauma or breakdown in the face
     of infertility.
(6) Sharing of feelings with others in similar situations – great relief is
     accomplished by simply knowing that others are in a similar posi-
     tion.
(7) Emotional pacing.
(8) Easing of judgement, guilt and blame.
(9) Exploration of other emotional outlets to avoid the quest for preg-
     nancy achievement becoming all-consuming.
(10) Facilitation of grief expressions and experiences.
(11) Psychosexual counselling if needed.
(12) Reduction of social withdrawal.
(13) Examination of life goals, dreams and aspirations.
(14) Dialogue on specific dilemmas brought about by individual treat-
     ment interventions.

Counselling sometimes centres around relief. Couples may have tried
many avenues and now need permission to give up trying and get on
with the rest of their lives. They may be consumed by the goal of
achieving a child and may have lost a hold on other avenues in their lives.
Some may have built up alternative avenues and feel guilty about this.
Counselling must also take into account the lack of social support many
women experience, together with the levels of anger, sadness and feelings
of helplessness which are, according to Fouad & Fahje (1989) 'very
realistic responses to the crisis'.

If a pregnancy is achieved, there may be specific counselling needs.

These may surround the nature of the interventions. Some treatments carry with them questions which will have a significance throughout the rest of the couple's lives. Artificial insemination, where sperm from a donor is used, means that the couple may struggle with the concept of the child as their true offspring. They may want to address questions of whether and how to tell the child of the circumstances of its birth.

Fertility treatment

There are a number of treatment options open to women, and fewer open to men. Most commonly, the female partner undergoes extensive investigations before her partner. Success rates for treatments are often low. These are sometimes improved after multiple attempts, with the corresponding elongation of psychological challenge. The data that exists is somewhat confused, with differences being drawn between pregnancy rate, live birth rate and survival (see Stacey (1992) for discussion). Furthermore, unforeseen complications (such as multiple births for 26.8 per cent of IVF treatments with allied problems of prematurity or congenital abnormalities) may solve one set of problems and herald another.

Table 3.1 gives some indication of the wide range of findings of 'success' rates which are often differently defined. Of note is the fact that they all exhibit a less than total success outcome, many with a very small likelihood of success.

Findings for the particular treatments are sometimes misleading given that many couples undergo multiple interventions. Leiblum, *et al.*, (1987) studied couples undergoing in vitro fertilization and found they expres-

Table 3.1 Success rates for various infertility treatments

Treatment	Estimate of success
IVF single attempt	13.0% (Soules, 1985)
IVF multiple attempts	37.0% (Guzick, Wilkes & Jones, 1986)
IVF (after 11 attempts)	2.3% (ILA 1991)
IVF live birth rate	8.6% (ILA 1985)
IVF live birth rate	11.6% (ILA 1989)
IVF pregnancy rate	15.4% (1989 rates in Stacey 1992)
Donor insemination	75.0% (Snowden & Snowden, 1984)
Frozen embryo transplant and IVF	14.0% (n = 15 392) (Huggins, 1991)
Gamete intrafallopian transfer	23.0% (n = 3651) (Huggins, 1991)
Zygote intrafallopian transfer	15.0% (n = 908) (Huggins, 1991)

Note: statistics vary because of outcome measures recorded. Some workers record pregnancy rates, while others record live birth rates (which may vary from pregnancy rates). See Stacey (1992) for a full discussion.

sed an optimistic bias regarding likelihood of achieving a pregnancy (a finding confirmed in almost all studies – Johnson, *et al.*, (1984), Glover, *et al.*, (1992); Daniels, (1989)). Few studies have examined the role of such optimistic bias or whether it is indeed a negative event. It may indeed provoke strong tenacity in couples enduring such stressful ongoing procedures. Leiblum, *et al.* documented specific drug related changes after the administration of menotropin to include fatigue, weight gain, headaches and mood fluctuation. Unsuccessful IVF attempts resulted in sadness, anger and depression, often more pronounced in the wives than husbands. Few couples regretted undergoing the attempt.

Blenner (1992) studied couples in treatment and found that professional competency, sensitivity and environmental comfort affected treatment stress directly. She describes a series of mental and action strategies which couples developed to mitigate the stresses of treatment. Some couples decide to terminate treatment, usually prompted by high stress, low hope and excessive frustration.

Daniels (1989) studied 61 couples awaiting in vitro fertilization and reported that most had considered adoption (with one third on adoptive waiting lists). Commitment to IVF procedures was equal. Many subjects expressed a desire for guidance and help from a social worker or counsellor.

Huggins (1991) reviewed studies on infertility treatments and reported that complications and adverse outcomes of IVF and embryo transfer were low. It was cautioned that poor outcomes may not be adequately reported. Of the 4736 births reviewed, 681 sets of twins, 182 sets of triplets and 16 sets of quadruplets were reported. They also found 47 documented chromosomal abnormalities and 53 reported cases of congenital anomalies – however these rates were not significantly greater than rates found in unassisted pregnancies.

There has been a general reluctance to treat women of 40 years of age or older (Sauer, *et al.*, 1992). This reluctance has been justified in part by concerns about increased obstetrical risks and the high miscarriage rate (as high as 50%) for women of advanced reproductive age (Sauer, *et al.* 1992). These workers studied 65 women over 40 who requested oocyte donation and compared them to younger women and older women undergoing a different fertility process. They found no age related decline in fertility with uncomplicated neonatal outcomes. Multiple births occurred in 24.1% of the sample.

The clinic visits

These play a key role in the course of infertility and fertility care. Ley (1988) has summarized the range of communication problems which may adversely affect any consultation. These may apply particularly to gynaecological and infertility consultations (Hunt, 1989). Women may be faced with a male doctor and may have to discuss intricate personal details covering taboo subjects such as menstruation, intercourse and ovulation. Although many women do not record a preference, Areskog Wijma (1987) noted that 4 per cent would prefer a male and 42 per cent would actively prefer a female doctor to carry out the procedure. Vaginal examinations are particularly difficult for women to endure. Men may be unused to genital examination and find these humiliating.

Psychological counselling interventions to provide information, to train relaxation and to focus on sensory information have been shown to ameliorate the problems experienced by women undergoing such procedures (Reading, 1982, Fuller, *et al.*, 1978). Generally, few clinics provide adequately, or at all, for the emotional needs of attendees (Owens & Read 1984).

An interesting study examined the role of power in patient/physician roles during the process of infertility treatment (Becker & Nachtigall, 1991) and discussed this in terms of uncertainty, medical competence and responsibility.

In male infertility, there are very few medical options available and the clinic visit often provides more by way of accurate explanations and information than miraculous cures. Glover, *et al.* (1992) found that attendees at a male infertility clinic showed high anxiety levels which persisted after the consultation. They also pointed out the extensive amount of investigations couples experience through the course of infertility treatments. Service is seen as less satisfactory when rated by couples if it is the male partner who is undergoing investigations (Owens & Read, 1984). Perhaps this reflects the underlying assumptions that emotional care is low on the priority list generally, but when available it should be focused on women who are seen as somewhat fragile and that men, being strong and unemotional, do not need such support. These stereotypes often hinder the provision of help and the funding for such facilities to be created in the first place.

Kedem, *et al.* (1990) examined the effect of infertility on psychological functioning of 107 male subjects and compared them to a small group not so diagnosed. Infertile men had lower self esteem, higher anxiety and more somatic symptoms. Infertility was linked to feelings of hopelessness, sexual inadequacy and stress.

Relationship problems

Relationship problems are often experienced by couples undergoing infertility treatments. These can either be associated with the problems of infertility in the first place, or can be secondary to the process of infertility investigations which place strain on relationships and sexual expression. Marital problems are more common when the male partner is undergoing treatment compared to the female partner (Connolly & Cooke, 1987).

Ulbrich, *et al.* (1990) studied marital adjustment in 103 couples undergoing infertility treatment. Although they found spouses similar in the way they perceived marital adjustment, they had arrived at their views by various routes. Acceptance of a childless lifestyle necessitates a greater adjustment for males. Greater stress associated with infertility undermined marital adjustment for couples. Adjustment in males was enhanced if wives were employed or had high incomes. Female adjustment decreased with time and the course of treatment.

Andrews, *et al.* (1991) examined the relationship between stress associated with the inability to have a child and aspects of marriage (n = 157 couples). The negative effects that were identified included marital conflict, sexual self esteem and sexual dissatisfaction for females.

Chandra *et al.* (1991) studied the impact of childlessness on the quality of marital life and found that one third of the subjects reported problems in marital functioning. Factors predictive of such problems were linked to residence, extended families and length of marriage.

Emotional trauma

Variations in emotional expression have been catalogued. Haseltine (1984) found a tendency for males to express more negative depressive mood symptoms than women whose anxiety levels were higher than their male counterparts. Women with unexplained infertility tended to experience greater emotional upheaval than those with explained infertility.

Many studies are cross sectional in nature and although they may highlight an array of issues in infertility, they do not give a complete understanding to the lengthy emotional experiences as time progresses. Berg & Wilson (1991) provided a study examining first, second and third year of infertility treatments. They showed that the level of emotional strain was raised in the first year, subsided in the second and dramatically increased by the third. Similarly, marital adjustment and sexual satisfaction were stable in the first two years, but deteriorated after the third year. These may be allied to both the passage of time, the cumulation of stress, or to the types of treatments at various stages.

Reading, *et al.* (1989) studied women during the process of IVF treatment cycles (n = 37). High clinical depression was identified. Stress levels and lowered mood increased over time. Pre-treatment level of worry was associated with post-treatment adjustment. Yet as a whole, psychological test scores were low.

Coping and adjustment

Coping and adjustment was studied by Stanton, *et al.* (1992). They found that when coping via avoidance was used, higher male distress was recorded. Women who coped via acceptance of responsibility also showed higher stress levels. There was a relationship between mobilizing support and decreased stress (although it was unclear if this is causative).

In an earlier study, Stanton *et al.* (1991) examined cognitive appraisal and adjustment. It was found that subjects assessed infertility as harmful and uncontrollable, yet with some beneficial aspects. Distress was associated with level of threat, challenge and perceived control.

Gender effects

Gender differences have been examined and recorded in many studies. Poorer studies simply enrol couples attending clinics and compare reactions. This may be appropriate when infertility causes are unknown. However, when infertility can be attributed to a biological finding in either partner, it may dramatically affect perceptions and reactions. Methodologically sophisticated studies ought to control for this to understand whether the psychological effects are truly gender specific or related to gender taking into account the fact that they are often the focus of the infertility.

Stanton *et al.* (1992) described females as less likely to use distancing, self control or problem solving strategies and more likely to mobilize support or use avoidance techniques. Women who used more self controlling strategies had more distressed partners. Again it is unclear whether these strategies resulted in male distress or resulted from/were reactive to male distress levels.

Abbey, *et al.* (1991) examined the role of gender in responses to infertility and found support for the notion that female lives were more disrupted by infertility than males.

Self esteem

Berg, *et al.* (1991) examined the effect of gender on sex role identification in infertility treatment seeking couples. They found no gender differences in emotional strain, marital adjustment or sexual satisfaction. Gender differences were identified in psychological distress measures. These authors conclude that the level of strain does not differ, but emotional expression may do so.

Interventions

Many interventions have been shown to alleviate emotional burden. Daniluk (1991) describes the role of counselling and support to allow the infertility experience to be one which allows for personal and marital growth. She summarizes the goals of counselling as:

- Helping clients navigate the grieving process.
- Helping clients relinquish and accept control as and when appropriate.
- To serve as a healing opportunity for damaged relationships.
- To provide a vehicle and opportunity for reassessing parenting motivations.
- To facilitate the decision making progress about future options.

Edelmann & Connolly (1987) examined the counselling needs of infertile couples (n = 843) and noted that one third felt the need for psychological support and guidance. These subjects did not differ systematically from those not requiring such support on medical factors.

Information
The passage through the clinic system itself is traumatic, and the provision of information can eliminate much distress. Some elements of information provision are simple to carry out, and include giving jargon free, clear information with opportunities to discuss treatment options and clarify understanding. The provision of factual information is enhanced when sensory data is provided as well as procedural data.

Environment
Care environments are important for all patients, but are particularly so for those undergoing infertility investigations. For example many men are required to produce sperm on demand and this can be an excruciatingly embarrassing experience when they are sent off to public toilets with specimen bottles.

Sensitivity
A procedure which is routine for a health care worker can often become depersonalized. Yet for the individual couple it is highly personal and workers need to remind themselves constantly of this, employing strategies to prevent routines developing which may depersonalize their clients. Clients may find it difficult to have a discussion during or immediately after an intimate examination, yet those are the very times which medics make available for questions. Clients may feel shy or embarrassed by who is present at such examinations and they should be allowed a choice in this, although the power imbalance may make real choice difficult. Permission should be sought by medical staff for any student presence (preferably not in front of the student concerned).

Results
Test results must be managed in a systematized way. Practitioners should

make sure the following stages are observed, in order for their clients to be well informed and reassured.

- Possible tests should be discussed.
- When tests are agreed upon, clarify understanding and consent.
- The clients should be told about the procedure, what is involved, how it is carried out and what it will feel like (Wallace, 1984).
- Clients should be warned of any side effects or unexpected sequelae.
- Ensure that clients know the timing of tests, procedures and, most importantly, the results. Many clinics have a poor record on result provision.
- Ensure as much feedback as possible is given during the procedure, in the wait for results, and at the time of provision of results.
- When results are provided, ensure that the clients have an interval to digest the information with a time available for discussion and queries.

Bromham, *et al.* (1989) reported on the psychological state of infertile couples and examined the differences between infertile and fertile couples, questioning both male and female partners. Findings revealed marked differences between the groups, pointing to some positive effects of pregnancy but also to some detrimental effects of childbirth among couples who were successfully treated for infertility.

Lalos, *et al.* (1985) interviewed thirty women in a microsurgical treatment programme for tubal infertility, together with their partners, both prior to the surgery and again at a two year follow up. Comparisons with reference to pregnant women and those requesting legal abortion indicated that interpersonal and intrapsychic motives dominated the responses for both the infertile women and their partners when questioned about motivations for a child. Essentially, the ultimate motivation was the expression of love that the child would signify. Such motivations were similar across all groups studied.

The effects on the children

Few studies have examined the impact of assisted reproduction on children. Blyth (1990) comments on the needs and rights of such children and how thought for their future should be incorporated when assisted reproduction is contemplated.

Daniels (1989) interviewed 61 couples awaiting in vitro fertilization and found that most expressed strong support for informing the child how she or he was conceived.

Daly (1989) described the preparation needs of infertile couples who sought to adopt a baby, based on interviews of 74 such couples. Couples experienced a feeling of loss of control, and often felt inadequately prepared for adoptive parenthood which was made worse by their social isolation.

Finally, much scientific progress has also heralded widespread ethical and social debate. Alder, *et al.* (1986) investigated attitudes to in vitro fertilization and human embryo research of 1716 women of reproductive age. The overwhelming majority approved of the techniques, and two thirds approved of research on human embryos prior to 14 days of age to improve IVF. A small number (10 per cent) endorsed research to avoid birth defects and nearly 80 per cent felt that women should be given the choice of donating ova for research.

When babies are born to previously infertile couples there may be a need for special care admission. However, Lind, *et al.* (1989) identified unique coping abilities among such parents.

Implications for intervention

Clearly pregnancy does not simply commence at conception and it is often the culmination of a series of decisions. Input can thus be usefully focused at specific levels in society, such as within educational systems, family planning and health education. It is also important to understand the hurdles experienced by couples who experience either transient or longer term infertility. Their desire to conceive must be respected and accommodation must be made for the wide array of psychological traumas which they come up against.

References

Abbey, A., Andrews, F. & Halman, L. (1991) Gender role in responses to infertility, *Psychology of Women Quarterly*, **15**,(2), 295–316.

Alder, E., Baird, D., Lees, M. & Lincoln, D. (1986) Attitudes of women of reproductive age to in vitro fertilization and embryo research, *Jnl. of Biosocial Science*, **18**,(2), 155–67.

Allen, I. (1981) *Family Planning, Sterilisation and Abortion Services*, The Policy Studies Institute, London no 595.

Andrews, F., Abbey, A. & Halman, L. (1991) Stress from infertility marriage factors and subjective well being of wives and husbands, *Jnl. of Health and Social Behavior*, **32**,(3) 238–53.

Areskog Wijma, B. (1987) The gynecological examination – women's experience and preferences and the role of the gynaecologist. *Journal of Psychosomatic Obstet. and Gynec.*, 6, 59–69.

Becker, G. & Nachtigall, R. (1991) Ambiguous responsibility in the doctor patient relationship: the case of infertility, *Social Science and Medicine*, **32**,(8), 875–85.

Berg, B. & Wilson, J. (1991) Psychological functioning across stages of treatment for infertility, *Jnl. of Behavioural Medicine*, **14**,(1), 11–26.

Berg, B., Wilson, J. & Weingartner, P. (1991) Psychological sequaelae of infertility treatment: the role of gender and sex role identification, *Social Science and Medicine*, **33**,(9) 1071–80.

Blenner, J. (1992) Stress and mediators: patients' perceptions of infertility treatment, *Nursing Research*, **41**,(2), 92–97.

Blythe, E. (1990) Assisted reproduction. Whats' in it for the children? *Children and Society*, **4**,(2), 167–82.

Bourne, G. (1975). *Pregnancy*. Pelican Books, London.

Boyle, M. (1991) Decision making for contraception and abortion. In *The Psychology of Health: An Introduction* (eds M. Pitts and K. Phillips) Routledge, London.

Bracken, M., Klerman, L. & Braken, M. (1978). Abortion, adoption or motherhood: an empirical study of decision making during pregnancy. *Am. Jnl. of Obstet. and Gynec.*, 130, 251–62.

Bromham, D., Bryce, F., Balmer, B. & Wright, S. (1989) Psychometric evaluation of infertile couples, *Jnl. of Reproductive and Infant Psychology*, **7**,(4) 195–202.

Callan, V. & Hennessey, J. (1989) Psychological adjustment to infertility: a unique comparison of two groups of infertile women, mothers and women childless by choice, *Jnl. of Reproductive and Infant Psychology*, **7**,(2), 105–12.

Cartwright, A. (1979) *The Dignity of Labour*. Tavistock, London.

Chandra, P., Chaturvedi, S., Issac, M. & Chitra, H. (1991) Marital life among infertile spouses, *Family Therapy*, **18**(2), 145–54.

Connolly, K. & Cooke, I. (1987) Distress and marital problems associated with infertility. *Jnl. of Reproductive and Infant Psychology*, 5, 49–57.

Coughlan, W. (1965) *Marital Breakdown*. Columbia University Press, New York.

Daly, K. (1989) Preparation needs of infertile couples who seek to adopt. *Canadian Jnl. of Community Mental Health*, **8**,(1), 111–21.

Daniels, K. (1989) Psychological factors for couples awaiting in vitro fertilization, *Social Work in Health Care*, **14**,(2), 81–98.

Daniluk, J. (1991) Strategies for counseling infertile couples. *Jnl. of Counseling and Development*, **69**,(4), 317–20.

Downey, J. & McKinney, M. (1992) The psychiatric status of women presenting for infertility evaluation, *Am. Jnl. of Orthopsychiatry*, **62**,(2), 196–205.

Dunn, S. (1988) A model of fertility decision making styles among young mothers, *Human Organization*, **47**,(2), 166–75.

Edelman, R. & Connolly, K. (1986) Psychological aspects of infertility. *British Journal of Medical Psychology*, 59, 209–10.

Edelman, R. & Connolly, K. (1987) The counselling needs of infertile couples, *Jnl. of Reproductive and Infant Psychology*, **5**,(2), 63–70.

Fouad, N. & Fahje, K. (1989) An exploratory study of the psychological correlates of infertility on women, *Jnl. of Counseling and Development*, **68**,(1), 97–101.

Fuller, S., Endress, M. & Johnson, J. (1978) The effects of cognitive and behavioral control in coping with an aversive health examination, *Journal of Human Stress*, 4, 18–25.

Glover, L., Sherr, L., Abel, P. & Gannon, K. (1992) *Male Infertility*. Paper presented to the British Psychological Society London Conference.

Guzick, D., Wilkes, C. & Jones, H. (1986) Cumulative pregnancy notes for in vitro fertilization, *Fertility and Sterility*, 46, 663–67.

Haseltine, F. (1984) Psychological testing of couples in the invitro fertilization programme: suggested dysphoria among the males and high anxiety component in the couples. Paper presented at World Congress of Infertility, Helsinki.

Hubner, M. (1989) Cancer and infertility: longing for life, *Journal of Psychosocial Oncology*, **7**,(4) 1–19.

Huggins (1991) In *Changing Human Reproduction* (M. Stacey, 1992). Sage Publications, London.

Hull, M., Glazener, C., Kelly, N. *et al.* (1985) Population study of census treatment and outcome of infertility. *BMJ* 291, 1693.

Hunt, M. (1989) Gynaecology. In *Health Psychology* (ed. A. Broome), Chapman and Hall, London.

ILA (1985) In *Changing Human Reproduction* (M. Stacey, 1992). Sage Publications, London.

ILA (1989) *The Fourth Report of the Interim Licensing Authority for Human In Vitro Fertilization and Embryology*, ILA, London.

ILA (1991) *The Sixth Report of the Interim Licensing Authority for Human In Vitro Fertilization and Embryology*, ILA, London.

Johnson, M., Sherr, L., Bird, D. & Shaw, R. (1984) *In Vitro Fertilization*. Paper presented at the Annual Conference of the British Psychological Society, Warwick University.

Kedem, P., Mikulincer, M., Nathanson, Y. & Bartov, B. (1990) Psychological aspects of male infertility. *B. Jnl. of Med. Psych.*, **63**,(1) 73–80.

Lalos, A., Jacobsson, L., Lalos, O. & von Schoultz, B. (1985) The wish to have a child: a pilot study of infertile couples. *Acta Psychiatrica Scandinavica*, **72**,(5), 476–81.

Lieblum, S., Kemmann, E. & Lane, M. (1987) The psychological concomitants of in vitro fertilization. *Jnl. of Psychosomatic Obstet. and Gynec.*, **6**,(3), 165–78.

Ley, P. (1988) *Communicating with patients*. In: Psychology and Medicine Series (Ed. Donald Marcer), Croom Helm, London.

Lind, R., Pruitt, R. & Greenfeld, D. (1989) Previously infertile couples and the newborn intensive care unit. *Health and Social Work*, **14**, 2, 127–33.

Morrison, D. (1985) Adolescent contraceptive behaviour: a review. *Psychological Bulletin*, 98, 538–68.

Najman, J., Morrison, J., Williams, G. & Andersen, M. (1991) The mental health of women six months after they give birth to an unwanted baby: a longitudinal study, *Social Science and Medicine*, **32**,(3), 241–47.

Oakley, A. (1980) *Women Confined. Towards a Sociology of Childbirth*. Martin Robertson, Oxford.

O'Moore, M. & Harrison, R. (1991) Anxiety and reproductive failure. *Irish Jnl of Psychology*, **12**,(2), 276–85.

Owens, D. & Read, M. (1984) Patients' experience with the assessment of subfertility testing and treatment. *Jnl. of Reproductive and Infant Psychology*, 2, 7–17.

Reading, A. (1982) The management of fear related to vaginal examination, *Journal of Psychosomatic Obstet. and Gynec.*, **1**,(3/4) 99–102.

Reading, A., Chang, L. & Kerin, J. (1989) Psychological state and coping styles across an IVF treatment cycle, *Jnl. of Reproductive and Infant Psychology*, **7**,(2), 95–103.

Ryan, G. & Sweeney, P. (1980) Attitudes of adolescents toward pregnancy and contraception. *Am. Jnl. of Obstet. and Gynec.*, 137, 358–66.

Ryan, I. & Dunn, P. (1988) Association of race, sex, religion, family size and desired number of children on college students' preferred methods of dealing with unplanned pregnancy. *Family Practice Rsrch. Jnl.*, **7**,(3) 153–61.

Sauer, M., Paulson, R. & Lobo, R. (1992) Reversing the natural decline in human fertility, *JAMA*, 268,(10), 1275–9.

Schellon, A. (1957) *Artificial Insemination in the Human*, Columbia University Press, New York.

Schinke, S. (1984) Preventing teenage pregnancy. In: *Progress in Behavior Modification* (ed. M. Hersen, R. Eisler, R. Miller) Academic Press, New York.

Seibel, M. & Taymor, M. (1982) Emotional aspects of infertility, *Fertility and Sterility*, 37, 175–82.

Shaw, P. (1991) Infertility counselling. In *Counselling and Communication in Health Care* (ed. A. Davis & L. Fallowfield) John Wiley and Sons, Chichester.

Shaw, P., Johnston, M. & Shaw, R. (1988) Counselling needs: emotional and relationship problems in couples awaiting IVF. *Journal of Psychosomatic Obstet. and Gynec.*, 9, 171–80.

Sherr, L. (1987) Evaluation of the UK Health Education Campaign on AIDS, *Psychology and Health*, 1, 61–72.

Sherr, L. & Strong, C. (1992) Safe Sex and women. *GU Medicine*, Nov, 113–15.

Sherr, L., Strong, C. & Goldmeier, D. (1990) Sexual behaviour, condom use and prediction in attenders at sexually transmitted disease clinics – implications for counselling. *Counselling Psychology Quarterly*, 3,(4) 343–52.

Sherr, L., Davey, T. & Strong, C. (1991) Anxiety and depression in AIDS and HIV/ Infection, *Counselling Psychology Quarterly*, 4,(1) 27–35.

Snowden, R. & Snowden, E. (1984) *The Gift of a Child*, Allen and Unwin, London.

Soules, M. (1985) The in vitro fertilization pregnancy note: let's be honest with each other. *Fertility and Sterility*, 43, 511–13.

Stacey, M. (1992) *Changing Human Reproduction*, Sage Publications, London.

Stanton, A., Tennen, H., Affleck, G. & Mendola, R. (1991) Cognitive appraisal and adjustment to infertility, *Women and Health*, **17**,(3) 1–15.

Stanton, A., Tennen, H., Affleck, G. & Mendola, R. (1992) Coping and adjustment to infertility. *Jnl. of Social and Clinical Psychology*, **11**(1) 1–13.

Ulbrich, P., Coyle, A. & Llabre, M. (1990) Involuntary childlessness and marital adjustment, *His and Hers Journal of Sex and Marital Therapy*, **16**,(3), 147–58.

Wallace, L. (1984) Psychological preparations: a method of reducing the stress of surgery. *Jnl. of Human Stress*, 10, 62–77.

Zelnick, M. & Shah, F. (1983) First intercourse among young Americans. *Fam. Planning Perspectives*, 15, 64–70.

Chapter 4

Staying Pregnant or Not

Pregnancies that do not progress to full term are pregnancies all the same. Of those that do not progress, some terminate spontaneously (miscarriage) and others are terminated by choice, either because of social factors, for psychological reasons, or because of medical factors in the woman or in the fetus.

Termination

Deciding to terminate

The decision to terminate a pregnancy will be one which is made fairly rapidly; but it will have lifelong consequences. Counselling given at such a time may offer help for the psychological adjustment for the future life of the woman, especially in terms of her childbearing experience. Although many centres specialize in terminations and are proficient at counselling, there are times when this input is merely incidental, or is overlooked or minimized in an effort to avoid discussion of painful decisions.

Decision making about termination has received some attention. Allen (1981) found that nearly three quarters of women who had a termination of pregnancy had sought this out prior to eight weeks pregnancy. Decision making models show that extensive social group dialogue is utilized by women to come to the initial decision to seek a termination and medical advice is then sought to support or confirm decisions, rather than to make them. This suggests that intervention needs to come early and that easy access to professionals is the only way to integrate this level of input into the formative stages of decision making.

Behavioural intentions were studied as predictors of pregnancy termination (Smetana & Adler, 1979), who questioned women attending for a pregnancy test (prior to pregnancy confirmation but obviously when pregnancy signs were possible). There was a high correlation with pre-result intentions and post-result behaviour. These workers emphasized the key role played by family and friends. This finding has been endorsed in other studies.

Decision making by professionals (whose permission is required to proceed with a termination) is also an interesting one for study. Hamill & Ingram (1974) showed varying trends for professionals. Professionals can certainly play a role in termination decisions for medical factors. Marteau (1989) and Sherr (in press) showed that the way the outcome probability is couched can affect termination decisions. Marteau fed back handicap probabilities to medical students in two different frames (positive, focusing on the per cent normality expected and negative, focusing on the per cent abnormality expected). It was found that negative frames were more likely to result in termination recommendations. This finding was true of pregnant women when considering terminations in the presence of HIV infection. If they were informed there was a 75 per cent likelihood of infection free infants, they were less likely to consider a termination than if they were informed there was a 25 per cent likelihood of infected infants. Boyle (1991) noted that source of care (health service or private) was associated with sterilization and abortion links. This may not necessarily reflect different policy or procedures, as it may well reflect different clients.

This chapter will outline the counselling approach and review the literature on short- and long-term consequences of termination.

Counselling and termination of pregnancy

Termination of pregnancy is not an option held open for all. For many people this option is unthinkable; for others it is simply not available. Termination counselling essentially requires workers to acknowledge that the decisions which have been made are those of the mother or parents and that they may be helped to come to that decision through the process of counselling, which may also help them to live with the consequences and plan a future. Good counselling also prepares them for any trauma that they may experience during the process of the termination and beyond. One in five pregnancies in England and Wales is terminated on therapeutic grounds (Kumar & Robson, 1984; Llewellyn Jones, 1982).

Emotional impact

There are few longer term studies on the impact of termination. Those that exist generally describe a range of short-term problems. They invariably describe the impact on the woman and no sound studies exist describing the impact on the male, short- or long-term. When follow up studies are carried out, few note longer term psychological difficulties, although follow up times are often limited. Comprehensive reviews (Blumentahl, 1991; Dagg, 1991; Alder, *et al.* 1990) generally show that psychiatric complications after abortion are rare. Indeed, the incidence of diagnosed psychiatric illness and psychiatric hospital admission after abortion is much lower after abortion than it is after childbirth itself. Brewer (1977) noted that post partum psychosis occurred after delivery in about 1.7 women per 1000 deliveries. Psychosis after abortion was considerably lower at 0.3 cases per 1000 women. Russo & Zierk (1992) followed over 5000 women for 8 years and found that abortion alone did not independently predict well being and that at 8 years there was no evidence of widespread trauma.

Certain groups are more likely to suffer psychiatric problems, particularly those with a history of psychiatric illness, those pressurized into abortion (Brewer, 1977) women who are young, of lower social support, the multiparous and those within a context where abortion is not endorsed (Zolese & Blacker, 1992). Most studies concentrate on psychological harm rather than psychological benefit, which certainly also exists (Greer, *et al.*, 1976; Shusterman, 1979). Indeed, Stotland (1992) notes that some women undergo transient feelings of stress or sadness which are qualitatively different from psychiatric illness. Although the prospective monitoring of termination is rarely carried out or reported, it has been studied both before the procedure and for a short duration afterwards (Friedman & Gath, 1989). Partridge, *et al.* (1971) followed up 207 cases and found that the overwhelming majority (94 per cent) reported improved mental health after abortion.

Many case descriptions of acute psychiatric disturbance after termination can be found in the available literature (e.g. Davidson & Clare, 1989). However, it is unclear whether the termination triggered the event, or whether the problems pre-existed.

Rizzardo, *et al.* (1991) studied 208 pregnant women, comparing 78 who were about to undergo voluntary termination, 63 who were threatening miscarriage and 67 who were routine antenatal attenders. They found that the subjects who were about to abort showed higher levels of psychological distress, whilst subjects with a threatened miscarriage showed an intermediate level of distress.

Kumar & Robson (1984) noted that there was a correlation between previous terminations and increased depression in early pregnancy subsequent to the termination. Depression in early pregnancy was associated with termination considerations.

Stotland (1992) noted that insensitive, negative or hostile behaviour or comments by staff or others encountered during the process of termination decision making could adversely affect psychological experience. Meikle, *et al.* (1977) showed that emotional distress was less frequent after legalization of abortion.

Psychological distress was linked with stigma associated with hospital admission, especially if care was on a gynaecological ward where other women were being admitted for infertility investigations (Zolese & Blacker, 1992). Women who presented for termination had additional relationship and social strain over and above the termination issue.

Press and media attention have attempted to describe an Abortion Trauma Syndrome, although the existence of such a syndrome has been refuted (Stotland, 1992). This writer very aptly describes that the emotional and physical effects of an abortion can only meaningfully be contrasted with the effects of an illegal abortion. Any psychological effects of the supposed Syndrome which are monitored may be due to the underlying reasons as to why the pregnancy was not desired in the first place, rather than being consequent upon the termination.

Termination counselling

There are many avenues of advice for women seeking terminations: mothers, fathers, grandparents, doctors, siblings, teachers and friends. Counselling differs from these sources in that it is the one place which is not concerned with telling people what to do.

People invariably come to counselling when the advice avenues around them are exhausted or ineffective. Counselling initially involves helping people make their own decisions. Once these decisions have been made, counselling should support people through their decisions and maximize their ability to cope.

All good termination counselling should commence with decision making about the termination itself. There are specific roles for the counsellor and basic counselling skills needed for termination counselling. Since termination of pregnancy may mark ongoing psychological problems, there are a wide range of associated support requirements.

Most workers feel that termination of pregnancy will involve considerable emotional reactions. Yet there are few prospective studies which systematically evaluate this and the literature is often very general and based on short-term studies. Overall, such studies have noted that psychological reactions to termination were common, but that severe long-term difficulties were unusual.

When longer term problems have been sought, few have been identified (Greer, *et al.*, 1976; Illsley & Hall, 1976; Donnai, *et al.*, 1981). Shusterman (1979) recorded that some women expressed relief after termination. Turell *et al.* (1990), in a review of the literature, marks a consistent finding of relief as the predominant feeling. Severe emotional trauma was not generally prevalent in any of these studies. The pattern seems to be one of short-term crises with a few, longer term, problems. This proportion seems to be in the region of one in ten. Yet extensive follow up is rare, and it may be that trauma is revisited many years later for more women. This is especially likely if subsequent fertility problems are experienced, either directly through physical problems resulting from the termination, or indirectly through guilt and emotional dissonance when a pregnancy is subsequently desired and contrasted with the termination.

There are both benefits and traumas associated with termination.

Workers should examine the literature to try to identify and predict factors which may be associated with longer term problems. Turell *et al.* (1990), Dunlop (1978) and Shusterman (1979) have recounted risk factors which could aid the focus of intervention as follows:

- Pressure or coercion in making the decision to terminate from many sources, including medical professionals, family, spouse or peers.
- Previous psychiatric history may be a predictor of subsequent coping problems. Thus a comprehensive medical and psychiatric history should be taken when women present for medical check-ups.
- Dunlop noted that terminations which are associated with medical reasons may create subsequent difficulties. It is unclear whether this is caused by the stress of facing up to the medical problem, or whether the medical problem recurs and that this contributes to psychological difficulties in the long term. It is important to differentiate between conditions where the woman does not want a pregnancy at all and those where a woman does want a pregnancy, but does not want this particular one.
- Carers should monitor the emotional reaction on discovering the existence of the pregnancy, as this has been found to be a useful predictor of subsequent distress. Essentially, those who feel ambivalence, immense anger and panic fare least well and may require special input.
- Social support is generally a positive factor and poor relationships, coupled with a lack of intimacy with a partner, have been associated with poor prognosis. It is unclear, however, whether it is the unfulfilling relationship which contributes to long-term difficulties rather than a termination in the presence of such a relationship. However, it does indicate that good counselling should primarily involve a comprehensive discussion on the nature and level of the relationship. The impact of the termination on the future of the relationship should also be incorporated into the dialogue. Although most discussions are held exclusively with the pregnant woman who is about to consider the termination, it is good practice to offer the possibility of contact with the male partner, or encourage the couple to enter into discussions.
- Shusterman (1979) found that dissatisfaction with termination decision was a predictor of poor emotional outcome. This finding points out the necessity to check the decision with the woman and to allow, at all times, for decisions to be re-examined and altered.
- Coping and well structured decision making styles (Turell, *et al.* 1990) were shown to be predictive of later emotional adjustment to abortion.
- Demographic variables have sometimes been correlated with the level of emotional response. Higher emotional reaction has been recorded in young women, those with no other children, those in the second trimester of pregnancy and those holding strong religious views.

From this data it seems that social support, plus the supportive decisions of others, are desirable ingredients for protection against future emotional disruption. When women think through their decision more clearly and feel in control of the situation, the prognosis is better. Counselling sessions which can provide or address these factors may help to equip women emotionally and protect them against short-and long-term distress. It also seems that couples vary in their reactions in coping with a termination. Counselling ought to address this, facilitating opening the dialogue between couple members and providing understanding and insight into what may be very differently paced reactions. This may prevent discord as a result of such differences and thus enhance coping. It may also diminish the differences, although it is unclear whether this is necessary or even desirable, given the importance for individuals to have their own reactions.

Counselling should therefore be a key element of termination decisions, providing both an occasion and an opportunity for full discussion and thought.

However, although many women find counselling beneficial, some also may not want assistance of this sort, or find it helpful (Marcus, 1979). Counselling should not be imposed on an unwilling recipient. In such circumstances it is important for medical and care staff to allow for considered and informed dialogue to take place prior to the termination. Counselling itself is not a panacea and subsequent contraception and termination problems are still apparent in some studies (Marcus, 1979).

Pacing the termination decision

Termination counselling is difficult. Counsellors need to understand that there are no right or wrong decisions. A decision which is right for one person at one time may be wrong for the same individual at another time. What is right for one individual is not right for all. Such decisions are highly specific. Termination counselling therefore needs to include the following elements.

Accurate factual information

The first step for anyone involved (client, counsellor or health staff) is to be fully informed. Accurate information is the basis for all effective decisions. Denial of such information effectively limits women's choice. Provision of such information must involve tailored, interactive dialogue, the free passage of information, the ability to apply the information to a personal situation and to go over information if it is unclear, forgotten or overwhelming.

Whilst counselling is clearly not simply imparting of information, the information itself should never be overlooked or undervalued. Those in possession of factual information sometimes feel they have no counselling skills and as they are intimidated by the counselling demands of their patients, they may feel reluctant to embark on anything vaguely resembling counselling. This is unfortunate as they have a major tool in their hands which if used wisely could benefit many clients.

Women also need to understand what the empirical data means in relation to their own circumstance. They also need to differentiate between the large body of data and their own personal situation.

Non-judgmental approaches

There is little room for strong opinions in counselling. The remit is to listen to the needs and thoughts of clients, help them come to the best decision for their circumstances and ensures that they have thought through all possible options.

The counselling process

Who should counsel?
Counselling can be carried out by the psychology, medical, midwifery or social work staff. If, however, the medical/midwifery staff are not involved they need to contribute and be informed of progress. Their involvement has advantages in that they may have an established trusting relationship with the woman and therefore may be ideally placed to offer ongoing help. The disadvantages may be the limitations on time and expertise. The obstetrician, for example, may have a different model of care and may be reluctant to allow the woman to explore decisions and options for herself. Although a learning procedure could help the obstetrician with this alternative model, this may be at some cost to the women concerned whose care will then be provided by an inexperience individual during their early learning process.

Essentially, counselling is a skilled procedure and anyone who has not acquired this skill should not presume that they can simply counsel. It requires training, insight, practice, critique and development.

Who should be counselled?
A counsellor needs to work out whether the mother should be seen alone or with her partner and should discuss this with the woman, who should be free to choose. Even if women choose to be counselled alone, their partners or family members may still have needs which ought to be addressed. Once these basic decisions have been made, the process of counselling should ensue.

Environment
The counselling venue is important. It needs to be comfortable, providing privacy for uninterrupted confidential conversation. It is important that normal social and work facilities such as coffee or tea, easy chairs, access to telephone, writing material and tissues are available.

Timing
Extensive delays always provoke anxiety. Termination counselling should occur as soon as possible after it is requested or required. Long waits in clinic waiting rooms should be avoided and clinic times should not coincide with any other clinics to the extent that they impede or upset the woman. As this particular type of counselling may result in a need to pause and think and with access to follow up information, timing should incorporate a facility for longer term commitment. The women can then be helped at multiple occasions to come to a decision and given support through that decision and beyond, whether she changes her mind or not.

Preparation
The first step in counselling should always come from the counsellor. The aims and goals of counselling must be clearly worked out prior to any interaction. Variations will, of course, occur according to individual needs. But counsellors need to be very clear about their role and responsibilities. The underlying goal of all counselling is to provide a non-judgemental environment where a woman can explore, in an open and unpressured way, the decision that she would like to make.

Some counsellors work alone, others work in pairs. However, a woman faced by too many counsellors may feel intimidated and most counselling is usually done in a one-to-one situation. Women should always be given the opportunity to choose whether they would like their partner or another particular person to be present with them. Counsellors should not have hard and fast rules. They need to be open to individual or couple counselling, and should not put pressure on clients to be seen with a partner if they prefer to be seen alone. The counsellor should give the women the opportunity to make this decision. This is often best done alone with the women who can bring her partner in later if she so chooses. At the same time, the wishes of the couple must be respected. If a woman is seen alone, she should be encouraged to enter a dialogue with her partner if he is available, prior to making any firm decisions.

Beginning the interview

Counsellors should always introduce themselves fully and ensure that they have the correct name of the person they are seeing and its proper pronunciation. Very importantly, the counsellor should be seen as helpful and friendly. The way an interview begins will often determine the extent to which this goal can be achieved. It is good practice to go out and fetch the person or couple, rather than have a receptionist call their names and let them find their own way to the room. Do not abandon normal social interaction such as greetings, introduction, seatings and ensuring comfort. It may be helpful to provide a place to hang coats, and to offer the provision of items which break social distance, such as a drink of coffee or tea.

However this is done, it is important to set out in the first instance what counselling means and what the session will entail. The woman, and her partner if present, needs to understand that you will be spending time exploring options, discussing the information that exists, and helping her (or them) come to a decision. She needs to know that she is not rushed for a decision and that she will be given as much time as she needs. There should be no pressure to come to any decisions at the end of the meeting. It may well take more than one meeting and the woman may want to go home and think about it before deciding.

The woman also needs to have a clear indication that the counsellor is impartial. If it appears that the counsellor is biased, this may colour the woman's decision or it may make it difficult, or even impossible, to explore her own feelings.

Basic background

At this stage the counsellor ought to establish basic background facts. These will form the basis of any subsequent information giving.

Reason for the termination
The underlying reason for the termination will have direct effects on the course of the interview. It may be that the pregnancy was unexpected or unplanned. It may be a much desired pregnancy where an abnormality has been discovered and although the woman desires a pregnancy, she does not desire this one. It may be that she is torn between a variety of factors. Problems relating to these factors may recur and this must be addressed within the sessions (for example genetic problems or sex linked abnormalities).

How far has the pregnancy progressed?
The legal limitations on termination vary from country to country. In any event, there are widespread accepted medical criteria which dictate safety limits for termination. Generally speaking, terminations should be aimed to take place prior to 16 weeks gestation. After that time, the risks to the mother do increase. The method of termination will also vary according to gestation of the fetus. In the UK, the legal limit for terminations has recently been brought forward from 28 weeks to 24 weeks gestation.

Parity
The counsellor should establish whether the mother has other children, has had other terminations in the past and whether she intends to have children in the future.

Social factors
The pregnant woman's social background may have many implications in her decision to terminate. Counsellors can never be available all of the time. One of the goals of counselling must be to establish other support networks that the patient can turn to if necessary. This will include both personal and community support, such as the woman's partner, parents, and friends on the one hand and professionals or agencies on the other. It is important to explain different forms of support, such as social support, professional support and financial support (Kincey & Saltmore, 1988). The timing of such support is also a key factor. If the correct ingredients of support are available in theory, but not readily available when needed, their efficacy will be reduced or even negated.

Other factors
Past psychiatric history, drug use, or any other behavioural patterns should be explored. Often such behaviours represent crisis coping and as termination decisions may well represent a crisis point for such an individual, these may recur or become more pronounced.

Discussing termination
The issue of the termination should be coached in terms of the pregnancy generally. This will allow for a fresh beginning so that the woman can go through the decision making process from start to finish without any presumed conclusions. It is necessary to explore the pregnancy with the patient and to understand what it means to them. They may want to discuss how they conceived, what they think about childbearing, their plans for the future and explore possible strategy outcomes. There are many possibilities for dealing with an unwanted pregnancy. At all times the woman's views must be respected.

The woman needs to know basic facts and information to help her come to a decision which is correct for her. It is at this point that the woman ought to be given the full facts in a simple and straightforward way. However, she also needs to appreciate, without ambiguity, that knowledge itself is often limited. There are simply no answers to many questions.

Facts wanted by women at this time include:

- The future and prognosis.
- The effects on any subsequent pregnancy.
- Personal effects of termination, such as discomfort, pain.
- Practical information such as length of time for the procedure and the method of termination.

- Time limits – how long do they have to make a decision, can it be reversed?
- Details of medical care that is available.
- Anticipated emotions.

Decision making summary

It is important to underline that at the end of the day, women must be able to make their own decisions. They need to know they have time to make these decisions. No woman should be hurried into a decision because a session is nearing an end.

Once a woman has come to a decision to terminate, the counsellor should then discuss with her all the possible outcomes based on this decision. She should be assisted to explore how she may react in a variety of circumstances. She should try and think through the consequences of the decision and plan some of her responses and the avenues to which she would turn for support at such a time.

Longer term problems

Part of the counselling procedure can then be devoted to longer term problems. This involves a discussion of future conception and contraception.

Zabin, *et al.* (1990) noted that women who present for a pregnancy test and then test negative may be at high risk of a subsequent unplanned pregnancy. Such women would also benefit from counselling.

Concerns and anxieties

The appropriate details of termination need to be discussed with the woman. This should be done by a qualified member of staff. If the counsellor does not know the facts, it is a good idea to involve one of the medical practitioners who can give accurate factual information to the woman. Anxieties are most common in the face of the unknown. People are often much less anxious when they have accurate facts. This also allows for good cognitive rehearsal of stressful events and may often prepare the woman for the forthcoming procedure.

The method of termination may depend on the gestation of the fetus. Good history taking skills form an important part of the counselling procedure. When dates are unclear, it may be appropriate for a doctor to prescribe an ultrasound scan.

Procedural information

Many of the procedures involved with termination require pacing and timing. Such procedures need to be explained to the women at an early stage and should include information about availability of procedures, the forms these procedures will take, and an explanation of procedures, as well as practical details relating to the hospitals and dates which will be involved.

Planning

The counsellor needs to help women plan through both the practicalities of the termination and her emotional responses to it. She may want to discuss her anxieties, worries and concerns. She may want to express sadness or relief. The counsellor can ask both clear and ambiguous questions. It is often helpful to invite the patient to contemplate the outcome realistically and to explore how they think they would cope. Very often people simply shut out stressful or worrying thoughts. This leaves them unprepared when reality hits. By opening the door to such discussions, the counsellor may allow the patient to think worrying thoughts within a less worrying environment.

Subsequent pregnancies

One of the most common issues with termination counselling centres around subsequent pregnancies. Some workers have found heightened anxieties and concerns during pregnancy for women who have had previous terminations.

Opportunity to reflect

Towards the end of the interview, the counsellor ought to summarize and reflect back to the woman some of the process that she has gone through. This serves to confirm that the counsellor has fully understood the woman's thoughts and feelings. It also allows for an opportunity to ask questions.

Preparation for termination

Termination of pregnancy is a surgical procedure with an increased emotional component. There is a common association of anxiety and concern with surgery in anticipation of the event, during the procedure and often for extended periods afterwards (Johnston & Carpenter, 1980). Furthermore, there is a considerable amount of psychology literature which shows an association between pre-operative emotional state (including anxiety, cognitive preparation and satisfaction) with post-operative outcome (Johnston & Carpenter, 1980).

A series of studies have been carried out to decide which forms of information have the best effects (see Ley, 1988). Shortcomings in the research are the failure to use systematic measures, the utilization of vastly differing operative procedures, and the measurement of post-operative outcome by a variety of indices. The net result is that it is difficult to generalize from one study to the next.

However, the overwhelming finding is that there does seem to be a positive impact when information is provided on a variety of outcomes (Matthews & Ridgeway, 1981). A range of medical situations have been examined: gynaecological surgery (Johnston & Carpenter, 1980), laparoscopy (Wallace, 1984), ultrasound scanning (Reading & Cox, 1982) and labour (Enkin & Chalmers, 1982). Input has varied from instruction booklets, written information, oral information, brief psychotherapy, counselling, instructions, role-play, sensitization, procedural information and so on. Outcome measures have included pain ratings, satisfaction, analgesia uptake, length of hospital stay, psychological well being, anxiety, medication and psycho-social adjustment.

Generally, the literature indicates that the provision of information has an overall beneficial effect. An addition of information about sensory experience enhances the effect of any procedural information (Johnson & Leventhal, 1974). In conclusion, psychologists have pointed out the need to address the particular needs and fears associated with the given medical procedure. More recent work has developed these ideas to incorporate a tailoring of input to individual coping styles (Miller & Mangan, 1983, Steptoe & O'Sullivan, 1986).

Post termination

The following points should be borne in mind after a termination:

(1) Immediate feedback is usually needed. This should be spontaneous and should also allow for questions and queries.
(2) There are a wide range of physical and emotional experiences that women report, such as pain, sadness, worry, fear, fluctuating moods or even relief. Women need to be forewarned of these and staff should reassure them of their 'normality'.
(3) Pain management should be discussed and provided. This may relate to how the woman feels before, during and after the procedure.
(4) The woman will have queries about general information, basic facts, physical and emotional things to anticipate, simple advice and warning signs in case of problems. Verbal answers and dialogue should be supplemented with written information.
(5) Psychological reactions to termination should be anticipated by the

provision of support. Follow up meetings should be set up, using the time to discuss contraception, protection, relationship issues, and future behaviour. Emotional reactions may well be delayed, and after the event the woman may experience a range of emotions which may need venting.

After discharge

Follow up is vital. Immediately after a termination, someone may express one emotion and some days later may oscillate to a very different emotion. They should be prepared for this possibility and encouraged to explore how they might cope.

Self help groups can be very useful. Here women can gather support and discuss their experience with other women who have undergone a termination or faced such decisions.

Miscarriage or spontaneous abortion

When a baby under 28 weeks spontaneously aborts, this is termed a miscarriage. It is a surprisingly common event, which is understudied; few resources are devoted to the care and amelioration of the incident for the woman or the couple concerned. Cartwright (1984) reports a miscarriage frequency as high as one to four in six. Some women miscarry only once, but others may suffer from multiple miscarriages or sporadic miscarriage. Intervention and emotional support, if provided, is usually only available for women who miscarry late in pregnancy. Early miscarriage, however, can be equally traumatic (Turner, 1989, Jackman, *et al.* 1991).

Emotional responses

The studies that have been carried out catalogue the range of emotional effects (Friedman & Gath, 1989), the extent to which these continue with time (Seibel & Graves, 1980), and ameliorating factors. Cartwright (1984) reports on the long-term impact of the event and the specific effects it may have on approach and coping in a subsequent pregnancy. Moulder (1990) gives a graphic account of the experiences from a woman's point of view.

Interviews with women after miscarriage (Jackman, *et al.* 1991, Cartwright, 1984, Gannon, 1992) show that some aspects of medical care are unsatisfactory. These include:

● Little consultation maintained throughout.

- No involvement in decisions to view the remains of the fetus.
- No involvement in decisions to 'dispose' of the remains.
- Unsatisfactory staff reaction.
- Limited opportunities to talk over the event.
- Poor provision of information.
- Limited explanations which were highly desired.
- No space to grieve.
- Regret at not knowing the sex of the baby.

Jackman, *et al.* (1991) reported that most negative emotions dissipated with time. Clinical levels of distress can be high. Jackman *et al.*, found an interaction between levels of distress, the opportunity to discuss the miscarriage and medical management. Dissatisfaction with aspects of medical care were commonly reported. It was rare for any dialogue or discussion about the fetal remains to occur – especially about whether to view these or how to bury them. Although many negative emotions occurred immediately surrounding the miscarriage, most women said these became less acute with time, yet levels of notable psychological distress was still present in 44 per cent of the subjects a year after the miscarriage.

Cognitions surrounding miscarriage have been studied extensively. Many women have specific ideas about blame and cause. Madden (1988) studied 65 women to examine such cognitions some of which were predictive of depressive moods on follow up. Maternal age and presence of an older child was protective against depression. Day, *et al.* (1987) found that family resource variables were stronger predictors of crisis and recovery than community resources, therefore supporting the notions that family cohesion and support are helpful.

Informational needs

Information and support are key elements. In studies, although two-thirds are satisfied with the level of support they receive, immediately after the incident (e.g. Helstrom & Victor, 1987), this decreases to just over half with the passage of a few weeks. Counselling can help to shorten the period of grieving (Forrest, Standish & Baum, 1982). Moulder (1990) describes a number of situations common to many women:

- Symptom recognition.
- Raised hopes.
- Need for confirmation of miscarriage.
- The role of scans in confirming a miscarriage.
- The physical facts.
- Uncertainty about what to expect.
- Medical emergency which may surround the event.

- Physical effects such as bleeding or pain.
- Trauma of dilation and curettage (or ERPC).
- Asking about the loss.
- Giving birth – and dealing with the fetal remains.
- Burial (often termed callously 'disposal').
- After the miscarriage (mood, milk coming in).
- Outsider help and hindrance.
- Partner and family roles.
- Telling others (especially children).
- Grief – not only at the loss of a child, but a loss of role which is often not spoken about.
- The next pregnancy and its concerns.
- Recurrence of miscarriage.

Grief

Grief can be centred around a number of aspects, including:

- Unfulfilled need.
- Unshared loss.
- Underestimated duration of emotion.
- Recurrence of emotion at triggering events (expected date of delivery, anniversaries).
- Uncertainty often made worse by gaps in knowledge.
- Societal pressure.
- Ramifications on other children, especially in terms of overprotection.

As with all loss, the grieving process is hampered if the loss is not acknowledged. This may entail the creation of memories in order to focus the grief. The knowledge of the sex of the baby or other details can assist.

Multiple or recurrent loss represent acute trauma for women. Although staff may blur each loss, women see them as very separate. The trauma is greater than simply a single miscarriage multiplied.

Explanations for fetal loss may affect coping and adjustment. Dunn, *et al.* (1991) examined explanations given by men and women for fetal loss and found the following themes:

- Blaming the mother.
- Physical problems with the fetus.
- Physical problems with the mother.
- Fate.
- No explanation.

The process of understanding can be twofold, with parents taking in the doctor's explanations, but formulating their own hypothesis. They may hold these simultaneously or endorse one to a greater extent than the other. When good communication and helpful explanations were given by doctors (Dunn, *et al.* (1991), these were not only satisfying but details were recorded after two years.

Women vary in their subsequent need and desire for a new pregnancy. There are those who want to wait and those who do not. Clearly, respect and understanding for individual variation is important.

Management

Management of miscarriage is often compounded by the routines and systems set up to deal with it. For the doctors (usually junior doctors on short hospital stays) it is seen as a common clinical problem. The woman, however, has lost her baby. Currently there is a debate on comprehensive management, in which queries are being made whether women need to be hospitalized, which ward they should enter, and how follow up, information giving, and emotional support can best be delivered. The role of dilatation and curettage in particular needs examining.

'The convenient medical conundrum which wraps up miscarriage ... the thing that is done to you to take it all away ... the convenient box into which we can offload the unmentionable and the unspeakable ...'

Impact on fathers

Few studies examine the impact on the father who has to provide a supportive role, may have less 'permission' to grieve and may be focusing on what he is expected to give rather than any understanding of what he needs himself.

Way forward

The way forward must be to acknowledge that every miscarriage is a potential 'catastrophe'. The medicalization and hospital procedures may serve a ritual function. The experience is poignantly described by a woman who first knew she was miscarrying when the radiologist asked 'have you had a miscarriage before?' (Anonymous, 1993). This medical interview centred around the doctor's problems rather than the woman who reported that

'my baby was disengaging itself from my insides and cascading down my legs. I was in pain and I was frightened. The other avalanche of feelings were waiting, howling at the door and she [the obstetrician] was of no use to me'.

Tunaley & Slade (1992) propose an interesting theoretical model to account for adjustment and reaction to miscarriage. They examined the Taylor model (Taylor, 1983; Taylor, *et al.* 1984) which proposes cognitive adaption to threatening events as follows:

(1) *Search for meaning*   This involves an attributional search (what caused this to happen?).

(2) *Search for mastery*   This involves an attempt to regain a sense of personal control over the event, which adds the possible component of preventing it happening in the future.

(3) *Search for self enhancement*   This serves to raise self-esteem after the threatening event and uses mechanisms such as downwards comparisons (examining the event in contrast to others who may be worse off than self) and examination of the positive consequences of the event – even benefits.

In a small study of 22 women experiencing miscarriage Tunaley & Slade found some support for the model. Of the subjects 86 per cent made causal attributions (including medical problems, stress, self blame, blaming others, punishment or no explanations). Nearly all the women perceived an explanation as extremely important. There was also evidence of mastery and control attempts, with high numbers expressing a desire for a subsequent pregnancy. Evidence of self enhancement search was also present. Comparisons were drawn between those who had children besides this pregnancy and comments were made about improved personal relationships, life reappraisal, priorities, knowledge and planning.

Women's voices after pregnancy loss

Black (1991) studied 70 women undergoing elective abortions and 51 who lost their pregnancies following spontaneous miscarriages. These women shared much with their male partners and on the whole felt understood and supported by them. Yet many differed from their male partners in their response to the loss. Coping patterns varied in the face of these differences.

Demb (1991) interviewed six teenage girls a week after abortion. It was found that pregnancy was often a result of inconsistent birth control. Second trimester abortion was more common. Emotional reactions centred around sadness, guilt, thoughts of their own mothers and a spurning of adoption as an alternative. Feelings about abortion were intense and a post-abortion appointment was beneficial. Such appointments were used to discuss the abortion rather than as an opportunity to simply focus on future sexual behaviour or contraception.

Implications for intervention

Pregnancy loss, whether spontaneous or by choice, is an emotionally harrowing experience. It needs to be handled with full appreciation of the short- and longer term ramifications for the woman and her family. Counselling at such a time may ease the process and prevent or ameliorate subsequent difficulties. No decision to terminate or experience of miscarriage should go without input from a member of staff. This may range from straightforward examining of emotions and feelings, to more intense help through decision making. Any woman who presents with a pregnancy in the face of a previous loss may have special needs in the light of this history.

References

Alder, N., David, H., Major, B., Roth, S., Russon, N. & Wyatt, G. (1990) Psychological responses after abortion. *Science*, 248, 41–44.

Allen, I. (1981) Family Planning Sterilization and Abortion Services. The Policy Studies Institute, no 595, London.

Anonymous (1993) Ms Carriage – an account of a thoroughly modern miscarriage. *Maternity Care of the Mother and Child*.

Black, R. (1991) Women's voices after pregnancy loss. Couples' patterns of communication and support. *Social Work in Health Care*, 16,(2), 19–36.

Blumenthal, S. (1991) *An overview of research findings in Scotland: psychiatric aspects of abortion* American Psychiatric Press, Washington DC.

Boyle, M. (1991) Decision making for contraception and abortion. In *The Psychology of Health: an Introduction* (Eds. M. Pitts and K. Phillips) Routledge, London.

Brewer, C. (1977) Incidence of post abortion psychosis: a prospective study. *BMJ*, 1, 476–77.

Cartwright, A. (1984) *Miscarriage*. Fontana Books, London.

Dagg, P. (1991) The psychological sequelae of therapeutic abortion denied and completed. *Am. Jnl. Psychiatry*, 148, 578–85.

Davidson, K. & Clare, A. (1989) Psychotic illness following termination of pregnancy. *B. Jnl. of Psychiatry*, 154, 559–60.

Day, R. & Hooks, D. (1987) Miscarriage – A special type of family crisis. *Family Relations Journal of Applied Family and Child Studies*. 36,(3) 305–10.

Demb, J. (1991) Abortion in inner city adolescents: what the girls say. *Family Systems Medicine*, 9,(1) 93–102.

Donnai, P., Charles, N. & Harris, R. (1981) Attitudes of patients after genetic termination of pregnancy. *BMJ*, 282, 621–2.

Dunlop, J.Z. (1978) Counselling patients requesting an abortion. *Practitioner*, 220, 847–52.

Dunn, D., Goldbach, K., Lasker, J. & Toedter, L. (1991) Explaining pregnancy loss –

parents' and physicians attributions. *Omega Jnl. of Death and Dying*, **23**,(1) 13–23.

Enkin, M. & Chalmers, I. (1982) *Effectiveness and Satisfaction in Antenatal Care*. William Heinemann Medical Books, London.

Forrest, G., Standish, E. & Baum, J. (1982) Support after a perinatal death. A study of support and counselling after perinatal bereavement. *BMJ*, 285, 1475–79.

Friedman, T. & Gath, D. (1989) The psychiatric consequences of spontaneous abortion. *British Journal of Psychiatry*, 155, 810–13.

Gannon, K. (1992) Psychological factors in recurrent miscarriage – a review and critique. *Jnl. Reprod. Infant Psychology*.

Greer, H.S., Lal, S., Lewis, S.C. *et al.* (1976) Psychosocial consequences of therapeutic abortion King's Termination Study II, *B.J. Psychiatry*, 128, 74–79.

Hamill, E. & Ingram, I. (1974) Psychiatric factors in the abortion decision. *BMJ*, 1, 229–232.

Helstrom, L. & Victor, A. (1987) Information and emotional support for women after miscarriage. *Jnl. of Psychosomatic Obstet. and Gynec.*, **7**,(2) 93–98.

Illsley, R. & Hall, M.H. (1976) *Psychosocial aspects of abortion: a review of issues and needed research*. WHO Bulletin, **53**, 85–105.

Jackman, C., McGee, H. & Turner, M. (1991) The experience and psychological impact of early miscarriage. *Irish Jnl. of Psychology*, **12**,(2) 108–20.

Johnson, J.E. & Leventhal, H. (1974) Effects of accurate expectations and behavioural instructions on reactions during a noxious medical examination. *Jnl. of Personality and Social Psychology*, **29**,(5) 710–18.

Johnston, M. (1979) Anxiety and surgery in surgical patients. *Psychological Medicine*, 10, 145–152.

Johnston, M. & Carpenter, L. (1980) Relationship between pre operative and post operative state. *Psychological Medicine*, 10, 361–70.

Kincey, J. & Saltmore, S. (1988) Stress and surgical treatments. In: *Stress and Medical Procedures* (Eds M. Johnston and L. Wallace) Oxford University Press, Oxford.

Kumar, R. & Robson, K. (1984) A prospective study of emotional disorders in childbearing women. *B. Jnl. Psychiatry*, 144, 35–47.

Lask, B. (1975) Short-term psychiatric sequelae to therapeutic termination of pregnancy. *B. Jnl. Psychiatry*, 126 173–77.

Ley, P. (1988) *Communicating with Patients*, Psychology and Medicare Series, Croom Helm, London.

Llewelyn Jones, D. (1982) *Everywoman – a Gynaecological Guide for Life*. Faber and Faber, London.

Madden, M. (1988) Internal and external attributions following miscarriage. *Jnl. of Social and Clinical Psychology*, **7**,(2–3) 113–21.

Marcus, R.J. (1979) Evaluating abortion counselling. *Dimensions in Health Service*, August 16–18.

Marder, L. (1970) Psychiatric experience with liberalized therapeutic abortion law. *Am Jnl. Psychiatry*, 126, 1230–6.

Marteau, T. (1989) Health beliefs and attributions. In *Health Psychology Processes and Applications* (ed. A. Broome). Chapman and Hall, London.

Matthews, A. & Ridgeway, V. (1981) Personality and surgical recovery: a review. *B. Jnl. of Clinical Psychology*, 20, 243–60.

Meikle, S., Robinson, C. & Brody, H. (1977) Recent changes in the emotional reactions of therapeutic abortion applicants, *Canadian Psychiatric Assoc.*, 22, 67–70.

Miller, S.M. & Mangan, C.E. (1983) Interacting effects of information and coping style in adapting to gynecological stress; should the doctor tell all? *Jnl. of Personality and Social Psychology*, **45**,(1) 223–36.

Moulder, C. (1990) *Miscarriage: Women's experiences and needs*. Pandora Press, London.

Partridge, J., Spiegel, T., Rouse, B. & Ewing, J. (1971) Therapeutic abortions: a study of psychiatric applicants at North Carolina Memorial Hospital. *North Carolina Medical Jnl.*, 32, 132–6.

Reading, A. & Cox, D. (1982) The effects of ultrasound examination on maternal anxiety levels. *Journal of Behavioural Medicine*, 5, 237–47.

Ridgeway, V. & Matthews, A. (1982) Psychological preparation for surgery. A comparison of methods. *B. Jnl. of Clinical Psychology*, 21, 271–80.

Rizzardo, R., Novarin, S., Forza, G. and Cosentino, M. (1991) Personality and psychological distress in legal abortion, threatened miscarriage and normal pregnancy. *Psychotherapy and Psychosomatics*, **56**,(4) 227–34.

Russo, N. & Zierk, K. (1992) Abortion, childbearing and women's well being. *Professional Psychology*, 23, 269–80.

Seibel, M. & Graves, W. (1980) The psychological implications of spontaneous abortion. *Journal of Reproductive Medicine*, 25, 161–5.

Sherr, L. (1993) Ante-natal HIV Testing. In: *AIDS Women and Psychology*. (ed. C. Squire), Sage, London.

Shusterman, L.R. (1979) Predicting the psychological consequences of abortion. *Social Science and Medicine*, 96, 683–9.

Smetana, J. & Adler, N. (1979) Decision making regarding abortion: a value times expectancy analysis. *Journal of Population*, 2, 348–55.

Steptoe, A. & O'Sullivan, J. (1986) Monitoring and blunting coping styles in women prior to surgery. *B. Jnl. of Clinical Psychology*, **25**,(2), 143–4.

Stewart, D. (1992) *Abuse in Pregnancy*. Paper presented at the Annual Conference, Society for Reproductive and Infant Psychology, Glasgow.

Stotland, N. (1992) The myth of the post abortion trauma syndrome. *JAMA*, **268**, 2078–9.

Taylor, S. (1983) Adjustment to threatening events; a theory of cognitive adaptation. *American Psychologist*, 38, 1161–73.

Taylor, S., Lichtman, R. & Wood, J. (1984) Attribution, beliefs and control and adjustment to breast cancer. *Jnl. of Personality and Social Psychology*, **46**,(3) 482–502.

Tunaley, J. & Slade, P. (1992) *Cognitive adaption to miscarriage: a preliminary report*. Paper presented at the Annual Conference Society for Reproductive and Infant Psychology, Glasgow.

Turell, S., Armsworth, M. & Gaa, J. (1990) Emotional response to abortion. A critical review of the literature. *Women and Therapy*, **9**,(4), 49–68.

Turner, M. (1989) Spontaneous Miscarriage: this hidden grief. Editorial. *Irish Medical Journal*, 82, 145.

Wallace, L. (1984) Psychological preparation for gynaecological surgery. In *Psychology and Gynecological Problems* (Ed. A. Broome & L. Wallace), 161–88 Tavistock Publications, London.

Zabin, L., Hirsch, M. & Boscia, J. (1990) Differential characteristics of adolescent pregnancy test patients. Abortion, childbearing and negative test groups. *Jnl. of Adolescent Health Care*, **11**,(2) 107–13.

Zolese, G. & Blacker, C. (1992) The psychological complications of therapeutic abortion, *B. Jnl. of Psychiatry*, 160, 742–9.

Chapter 5

Communication and Interactions in Antenatal Care

Communication is the key element in establishing a therapeutic relationship, in gathering adequate and accurate background information and in ongoing care. Effective communication is vital. It is used:

- To gather information – most notably at booking clinics and during various procedures.
- To allay anxiety – during all aspects of childbirth, but particularly during interventions, labour and delivery.
- To ease distress – at all stages of childbirth, but most notably preceding any potentially distressing event, such as a medical consultation, vaginal examination, invasive procedure such as amniocentesis, labour and delivery.
- To assist preparation for labour and delivery.
- To promote compliance with medical advice during pregnancy (such as smoking and alcohol adjustments).
- To promote recovery. This can be before, during or after a procedure to promote anticipatory coping, rehearse coping skills and enhance adjustment.
- To help with pain management.
- To persuade. Persuasion may be necessary at many stages: from the first decision about where to have the baby, to pain management, alcohol reduction, smoking cessation.
- To promote personal uniqueness in the large and often impersonal care system.

The majority of births in the west are overseen by the medical and midwifery professions. Any interaction between professionals and a woman has implications for satisfaction, compliance, anxiety and coping. The doctor/patient literature continually examines the numerous contact points during childbirth – be they with the medical, midwifery, nursing or other professions. The face-to-face encounter between practitioner and patient forms the fundamental core of all interactions. The skilled performance of the initial contact interview is the factor which determines information flow, satisfaction and often compliance and emotional feelings of well being. Ley, *et al.*, (1977, 1982, 1988) have noted serious communication dissatisfaction in a third of all samples questioned, despite satisfaction with medical care generally.

It is not surprising that extensive shortcomings in the abilities and proficiency of professional communication have been catalogued. Communication training is a relatively new innovation, time pressures devalue communication demands, and skills may be lacking and motivation may be low. Few studies examine the general situational factors which may confound communication expertise. Any medic working in an overcrowded situation for unreasonable lengths of time, carrying out repetitive work, in poor environmental conditions and with limited rewards will experience a drop in communication proficiency and motivation. Motivation will recede, as will production. Antenatal care is often typified by such settings. Large depersonalized clinics, often understaffed and overstretched, provide the worst possible conditions under which good personal relationships can be fostered and where time can be devoted to communicate.

Women can be extremely aware of such conditions, and this conspires to make them reluctant to ask questions, to 'waste' time on small items which may be considered trivial, or even to be bold enough to have hope for good communication. Indeed, patients often feel embarrassed if they take up too much time asking questions.

Given this counter-productive environment, communication skills may be notable only by their absence. Although communication training has been an innovation in the last decade (Novack, *et al.* 1993), many programmes have not fully integrated such training into the curriculum and there is much still to be learned. Staff selection rarely invokes communication skills as criteria for acceptance.

There are numerous benefits to improving communications. When these are utilized, not only satisfaction, but successful recall, compliance and informed consent can be increased. Furthermore, studies examining varied communication factors have shown improvements in adjustment, stress level, feelings of control. These often lead to other benefits. Studies (Ley, 1988) have measured as additional outcomes, reduced medication, reduced hospital stays, increased speed of recovery, lowered pain levels and quicker mobility.

However, problems arise when:

- Expected communication fails to occur.
- Communication is unsatisfactory.
- Communication does not have the desired impact.

Communication skill acquisition

Communication skills are often poor, whether one is assessing trainees or those who have been qualified for substantial amounts of time. Much research is carried out on doctors (e.g. Ley, 1988), but the problems are also clearly documented for other professions, particularly nursing (Maguire, *et al.* 1986; Macleod Clark, 1985) and other paramedical professions (Ley, 1988). The results of such problems include general incompetence (Platt & McMath, 1979) and the following poor communication skills:

● Staff interrupting patients (within 18 seconds in Beckman & Frankel, 1984).
● Ignoring emotional/psychiatric problems (Schulberg & Burns, 1988).
● Lack of understanding.
● Lack of recall.
● Overuse of jargon (Korsch *et al.*, 1968).
● Poor interviewing skills (Maguire & Rutter 1976; Maguire *et al.* 1986).
● Missing the main problem (Maguire & Rutter, 1976; Stewart, *et al.*, 1979).
● Asking too many questions (Weiner & Nathanson, 1976).
● Dominating with questions and interruptions (Waitzkin, 1984)
● Lack of feedback of test results (Maguire, *et al.*, 1986; Freeling, *et al.* 1985).

Satisfaction with communications

Communication is seen as a key element in satisfaction with medical care. Approximately one in three patients, in an analysis of many satisfaction surveys are dissatisfied with the level of communication they have experienced (reviewed by Ley, 1988). Satisfaction is also a key correlate of other outcome measures, such as general satisfaction, rating of a clinician's competence (DiMatteo, *et al.*, 1978), compliance, information recall (Ley, 1988), anxiety and accuracy of recall (Sherr, 1989). Unsatisfactory communications can be explained by a number of factors:

Insufficient training
Clearly this is a major factor and one that has been taken into the curriculum of many medical schools. The midwifery and nursing professions are now addressing the need to incorporate communication training into their programmes, but all too often these sessions are seen as add-ons. When they are taught with relevance to applied settings, they are often not taken seriously.

Insufficient time
Lack of time may well result in unsatisfactory communication. Workers have shown that sacrificing communication in favour of time is a false economy as dissatisfied clients often return and in the long term take up

more time. Korsch, *et al.* (1968) found that length of time spent in the interview was not related to satisfaction. However, other researchers have noted that time spent was a factor in satisfaction (Smith, *et al.* 1981), as was information provided. It seems to follow that it is not simply the amount of time, but what occurs during that time that is the key to successful communication.

Lack of motivation
Some health workers lack motivation to communicate well with their patients. Simply altering levels of motivation, without supplementary skills is insufficient. Houghton (1968) carried out an investigation in a maternity ward where one group tried hard with their communication skills, wore name badges, set aside time and focused on communication – to no avail in terms of dissatisfaction ratings.

The content of the communication
Some argue that if bad news is to be communicated, dissatisfaction is inevitable. Ley (1989) has shown that this is not so – indeed, many patients have specifically noted a desire for more accurate and comprehensive communications in the presence of bad news, poor diagnosis and life threatening illnesses.

Difficult patients
There is an argument that some patients constantly complain and no matter what communications they receive, they will always be dissatisfied. Ley (1988) argues that this is probably inaccurate as studies showing dissatisfaction with communication invariably show high satisfaction with medical care. The disgruntled patient hypothesis would entail dissatisfaction with all aspects of care.

Misunderstandings
Another argument put forward to account for dissatisfaction is that although communication does occur it is not understood. This may well contribute to the problems, given that medical staff often overuse jargon or presume knowledge bases which may not be present.

Expectations
Expectations are often not met and this can be a source of apprehension (Morcos, *et al.*, 1989). In this study, the majority of prospective parents had desires and expectations which they felt would not be accommodated.

It is therefore extremely important to understand what contributes to satisfactory communication. Findings in the literature suggest:

Factors associated with the message
These include the extent to which the message can be understood, how

forthcoming it was, how relevant it is, the content and implications of the message and the context in which it may be given.

Factors associated with the recipient
The recipient brings a host of variabilities to the situation. They may have personality variables which interact with communication, together with other factors such as social class, expectations, prior knowledge levels, understanding and willingness, which may all interact within the situation.

Factors associated with the messenger
The doctor or health worker needs to supply the information, but to also utilize their position to allow the recipient the time and opportunity to feed in their specific information, their understanding of the situation and their queries. There may well be verbal and non verbal aspects to communication. Larsen & Smith (1981) showed that non-verbal factors such as eye contact, relaxed muscle tone, body orientation and touch were related to increased satisfaction.

Factors associated with the situation
Communication does not occur in a vacuum and comprises a moving process rather than a static event. Thus situational factors and the way in which the process unfolds will continuously feed into the cycle.

The effects of poor communications

If communication is faulty, it is not only satisfaction which is affected. Other problems may result, such as:

- Missed diagnosis.
- Increased legal action, litigation or suing (most suits involve communication and not medical competency (Simpson, 1991)).
- Poor knowledge transfer.
- Limited future health education.
- Non-compliance.
- Failing to seek medical care.

Effective communication is of profound importance for the psychological well-being of the patient (Simpson, 1991). In childbirth related studies, the quality of communication has been shown to affect anxiety levels (Sherr, 1989), satisfaction (Sherr, 1989; Ley, 1988), blood pressure, compliance (Reading, 1982) and distress (Fallowfield *et al.* 1986).

Rutter, *et al.* (1988) studied the effect of satisfaction with maternity care on outcome. They found that knowledge played no part in satisfaction, but attitude (towards medicine and hospital care in particular) was the best predictor of satisfaction.

Communication training

Communication training is often low on the agenda of a typical health care department. It is often believed that good communication simply comes from observation and practice. In reality, observation is only one of a number of techniques needed to acquire such a behavioural skill and is in fact one of the less effective techniques. 'Role modelling' depends on adequate skill transfer and excellent role models. Poor role models may perpetuate poor skills if this is the only method of teaching. Observation and mimicking can never provide sufficient feedback for the student. If the experience is negative, the student may avoid such attempts in the future rather than face up to the factors which cause the difficulty and practise (in a non-relevant circumstance) how to adjust their own individual styles.

Communication in a medical setting is often given low priority as it is a time consuming activity which requires a certain amount of training at multiple points including before, during and after the applied situation. When training does occur, it is invariably focused at the student level, prior to client exposure. Thus, as the years go by, bad habits may become entrenched.

An examination of the methodology used for communication training is also uninspired. The traditional models of education use a passive transfer of knowledge. This may be fine for pure information based learning, but for skill-based knowledge, practice is vital to complement the informational components. More counselling, listening and empathy skills are slowly filtering into the better training programmes.

There are multiple costs involved in good communication care. These are often seen in terms of time spent, but few workers analyse the time wasted through unsatisfactory communications. In addition, the medical and nursing professions are often constructed in hierarchies of power, and such organization often impedes communication progress and attention.

When time is short, communication may be seen as unimportant and superfluous. If something has to give, it is usually communication which goes first.

Few researchers take into account the boring repetitive nature of the schedules of the medical profession. This situation can lead to depersonalization and poor communication encounters. This is exacerbated by organizational barriers which may impede the flow of patient contact through disrupted continuity, understaffing and competing needs.

Finally, research often fails to examine the fact that simple fatigue may also inhibit communications – a factor of special note where junior doctors are concerned. Essentially, the staff who do the longer hours are those who have to communicate the most and this may result in incoherent, unsatisfactory contact.

The psychology of communication

Reluctance to ask
The literature on communication shows a regular finding that patients are reluctant to ask questions. They think of questions and want information, but even those who have clear informational needs often fail to verbalize these into questions to pose to their carers. Such passive behaviour can possibly be understood in terms of a variety of psychological models ranging from power structures to models of deference, embarrassment, fear, being overwhelmed or role models which teach acceptance and frown on questioning. Certainly patients who have tentatively posed questions and had their efforts rejected will be less likely to ask questions in the future. Roter (1979) found that patients could be trained and encouraged to ask more questions by pre-consultation intervention which included rehearsals, prompting and, by the very presence of the study, an implicit 'permission' to ask. This study reported that patient training did result in increased questioning. However, doctors appraised 'questioning patients' more negatively than 'passive patients'.

Understanding
Numerous studies have elaborated on the limitations patients may have in basic levels of understanding. This includes knowledge of their own body, knowledge of disease and treatment and knowledge of medical terminology. Such findings are of particular note within pregnancy. Sherr (1989) reported that pregnant women had many misconceptions about their reproductive body parts, as well as about aspects of pregnancy and birth, and about care and the interventions that they may face during labour and delivery. Furthermore, when doctors and midwives were questioned, they overestimated women's knowledge. They expected multiparous women to have gathered expertise. In reality, experience did not confer expertise – indeed, it sometimes led to entrenched errors and misunderstandings. Doctors and midwives also assumed that middle-class women were more knowledgeable. This was not borne out by the facts. However, middle-class women were more efficient at gaining information from their doctors and midwives.

Such problems are aggravated by the overuse of jargon and a reluctance on the part of some practitioners to explain, and corresponding reluctance for patients to ask or clarify.

Cognitive factors and communication
The most widely used theoretical model relating to medical commu-

nications is one proposed by Ley (1982, 1988). This is essentially a cognitive model. Ley (1988) proposed that there is a direct link between understanding, memory satisfaction and compliance. This also goes some way to explaining the finding that, despite increased communication training, patient dissatisfaction is still as high as ever. It may be that not only does staff behaviour need to change, but a more complex understanding of the communication process is also required, in which patient factors and communication impediments need understanding.

The solution does not simply lie in the provision of information. Early simplistic models of communication examined communication acts in terms of the communicator, the recipient and the message itself. Such models are perhaps over-simplistic as they take little account of social circumstance, normative influence, cumulative experience and so on. However, as an analysis tool, they allow an examination of communication from these three angles. Cognitive factors for each should address:

The recipient

The recipient may facilitate or hinder communications and rarely plays a passive role. Passive roles are imposed when communications are in writing (thus avoiding interaction) or when the recipient is rendered passive (which may be the case during labour, under anaesthesia or while asleep or drugged). However, passive states can be engendered by the exertion of control, the implementation of social rules (such as those which hinder questioning) or by the manner and availability of the communicators who simply do not respond to the recipient's needs.

From the recipient's point of view, memory limitations as well as processing problems may join together to contribute to high levels of forgetfulness. Social norms and social learning may determine information, affect understanding or even result in misunderstandings. Emotional state can also mitigate against communications: raised anxiety, fear, panic, worry, elation, crying and even depression can affect the amount of information the woman can accept, process and integrate, irrespective of how much is offered.

Humans are constantly seeking to understand, rationalize and explain cognitive factors and new environmental input. Thus, new information is inevitably integrated into existing schemata. Women may thus attend to information selectively, sift out bits they are seeking or which accord with their explanations of events, and at times twist the information to accommodate it within their own understanding. Doctors may well do likewise.

The message

The message itself is certainly not passive and will have considerable effect on the communication process. Simply the amount of information which is presented can affect recall, with a linear relationship between amount and subsequent recall shown in studies (Ley, 1989). However, the picture is not straightforward. Information that can be offered in 'chunks' allows for greater recall. Memory studies predict a primacy and recency effect in recall: information given at the beginning and end of a conversation is recalled with greater ease than any other information. However, a typical antenatal interview often consists of niceties and social chatter in the beginning and end, with the bulk of real information being given during the middle. Psychological models examining such interviews would not only predict that information in the middle would be forgotten, but would show that decision-making and appraisal would be made on what is recalled, i.e. the social chatter. Thus quality and competence are often judged on social parameters rather than medical ones.

Figure 5.1 sets out the information flow and recall periods present in interviews.

The content of the information has a dramatic effect on recall. Ley & Spelman (1965) showed that patients recalled diagnosis statements best and tended to recall instructions worst. Patients are not passive receivers of information and may have set ideas prior to receiving information. They may then differentially recall items which endorse their understanding or explanation of an event, and reject conflicting information.

Messages are provided in different ways. Messages given or endorsed by high status individuals have greater salience and may therefore be recalled to a greater degree. Thus, information from the student nurse may be attended to less than information from the senior doctor. The format of messages may also affect the effectiveness of the communication. Messages can be given verbally, in writing, audio-visually or by a combination of ways. Obviously, the way to maximize the efficacy of the communication is to use multiple input channels. Written messages should be supplemented with graphics. Colour contrast and novelty should be exploited to maximize interest and attention and thereby to enhance recall. Repeated messages are more likely to be recalled than messages given once. Messages that are understood are more likely to be recalled. Simply floating information past a woman is insufficient. If she can ponder the information, discuss it, raise questions or even hear the arguments, recall and understanding will be enhanced. Specific and structured information is superior than general information. Messages which are perceived to be of importance are more likely to be recalled. Thus emphasis and highlighting, pointing out, and repetition of a key message will promote the communication process.

Simple lessons about recall and understanding can be incorporated into communications. Repetition, high personal relevance and background medical knowledge all enhance communication and message recall. Thus, practitioner behaviour should incorporate these lessons, repeat information, emphasize the personal relevance if this is unclear. Early health

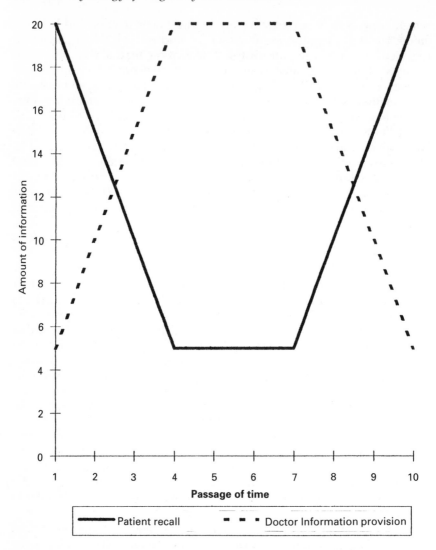

Fig. 5.1   Primacy and recency effects in medical interviews.

education enhances the process. Antenatal classes and basic literature both contribute to the process.

The communicator

The communicator can set the pace, determine the content and influence the outcome of an interview greatly. Initially, there has to be a motivation to communicate. However, there needs to be an understanding that the will to communicate, although necessary, is not sufficient on its own for effective communication. The motivation of the communicator is vital. In general, the interpersonal behaviour of professionals is an element which consistently attracts criticism (Davis & Fallowfield, 1992).

Basic communication skills are only now being integrated into medical training. Older (and thus more senior) medics have not had these training opportunities and consumers may have to wait a generation before the effects of current training programmes filter through. Criticism is difficult to take, yet many studies have commented on the poor or even appalling levels of interpersonal skills which not only affect patient satisfaction but dramatically affect information flow, thus directly affecting the ability to make competent medical judgements. Studies such as Maguire & Rutter (1976) showed deficiencies in first interviews of medical students. Weiner & Nathanson (1976) described how postgraduates posed too many questions, used vague statements and responded inadequately to patient questions. Maguire (1986) followed up trainees and found entrenched difficulties in beginning and ending interviews, handling information, and asserting accuracy. Often simple social rules (such as greetings, introductions, farewells and assurances) were missing (Platt & McMath, 1979, Waitzkin, 1984). Controlling doctor-centred styles of communication have frequently been documented (Korsch & Negrete, 1972; Byrne & Long 1976; Maguire, 1976). This controlling type of communications can lead to impersonal meetings, lack of empathy, inadequate history taking, which often results in patients failing to divulge their main concerns. Coupled with patient's reticence in asking questions, many poor quality interactions occur.

Davis & Fallowfield (1992) point out that there are wide ranges of performance, with some practitioners showing consistently talented communication abilities while others varying in their skills with some interviews being of high quality and others of low. They attribute inadequate communications to six factors:

(1) Medical ethos
Technological advances and a focus on health rather than on the individual, act as a barrier to communication.

(2) Power
There is an enormous level of power associated with medicine and its practitioners. Feedback, dialogue, argument and emotional acknowledgement may be discouraged in order to maintain such power (Waitzkin & Stockle, 1972).

(3) Expert roles
This explanation relies on the medic's need to be an expert and the collusion of the patient in this role. It may be a reassuring function but runs the risk of disappointment when proved inadequate.

(4) Political models of service
This explanation examines the way in which services evolve and finds they are usually a result of professional, political or high level innovation, and rarely in direct response to consumer desires.

(5) Theoretical models of service
This elaborates the fact that much of medicine is disease-centred rather than holistically centred. This often leads to compartmentalization of problems, with insufficient or inappropriate attention to the socio-emotional ramifications of disease.

(6) Self-perpetuation
This explanation simply elaborates on the problems that self-selection of future medics may effectively perpetuate ineffective styles and approaches. Such selection and input into training limits change.

Models of doctor/patient relationships

It is trite to presume that all doctors and all patients behave in a standard way. Indeed, the situation is much more complex with individuals adjusting their interactions according to situational factors (such as medical condition, time constraints, environmental factors, perceived patient factors) and a complex series of personality factors (including disposition, motivation, training, expertise, biases, motives and goals). Emanuel & Emanuel (1992) differentiate four types of relationships, paternalistic, informative, interpretive and deliberative.

Communication and health education

Health education has been used comprehensively in pregnancy related contexts. Often this is simply a 'leaflet panacea' where information booklets are supplied to women with little thought on content, impact or implications. Ley (1989) notes that there are advantages to written information, which can be constructed out of the clinical encounter and which allow time and effort to present a carefully thought out and formulated piece. There is general positive response to written information (Morris & Groft, 1982). Yet the efficacy of such information in altering understanding or behaviour must depend on the standard of the content, the extent to which it is noticed, read, comprehended, recalled and believed (Sherr & Hedge, 1990). When written material is provided, there are usually high levels of reading (Ley 1988 – 49 per cent–95 per cent; Kanouse, *et al.* 1981 – 72 per cent). Many people keep their written information for future consultation. Health education efforts have been used to promote a variety of regimes, to raise awareness of childbirth related problems (notably genetically conveyed disorders), to explain antenatal care and procedures and to supplement background mother/baby knowledge.

Waterson *et al.* (1990) examined three methods of information provision to encourage a reduction in alcohol consumption during pregnancy. At the first clinic visit 2100 mothers were studied. The first group were given written information only, the second group was given information reinforced by personalized advice from the doctor and the third group was given written information supplemented by a video taped message. There were no significant differences between the groups in terms of behaviour change.

Compliance

There is a wide debate surrounding compliance with medical advice. Often medical advice is not complied with, drug regimens are not adhered to, protocols are adapted or overlooked and errors subsequently occur. Lack of compliance is usually seen as a failing on the part of patients. However Ley (1988) has clearly shown that medics suffer from compliance problems with their own standards, routines and protocols.

Compliance evokes much ethical debate about power, persuasion and domination. In order for a pregnant woman to comply with advice, there is an underlying assumption that 'accurate' advice should go unquestioned. Notwithstanding, there are some elements of advice that can cause consternation to women such as avoidance of smoking or alcohol during pregnancy. Ley (1988) concludes that compliance is a difficult concept to measure as different methods of recording result in variations in frequency of recorded non-compliance.

Ley (1988), records that health professionals often do not comply with a variety of basic procedures, such as informing patients about medication, complying with regulations, adhering to procedures such as drug issuing, prescribing medications which may be of questionable use, using safety procedures on all occasions and keeping up to date and proficient with basic techniques. Studies to examine causes or triggers for such non-compliance record findings remarkably similar to those involved in patient non-compliance. The usual accounts include information or memory gaps, personal job satisfaction and normative influences.

Few studies are carried out in any area of maternity care, but factors which are associated with non-compliance outside of maternity care are linked with satisfaction, expectations, complexity of the action, duration of the behaviour involved, amount of supervision required (and supplied) and social/normative influences. Compliance can be improved by better communication, raised information recall and reminders.

Written information – the leaflet panacea

There is a well established role for written information in many aspects of medical care generally and especially in maternity care. However, as with any intervention, written information has strengths and weaknesses, advantages and limitations which vary in impact according to recipient factors.

There is a wide array of literature available for pregnant women covering many aspects of their pregnancy, birth and parenting experience. Written material is widely used to enhance or support verbal interactions.

Written material that is not consulted is worthless. In any given population there are always people who are unable to utilize written material, such as those who are illiterate, those who are visually impaired (unless it is specially prepared in braille) and those who cannot speak the language of the document.

For written material to be effective it has to be:

- Attended
- Consulted
- Understood
- Recalled

Only after these challenges have been met, can the content of the leaflets be addressed.

There is much research available on leaflet presentation, and of factors which hinder or promote understanding, recall or usefulness. Complex material is less often consulted or recalled than simple jargon-free material. The visual impact and presentation of material may affect the extent to which it is initially consulted and the impact it subsequently has. Written information should be supplemented by graphics (either in the form of pictures, charts or tables) to assist assimilation of information and understanding.

If written information is to be heeded, it must be salient and believable. The use of generalized statements and advertising diminish its salience, whereas the use of high status endorsement and multiple points of view increases attention. There is clear evidence that the provision of written information enhances the communication process from the aspect of understanding, increasing knowledge, recall, compliance and satisfaction. If communication is personalized it is endorsed more highly than if it is not.

Experimental studies on manipulating information and measuring differential outcome have shown that procedural information is best supplemented by information on sensations. Literature which arouses fear does not necessarily change behaviour. Recall and recognition is greater for humorous material than anxiety-laden material.

Interventions

The provision of information has been one of the major intervention methodologies. Studies have examined the effects of various forms of information with a wide variety of outcome measures. It is unclear whether such information is beneficial, and if so, which are the optimum kinds of information. Some reviewers (Averill, 1973; Thompson, 1981; Miller & Mangan, 1983) put forward the ideas that information may not always be helpful if it creates more problems. The majority of studies have focused on different outcomes dependent on sensory or procedural information. Outcomes have been the subject of numerous major reviews (Suls & Wan, 1989; Anderson & Masur, 1983). Overall, it appears that both types of information are superior to no input at all. Sensory information alone is most helpful, but if this is combined with procedural information the best results are yielded. Suls & Wan propose that this is because procedural details can provide a map of specific events, while sensory information can promote interpretation as non-threatening. They therefore advocate a combination of the two.

It seems that these overviews and reviews are pointing the way forward. However, more sophisticated understanding of information packages allows for the complexity of information flow, retrieval, understanding and interpretation to be integrated into studies. These no doubt ramify into cognitive mapping and coping by recipients and manifest in a variety of outcome measures.

Criticism of the Ley Model of communication

Although the various aspects of the model proposed by Ley are extremely helpful, they also have limitations. The model proposed by Ley is essentially flat, one dimensional and does not take into account a number of aspects of the situation which may well have direct and indirect effects on communication. The model has many strengths in the empirical support for the cognitive factors, but overlooks a number of other psychological mechanisms which may well contribute. These are:

Motivation
There is an entire literature on the effects of motivation on actions. The ability to mount, sustain and succeed seems to be directly influenced by motivational factors.

Attribution
Again, there is much literature in social psychology which explains behaviour in terms of attributions that people make, and how this affects their judgement, decisions and behaviour. In maternity care, this can be seen with the role of social class. Attributions of class may not only affect

practitioner behaviour, but the experiences and expectations of women they treat. Social class is difficult to measure in women in studies, given that it is usually the spouse's occupation which is recorded. 'Housewife' and other female occupations such as 'mother' or 'child carer' are not even entered in the registry of professions.

Personality
Personality theories can never be overlooked when communication is being examined. This applies to the personality characteristics of both the communicator and the woman. It may apply to real or perceived personality attributes. This may feed into role norms, role aspirations, role models and may affect the quality, content and existence of any dialogue.

Social context
There may well be an impact on communications emanating from the social context within which they occur. This is particularly valid in the area of obstetrics. The tenets of Ley's theories often utilize interchangeable notions of disease and illness. Findings from dental clinics are applied to cancer patients. Experiences of people with ulcers form the basis for interventions applied to gynaecology clinics. There may simply be some aspects of communication which are condition specific. Maternity care may well be a prime example. Although good theories should generalize across conditions, there is always a need to check this out. Few studies have examined all the factors within the cognitive theory as they apply to obstetrics.

Communication aspects of pregnancy care

Routines of care are often constructed to hinder the flow of communication. This results in a depersonalization of the recipient and may set up spirals of discontent. The long term impact may be disastrous and may never be correctly attributed to simple early communication breakdown.

Dragonas (1987) studied 21 156 Greek women before and after the birth of their infants and found that subjects wanted more personal care, more time, continuity of care, information about their pregnancy and less distance from their doctor. They expressed a consistent need for emotional support.

Barton, *et al.* (1987) showed that the quality of communication and feedback determined postscan anxiety level and satisfaction for high risk women undergoing fetal echocardiography. Korsch, *et al.* (1968) found that satisfaction with the consultation generally was associated with five key factors:

(1) The manner of the doctor (friendly, in preference to business-like).
(2) The empathy of the doctor in understanding the patient's concerns.

(3) Meeting of expectations (whatever these may be).
(4) An appreciation of the communication skills of the doctor.
(5) The informational component of the interview.

Methuen (1989) studied 43 booking clinic interviews and provided a systematic analysis of the skills employed, the areas covered and related outcomes. She found:

- Extensive use of closed questions which served the purpose of tightly controlling the interviews (at times at the expense of accuracy).
- Excessive use of leading questions which encouraged women to tailor their responses.
- In the transcripts of 40 interviews, only three instances of open questions were monitored.

When judged against the Rutter & Maguire standards for medical student interviews, midwives were shown to exhibit poor devices for conversation development or fact probing. In general, the interviews were almost totally circumscribed by checklist prompts emanating from standardized forms. The overpowering need to complete such standard forms obstructed any attempts to examine anxiety, emotions, feelings, worries or concerns. This was compounded by an inflexible approach to the interviews which inhibited women from venturing to pose questions.

Some fundamental flaws in interviewing technique were also observed. Only one midwife introduced herself and only three midwives addressed their clients by name during the entire interview. Not surprisingly, over half the women questioned were not even able to identify the fact that the interviewer had been a midwife. Interviewing skills were also limited when it came to terminating the encounter. Thirty-three of the 40 interviews ended with the midwife simply ushering the woman to the next phase of her appointment, and four midwives simply left the interview with no farewell or explanation at all.

Porter & Macintyre (1989) reported that 60 per cent of antenatal attenders asked no questions during their interview. Of the 40 per cent who did ask a question, half of these ventured to ask a single item only. In nearly two thirds of the interviews there was no discussion beyond basic questions and answers surrounding the factual data. Porter & Macintyre measured topics raised during the interviews and found that in over half the interviews no topics were raised (for even the briefest of discussion). This reluctance to ask was revealed when half the women reported that they had questions they wished to pose but felt inhibited, put off, lacked the opportunity or were too overwhelmed to ask.

Thus it seems that questioning and dialogue are not simply a function of desire, but emanate from a much more complex base relating to opportunity, time, atmosphere, facilitation and relevance. The short amount of consultation time (on average five minutes in this study) may render such opportunities impossible, and, indeed, many key questions were posed as the doctor exited the room. Those who did manage to ask questions were met with hostile reactions, patronizing replies and labelled 'neurotic', 'troublesome' or 'insecure'.

Society's perception of the pregnant woman

Many people believe that women are basically less responsible and/or intelligent than men. These beliefs are often enhanced by notions surrounding the control of women by their hormones, the unpredictable nature of their reproductive functioning and society's attitude (Ussher, 1990). Corse (1990) studied reactions of subjects to a pregnant and non-pregnant manager in a workplace conflict situation and found that there were more negative impressions and lower satisfaction with the pregnant manager, irrespective of the gender of the judges.

What the women say

The words of women speak loudest in terms of their communication experiences during antenatal care, labour and delivery. These can be categorized according to some of the criteria raised in the communications literature generally. A series of comments by women interviewed (Sherr, 1989) will serve to highlight many of the points discussed in this chapter.

(1) Brevity of interactions

One possible explanation or dissatisfaction with communication may be the brevity of an interaction (Ley, 1977; Byrne & Long, 1976). Half the women in a study (Sherr, 1989) noted brief interactions.

'The doctor at the hospital sort of just comes along, does what he has got to do and is off again.'

(2) Quality of interactions

Quality is often seen as an index of satisfaction (Ley, 1988). There were not 'negative' and 'positive' women; rather all women reported some positive interactions, but also reported negative interactions to a greater extent. Examples of comments on such interactions are:

Positive: 'He was very helpful [GP] told me everything I wanted to know'.

Negative: 'You get prodded around by a student who then reports to whatever doctor comes in what he has seen – and the doctor informs you'.

'In hospital they just handed me a bottle and walked off.'

(3) Provision of explanatory information
Cognitive coping, especially with new or frightening experiences, often hinges on the provision of comprehensive and understandable information. Comments on this factor include:

'They did a scan again two weeks after – why, I am not sure.'

(4) Communication factors
Communication factors were key elements in the appraisal of the experience. Both positive and negative statements were given about these factors.

'They were incredibly nice, they really were. A nurse came and sat with me and told me how her mother makes coffee. I mean they just really wanted to distract me, I had the feeling; to help to make it pleasant.'

(5) Misunderstandings
Many misunderstandings abound which can impede communications and understanding, as may be seen in this disturbing quote:

'It looked terrible and I didn't realize it was dry blood – it was like scabs really.'

(6) Questions to the interviewer
Some women *still* had unresolved issues, which they addressed to the interviewer. This was a finding documented by Cartwright in her study and it serves as a reflection of the long term effects of poor communication and confusion.

'They decided he was lying the wrong way round. [To the interviewer] Which way should they be?'

(7) Anxiety
Communication factors play a key role in anxiety and can be used to ameliorate stress and anxiety. At times of anxiety, women seek out high quality communication to aid coping and reassurance. Some comments from women include:

'I couldn't find the bell, I was shouting for the nurse. No nurse appeared and I was ringing the bell frantically when I did find it.'

'I started to get frantic, I was very panicky and I said "I want my husband." '

(8) Upsetting incidents
Most women reported something which upset them. This often involved communication aspects of their experience. For example:

'The tea lady – well, she came in and said "Only two visitors to a bed." And I said to one of the visitors, "Oh, you should go." And afterwards we realized, well, she was only a tea lady.'
   'So I went to the doctor who said I had come too soon. It amazed me.'

(9) Rules and institutionalization
It is via communication (or the lack thereof) that the social rules surrounding childbirth are conveyed to women. Many report the strictures of such rules and the realization of the rules, often in the breach thereof. Communication was a thread running through many of these comments:

'They had fathers visiting in the evenings. My mother was absolutely dying to see the baby, she came up straight from London and the ward clerk initially would not let her in.'

(10) Passivity
Many women were fairly passive, and did not question much. As noted in the literature, women were often reluctant to ask their carers. Some statements include:

'But again, I really did not ask anything. I really did not, I just left it ...'

'I had to have an injection to make me sleep. And I wondered then – I don't need an injection to make me sleep ... but I don't like injections and I said "Do I have to?" and they said "Yes", so, anyway, I had the injection.'

Implications for practice

The importance of communication cannot be underestimated. Specific individual focus forms the cornerstone of good quality care. If a patient does not perceive they have received this they feel neglect, uncertainty, mistrust and fear. The quality of communication aspects of care hinge on the availability of communication, the content and style of its delivery, the time and importance accorded to it, the source from which it comes and the relevance to the individual.

Numerous remedies have been proposed for affecting communications (Ley, 1989). These include:

(1) Recall for information presented initially and finally is greatest. Ensure that the key elements of communications are told initially and repeated finally.

(2) Simple repetition enhances recall. Thus stressing important items and repeating important instructions will have an increased likelihood of working.

(3) Jargon is problematic. Utilize clear, plain language, and ensure that technical terms are understood by asking patients directly what they think they mean. If patients are asked whether they understand they will usually say 'yes' whether they do or do not, as misunderstandings, by their very nature, are unintentional.

(4) If material is to be presented, communication can be enhanced if it is categorized.

(5) Earmark key items. Before key items are discussed their importance should be stressed and the patient's attention specifically drawn to them.

(6) Global statements are less likely to be effective than specific statements. For example 'increase your exercise' is more general than 'try to swim 4 lengths each day'.

(7) Supplement verbal communications with other modes of communication, such as:
- Written information
- Audio visual information
- Group discussion
- Audio information

Of these aids, written information is the most widely used. Generally, clear, easy to understand information forms a welcome addition to medical encounters. However, some centres go overboard and ply their clients with such overwhelming amounts of literature that their usefulness can be questioned. Personalized information is preferable to general information. Information with commercial information (such as baby milk promotions) is less believable than information from pure medical sources.

There is a practical requirement to examine the training needs for future generations. Communication training should play a key role during qualification training, in the early years of experience, and during ongoing education. This will ensure cross fertilization of new ideas, help maximize learning from experience and errors and minimize damaging communication experiences for vulnerable patients.

References

Anderson, K. & Masur, F. (1983) Psychological preparation for invasive medical and dental procedures. *Jnl. of Behavioural Medicine*, 6, 1–40.

Averill, J. (1973) Personal control over aversive stimuli and its relationship to stress. *Psychological Bulletin*, 80, 286–303.

Barton, T., Harris, R., Weinman, J. & Allan, L. (1987) Psychological effects of prenatal diagnosis; the example of fetal echocardiography. *Current Psychological Research and Reviews*, **6**,(1), 57–68.

Beckman, H. & Frankel, R. (1984) The effect of physician behaviour on the collection of data. *Annals of Internal Medicine*, 101, 692–6.

Byrne, P. & Long, B. (1976) *Doctors Talking to Patients*, HMSO, London.

Corse, S.J. (1990) Pregnant managers and their subordinates. The effects of gender expectations on hierarchical relationships. *Jnl. of Applied Behavioural Science*, **26**,(1), 25–47.

Davis, H. & Fallowfield, L. (1992) *Counselling and Communication in Health Care*. Wiley, Chichester.

DiMatteo, M.R., Prince, L.M. & Taranta, A. (1978) Patients' perceptions of physician behaviour. *Jnl of Community Health* 4, 280–9.

Dragonas, T. (1987) Greek womens' attitudes toward pregnancy, labour and infant. *Infant Mental Health Journal*, **8**,(3), 266–76.

Emanuel, E. & Emanuel, L. (1992) Four models of the physician patient relationship. *JAMA*, **267**, 2221–6.

Fallowfield, L., Baum, M. & Maguire, P. (1986) Effects of breast conservation on psychological morbidity associated with diagnosis and treatment of early breast cancer. *BMJ*, 293, 1331–34.

Freeling, P., Rao, B., Paykel, E., Sireling, L. & Burton, R. (1985) Unrecognized depression in general practice. *BMJ*, 290, 1880–3.

Houghton, M. (1968) Problems in hospital communications. In *Problems and Progress in Medical Care* (Ed. G. McLachlan), Oxford University Press, Oxford.

Kanouse, D.E., Berry, S.H., Hayes Roth, B. (1981) Informing patients about drugs. *Summary Report*, Rand Corporation Santa Monica CA.

Korsch, B. & Negret, V. (1972) Doctor patient communication. *Scientific American*, August, 66–73.

Korsch, B., Gozzi, E. & Francis, V. (1968) Gaps in doctor patient communication. Doctor patient interaction and patient satisfaction. *Paediatrics*, 42, 855–71.

Larsen, K. & Smith, C.K. (1981) Assessment of non verbal communication in the patient physician interview. *Jnl. of Family Practice*, 12, 481–8.

Ley, P. (1977) Psychological studies in doctor patient communication. In *Contributions to Medical Psychology Vol 1* (Ed. S. Rachman) Pergamon Press, Oxford.

Ley, P. (1982) Satisfaction, compliance and communication. *B. Jnl. of Clin. Psych.*, 21, 241–54.

Ley, P. (1988) *Communicating with patients*. Psychology and Medicine Series. Croom Helm, London.

Ley, P. (1989) Improving patients' understanding, recall, satisfaction and compliance. In *Health Psychology* (Ed. A. Broome), Chapman and Hall, London.

Ley, P. & Spelman, M. (1965) Communications in an out patient setting. *B. Jnl. of Social and Clinical Psych.*, 4, 114–16.

Macleod Clark, J. (1985) The development of research in interpersonal skills in nursing. In *Interpersonal Skills in Nursing* (Ed. C. Kagan), Croom Helm, London.

Maguire, P. (1976) The psychological and social sequelae of mastectomy. In *Modern Perspectives in the Psychiatric Aspects of Surgery*, (Ed. J. Howels), Brunner Mazel, New York.

Maguire, P.P. & Rutter, D. (1976) History taking for medical students, deficiencies in performance. *The Lancet*, Sept. 11, 556–8.

Maguire, P., Fairburn, S. & Fletcher, C. (1986) Consultation skills of the young doctor. *BMJ*, 292, 1573–78.

Methuen, R. (1989) Recording an obstetric history or relating to a pregnant woman? A study of the antenatal interview. In *Midwives Research and Childbirth Vol 1*, (Ed. S. Robinson & A. Thomson), Chapman & Hall, London.

Miller, S.M. & Mangan, C. (1983) Interacting effects of information and coping style in adapting to gynaecologic stress; should doctors tell all? *Jnl. of Personality and Social Psychology*, 45, 223–36.

Morcos, F., Snart, F. & Harley, D. (1989) Choices, expectations and the experience of childbirth. *Canada Mental Health*, **37**,(1) 6–8.

Morris, L.A. & Groft, S. (1982) Patient package inserts: a research perspective. In *Drug Therapeutic Concepts for Clinicians* (Ed. K. Melmon) Elsevier, New York.

Novack, D., Volk, G., Drossman, D. & Lipkin, M. (1993) Medical interviewing and interpersonal skills teaching in US medical schools. *JAMA* **269**,(16) 2101–5.

Platt, F. & McMath, J. (1979) Clinical hypocompetence: the interview. *Annals of Internal Medicine*, 91, 898–902.

Porter, M. & MacIntyre, S. (1984) What is must be best. A research note on conservative or deferential responses to antenatal care provision. *Social Science and Medicine*. 19, 1197–200.

Porter, M. & McIntyre, S. (1989) Psychosocial effectiveness of antenatal and postnatal care. In *Midwives Research and Childbirth Vol 1* (Ed. S. Robinson, & A. Thomson) Chapman and Hall, London.

Reading, A. (1982) How women view post episiotomy pain. *BMS* 284, 28.

Roter, D. (1979) Altering patient behaviour in interaction with providers. In *Research in Psychology and Medicine Vol 2*, (Ed. D. Osborne, M. Gruneberg, J. Eiser), Academic Press, London.

Rutter, D., Quine, L. & Hayward, R. (1988) Satisfaction with maternity care: psychosocial factors in pregnancy outcome. *Jnl. of Reproductive and Infant Psychology* **6**,(4) 261–68.

Schulberg, H. & Burns, B. (1988) Mental disorders in primary care. *General Hospital Psychiatry*, 10, 79–87.

Sherr, L. (1989) *Communication and Anxiety in Obstetric Care*. Unpublished PhD Thesis, Warwick University.

Sherr, L. & Hedge, B. (1990) The impact and use of written leaflets as a counselling alternative in mass antenatal HIV screening. *AIDS Care*, **2**,(3), 235–46.

Smith, C., Polis, E. & Hadac, R. (1981) Characteristics of the initial medical interview associated with patient satisfaction and understanding. *Jnl. of Family Practice*, 12, 283–8.

Stewart, M., McWhinney, I. & Buck, C.W. (1979) The doctor patient relationship and its effect upon outcome. *Jnl. of R. C. of Gen. Pract.*, 9, 77–82.

Suls, J. & Wan, C. (1989) Effects of sensory and procedural information on coping with stressful medical procedures and pain: a meta analysis. *Jnl. of Consulting and Clinical Psychology*, **57**(3), 372–79.

Thompson, S. (1981) Will it hurt less if I can control it? A complex answer to a simple question. *Psychological Bulletin*, 90, 89–101.

Ussher, J. (1990) *The Psychology of the Female Body*. Routledge, London and New York.

Waitzkin, H. (1984) Doctor patient communication. Implications of social scientific research. *JAMA* 252, 2441–6.

Waitzkin, H. & Stoeckle, J. (1972) The communication of information about illness; clinical, sociological and methodological considerations. *Advances in Psychosomatic Medicine*, 8, 180–215.

Waterson, E., Murray, L. & Iain, M. (1990) Preventing fetal alcohol effects. A trial of three methods of giving information in the antenatal clinic. *Health Education Research*, **5**,(1) 53–61.

Weiner, S. & Nathanson, M. (1976) Physical examination, frequently observed errors. *JAMA*, 236, 852–55.

Chapter 6

Antenatal Period

'I had been kept waiting in this little cubicle for up to three quarters of an hour on occasion, sitting and thinking – have they forgotten me, what has happened, where has everyone gone? And there is no one you can see.'

Antenatal care is something of a twentieth century invention. Despite the fact that there are criticisms of some aspects of care, this century has also marked the safest time for women to conceive and have babies. Obviously the way forward is to integrate new procedures with caution, to change or abandon where necessary and, at all times, to maintain a sense of individuality for every woman. This ideal is difficult to achieve but when good levels of care are delivered, much gratitude and appreciation is expressed. Indeed, the actual behaviour of most women demonstrates their respect for and belief in a system in their overwhelming attendance at antenatal clinics.

It is surprising that so much study has been devoted to the few hours of antenatal clinic attendance and so little to the remainder of the nine month experience. Women have been questioned in detail about their clinic experiences, yet very little is known of their day-to-day feelings and changes during pregnancy. Much of the research is either medically biased (concentrating its attention on such areas as nausea and gait), economically biased (examining limitations imposed by work or its cessation), or socially biased (looking at the roles and expectations of a woman, her family and friends). There also is much literature on the common 'presumptions' of pregnancy (that it is enjoyable, desirable and feeds into a 'natural state' for women) despite a growing view which criticizes this opinion (Ussher, 1989). Very little is psychologically based.

Wolind & Zajicek (1981) describe some of the physical burdens that pregnant women experience, including minor complaints such as indigestion, lack of energy, cramps and aches, breathlessness, and frequency of micturition. Worries and anxieties are commonly sought and described. Explanations for these vary from 'hormonal changes' via 'the frailty of pregnancy', to the 'psychological imbalance of women', right down to pragmatic concerns, such as worries about the baby and miscarriage, fears about economic and role changes and, notably, concerns about impending hospital visits (Green, 1990; Elliot, 1984).

Antenatal care is typified by multiple clinic attendance. These are either specialist or general clinics, usually hospital based, but increasingly general practitioner based for at least some of the time. Hall & Chang (1982) recorded that in an average pregnancy a woman would attend up to 11 clinics. McIntyre (1977) noted that most women when questioned felt that their pregnancy would be affected in some way if they did not attend, but could not explain these suspicions further. After the visit only 17 per cent felt they had learned anything and only 31 per cent felt they had enjoyed their visit. Green (1990) noted that over 1 in 10 women were specifically worried about hospital attendance.

Many consumer complaints of antenatal care have been recorded (Reid & McIlwaine, 1980; O'Brien & Smith, 1981; Hall, *et al.* 1985). Some women report the experience as 'alienating and unpleasant' (Porter & MacIntyre, 1989). The Short Report (1981) points out that dissatisfied consumers make irregular attenders. When complaints emanate from such groups of women, it is unclear whether it is a minority who are dissatisfied or whether they are the spokeswomen for the silent majority. It seems the latter explanation is more likely, as systematic consumer studies have documented considerable consumer dissatisfaction as well (Garcia, 1982; McIntyre, 1979). These complaints often occur, despite acceptable levels of medical care (Garcia, *et al.* 1990). In essence, complaints centre around:

- Poor levels of communication (see Chapter 4).
- Disruptions in continuity of care.
- Abhorrence of the mass approach to antenatal care, which results in a production line atmosphere and inevitable depersonalization, at the very time when the uniqueness of any woman should be paid greater attention (Sherr, 1989; Cartwright, 1979).
- Criticism of certain procedures such as episiotomy, induction.
- Testing, results and feedback for antenatal procedures.
- Discrepancies between the expectation and experience of care.
- Poor timing of clinics and inadequate organization.
- Discomfort with vaginal examinations (especially at first visits, with which one in three can be dissatisfied – Oakley, 1979).

Much of this dissatisfaction can be attributed to a 'conveyor belt' approach to care which inevitably engenders a perceived lack of control for patients, bolsters a sense of passivity, blurs individualization and hinders elements of care which are crucial for therapeutic relationships, such as continuity of care, adequate appreciation of problems, high level reassurance and pacing. Some studies do show high levels of satisfaction, but this declines when women are questioned over a long period of time and have the opportunity to reflect (or the freedom to report their feelings without fear of recriminations within the hospital setting – Garcia, *et al.*, 1990). Reid & McIlwaine (1980) randomly selected 90 women attending a Scottish antenatal clinic and noted that the difficulties they experienced included long travelling distances to the clinic and excessively long waits to be seen. The women in this study saw a different doctor each visit, despite the finding that 85 per cent would have liked to see the same doctor and 39 per cent reported they did not find out all they wanted to know.

There is a assumption that antenatal attendance is a 'good' thing and indeed, the Spastics Society has produced statistics correlating poor obstetric outcome in childbirth with poor or late antenatal attendance. Hall & Chang (1982) however, encourages caution as the factors responsible for such late bookings or non-attendance may account for obstetric outcome rather than the simple absence of antenatal care. Such causes may be unwanted pregnancy, poor socio-economic standard, teenage pregnancy or drug use. Indeed, an analysis of the data shows that women go to considerable lengths to attend their clinics: O'Brien & Smith (1981) showed that only 2 per cent of their sample received no antenatal care. The Royal Commission's report on the health service noted that over half their sample arrived within 5–10 minutes of their appointment time, with 40 per cent arriving early. Additionally, late arrival was invariably associated with hospital transport failures. Despite such meticulous attendance, Garcia (1982) notes that women wait to be seen for an average of 156 minutes (this figure is lowered to 69 minutes for general practitioner care).

Porter & MacIntyre (1989) questioned the extent to which the 'promise' of antenatal care is delivered. The majority of respondents in this study could not specifically identify benefits of antenatal attendance, with only 5 per cent stating they were 'useful'. Given this lack of benefit, one needs to analyse whether such attendance has the potential for causing harm. Porter & MacIntyre not only reported that 46 per cent of their subjects 'got nothing at all' out of attending but they also found their check-up unpleasant or upsetting. Yet few women missed their appointments.

Screening

Pregnancy inevitably involves exposure to a wide range of antenatal screening tests. These are carried out to ensure the 'normal progression of pregnancy', yet there is often a high psychological cost. Marteau (1989) noted that most testing procedures and results were associated with negative emotions. The efficacy and usefulness of many of the tests is under constant review (Enkin, *et al.* 1989), together with the manner in which they are administered. Psychological factors need to be considered in the decision to test, the procedure of testing, the preparation for testing, the provision of test results, and to assist women in coping with the uncertainty after test results.

In the final decade of the twentieth century, antenatal care has seen an advancement of technological progress, together with improved knowledge of potential problems. These factors have contributed to an altered nature of care offered to pregnant women. However, such advances in technology provide disturbing questions for women under examination. For instance, the advantages of detecting forms of fetal abnormality need to take consideration of the psychological well-being of the pregnant mother who undergoes the procedures. The focus in the literature relates to the anxiety created in women's minds by the initial decision to enter such a screening programme, the wait for the results and, of course, the implications of any results which bring to light any abnormalities. There are both advantages and adverse aspects of antenatal screening. Interventions available for the adjustment or minimization of the physical problems detected by tests must be weighed in the cost-benefit analysis of the test and the extent of its implementation.

Hall & Chng (1982) revealed that the majority of antenatal admissions for pregnancy-related problems arose despite routine antenatal care which 'neither detected nor prevented' such conditions. They felt that 'the expectation of what can be achieved was unrealistic'. For example, in this study, intrauterine growth retardation was detected by the clinicians in under half the cases. Overdiagnosis was the cost of many procedures, with a case of inconsequential transient hypertension diagnosed for every case of sustained hypertension; with 2.5 inaccurate predictions of growth retardation for every accurate prediction. Such findings lead to scepticism of the mass approach to antenatal screening, where the risk of over-investigation may result in high financial and psychological costs.

Richards (1989) notes that there are many social, psychological and ethical effects related to such tests as ultrasound screening, fetoscopy, amniocentesis, etc. The issues which such testing raises relate to the role of termination of pregnancy, and the difficulty of health care moving towards the 'promise' of a 'perfect' baby. Such tests occur in social settings, and class and ethnic differences for example may account for systematic differences, both in terms of reactions to screening, experience of screening and outcome of the procedures, let alone staff reaction and handling of the individuals concerned. Tests also emphasize the dilemma of balancing the interests of the mother and the interests of the baby, and highlights attitudes towards disability which may prove problematic.

Studies which have monitored such antenatal procedures have attempted to quantify the psychological impact of screening procedures and to evaluate the emotional effects with varying protocols and forms of delivery. Reading (1982) showed that the provision of feedback during a scan could increase levels of reassurance, information, involvement, and health related behaviours such as smoking reduction and alcohol cessation. Social support has been shown to reduce anxieties for women undergoing screening for neural tube defects (Robinson, *et al.*, 1984). Risk levels of the individual pregnant woman may contribute to pre- and post-screening anxiety and adjustment (Fearn, *et al.* 1982). Emotional reactions may be a function of quality of feedback. Poor preparatory information and delayed feedback were associated with higher anxiety levels and adverse emotional alterations (Field, *et al.*, 1985; Nielsen, 1981; Robinson *et al.* 1984). The element of choice may be a determining factor in anxiety and adjustment (Barton, *et al.*, 1987). This study also showed a persistence of raised anxiety, even after reassuring results had been relayed. Fearn *et al.* (1982) noted that raised levels of Alpha feto protein (AFP) were associated with high levels of anxiety.

Marteau, *et al.* (1988) found that a sizeable minority of subjects incorrectly identified which tests they had undergone in a recent pregnancy. When Marteau, *et al.* (1989) monitored a group of subjects who had either undergone amniocentesis to detect Down's Syndrome, or were screened for fetal neural tube defect, they found that these subjects exhibited significantly lower anxiety levels in the third trimester and a more positive attitude towards the pregnancy in the second trimester. Studies often do not include those women whose tests actually did identify neural tube defects or Down's Syndrome, so the full picture is not complete.

Any screening programme needs to take into account the psychological factors associated with the decision on whether to implement testing or not in the first place, and subsequently, if testing is implemented, on the way in which the procedure is carried out so as to minimize psychological trauma.

A number of issues need to be analysed prior to mounting a screening programme, as well as while auditing and evaluating such programmes. These are as follows:

- Routine, as opposed to selective, screening.
- Specific criteria for selection, such as risk group, age.
- Counselling implications at all levels (entry to the procedure, initial test, subsequent test, results, especially surrounding any decision to terminate).
- Cost benefit analysis.
- Accuracy of any test.
- Emotional cost of reassurance to the women.
- Psychological cost of not detecting any disorder or illness.
- False positive rate/error and inaccuracy factors in the procedure.

Psychological factors associated with implementation policy

Screening decisions do not take place in isolation. Once a programme has been initiated, there are a number of functional variables which should be constantly examined. If a screening programme is not introduced, the issue whether to do so should be constantly re-examined. Factors for consideration include:

- Manner of implementation of the programme.
- Counselling and informed consent at all testing stages.
- Protocol handling.
- Speed of results.
- Provision of results.
- Funding of counselling care.
- Ongoing evaluation and research.

Problems

Whichever course of action any unit embarks upon, there will always be problems. These should be anticipated, incorporated into future action and utilized to generate subsequent change and adaptation. Procedures should incorporate analysis of the following:

(1) Results associated with negative emotions engendered by the process, whatever the outcome.
(2) False positive problems where a woman is given a positive test result when the result is in fact negative. Reconfirmation may confirm this, but once anxieties and worries have been initiated there may be continued doubt and questioning on the part of the woman.
(3) Conversely, false negative problems occur when a problem is missed or a test fails to pick up a positive case.
(4) Handling of tests. The handling procedure must be individualized and information transfer maximized. There is always a risk with a routine procedure that the individual needs, worries and concerns of the woman concerned may become swamped.
(5) Decisions after the test. Tests are a means for supplying information based on which decisions are made and as such are not 'final'. These decisions are traumatic and agonizing in their own right. Any unit policy which involves testing ought to have a clear methodology for accommodating decision making processes which are based on test outcomes.
(6) Impact of the tests. Tests may have a widespread impact on staff carrying out the procedures, the women who undergo them, as well as their partners and family and the unborn fetus.
(7) Effects on relationships of test outcomes. Workers must take on board the impact that certain tests may have on the relationship of the couple. For example, a positive Wasserman test or HIV test may raise all sorts of questions about the couple's sexual behaviour, mutual trust and the future of the relationship. Partners may also

have different views on steps to be taken as a result of some test outcomes and this may well trigger friction.

(8) Intervention to ameliorate testing effects. If testing is seen as desirable, staff should seek access to the comprehensive body of literature which can be used to understand or ameliorate any negative effects which such tests may produce. This ranges from the protocols of test handling, the construction and provision of test information, the availability of staff to discuss testing decisions, procedures and outcomes and the way in which the test procedure are carried out. For example, women who are given feedback while viewing a scan have a more positive experience than those who are not allowed to see the screen and are not told what is being observed.

(9) Pre-test strategy. The way a test is introduced can have significant bearing on the level of emotional trauma which women subsequently experience.

(10) Sample gathering. Some tests involve blood or urine samples while others require more invasive techniques such as the gathering of amniotic fluid, which involves a needle insertion into the amniotic sac. Fears and worries around the process may be overlooked while staff think about fears and worries about the outcome.

(11) Post-test strategy. Every testing procedure requires a well thought out post-test strategy, which should be explained to the woman prior to testing. This should cover the time which it will take to obtain results, the manner in which results will be given and the follow up. Generally studies have shown that pacing is very important, and that the wait for results is anxiety laden: the shorter this is the better.

(12) Feedback of results is a crucial component of testing. It is always preferable for results to be given in person rather than in writing or by telephone. There should not be a different procedure for positive and negative results.

Deciding who should be tested

Marteau *et al.* (1992) examined the procedure associated with attendance at alpha fetoprotein (AFP) screening in 1000 eligible pregnant women, of whom 902 were tested, 51 declined and 47 failed to undergo such tests. Decliners were significantly different in their ratings of perceived threat, attitudes towards termination of pregnancy, their knowledge levels and their attitudes towards doctors and medicine.

Provision of test results

The way in which results and feedback are handled in all these tests varies considerably, often depending on the technology involved, the personnel involved, the frequency or rarity of the procedure itself and the constraints imposed by the clinic, its staffing levels, space restrictions and the number of women attending. Feedback for routine tests is generally lacking. When given, it was always appreciated, whether it was positive or negative (McIntyre, 1977). In a controlled investigation (Sherr, 1989) antenatal attenders were given personalized feedback of routine tests together with brief explanatory information. Subsequent anxiety levels were significantly lower than a comparison group with no such intervention. Corresponding satisfaction was also higher with the intervention group.

There is a great divide between result feedback and result interpretation. The former may be fairly standardized, but the latter is open to clinical judgement and variation of interpretation. Thus communication problems may be found as a result of vastly different information provision. Marteau *et al.* (1989) reported that information provided for amniocentesis procedures was very varied. The rate of miscarriage as a result of the procedure was quoted from 1 in 100 to 1 in 400.

It is surprising to note that many women are reluctant to ask for results. Cartwright (1979) showed there was a lack of correlation between the desire to ask questions and questions which were actually asked. Sherr (1989) found that most women wanted full explanations and preferred medical professionals to give these, yet few asked, as they felt they could not approach their doctor. Social class was not a differentiating factor for women in their desire for knowledge, but it did differentiate in their success at receiving it (Sherr, 1989). It could be that the professionals are more prepared to give full feedback and proper explanations to middle-class women. Such information and explanations gaps often formed an ongoing saga where women were still seeking information and clarification during later interview studies (Sherr, 1989; Cartwright, 1979).

Negative results mark the end of a specific worry, yet a proportion of women continue to be anxious after results. This is intensified if false positive results are given, even if subsequent negative results are found.

Any protocol is faulty which relies on the assumption that a negative test result, as opposed to a positive result, does not need conveying to the woman. Such a protocol creates endless and needless worries. Many women cope with the wait this involves by creating their own arbitrary deadlines. When such deadlines arrive, they conclude that the institution would have contacted them if the result was poor. Farrant (1980) recorded increased uptake of alcohol and medication at such times of uncertainty and this is obviously counter-productive. Anxiety can be reduced if results (even if negative) are conveyed in person (Robinson, *et al.* 1984).

It is imperative that staff understand the underlying protocols about breaking both good and bad news. Both sets of protocols have much in common. How to convey bad news will be described in detail later on in this book. As good news is usually perceived as positive, little attention is given to the protocols. However, the following points should always be considered:

(1) Ensure women are always told the good news. It is surprising how often good news is simply marked in files and not directly fed back to women.
(2) Ensure that privacy is available. It is very tempting to break good news in public, but this may limit the number of questions or dialogue the women may want to make. It will also send chilling messages to those who are called in to private rooms for their news (they will make the assumption that being called in equals bad news).
(3) As with all news, tell the truth and tell it quickly.
(4) Even though the person breaking the news knows that it is good, the receiver will not. Many women fear the worst while others anticipate good news. Some women may be so pessimistic that they do not even hear the good news. Repeat it and ensure that the message is understood.
(5) Good news ought to be reassuring, but sometimes it is not. Do not assume that it will be, and ensure that underlying worries and concerns are aired and discussed.
(6) Explanations of the news are as important as the news itself. In some cases, women may desire a negative result, but are unsure of the meaning, implications and ramifications of such an outcome. For example, a negative HIV test does not mean that someone could not become infected in the future. A negative screening test for a specific abnormality does not exclude all abnormalities.
(7) Allow time for the news to be absorbed and for the individual to consider any questions they may have.

Pregnancy tests

The first time science raises its head is the moment when the pregnancy is diagnosed. Women no longer examine their bodies or their instincts – they gaze at rings in test tubes or wait upon the word (and convenience) of medical practitioners.

Home pregnancy testing kits are frequently used. Coons, *et al.* (1990) reported that of American student health attendees, one in six responders had used a kit at least once. The majority use such kits for reasons of speed and confidentiality, but in general they were utilized as a supplement to medical care, rather than as a substitute.

Routine screening tests

Most women can recount quite clearly that routine antenatal clinics will involve tests of blood pressure, blood tests, urine samples and weighing. McIntyre (1977) found the tests were so integrated into care management that few women questioned them. Results and explanations were seldom provided. This lack of dialogue and questioning does not reflect a lack of interest on the part of women.

Weight monitoring formed a key element of routine antenatal care, although the efficacy and usefulness of the procedure is under some debate (Hytten, 1980, Varma, 1984). Women are used to weight monitoring and the test itself is not invasive. It is, however, important to inform women of the reasons for weight monitoring and the implications of results. Feedback from weight monitoring is not difficult as most women can read scales. However, their differing interpretations of the measurement may be disconcerting. Many feel that weight gain is unpleasant merely serving to remind them of their changing body size and image and their departure from their former (slim) self. They often perceive weight gain as something which will be censured. Sherr (1989) found that many women thought their weight gain to be 'too much', despite the fact that the obstetric staff did not agree.

Specialized screening procedures

Specialized screening tools are now widely available. These will not be discussed here. Relevant medical textbooks should be studied for technical details. However, their psychosocial consequences should not be divorced from the biochemical procedures.

Ultrasound scans

Ultrasound can be carried out in women at low or high risk for certain problems, and its impact seems to vary accordingly. Consistent findings relate to problems with the provision of feedback. Michelacci, *et al.* (1988) found that anxiety, depression, somatic symptoms and hostility significantly decreased after video and verbal feedback were provided during the first ultrasound examination. These decreases were maintained at subsequent examinations.

Reading (1982) and Campbell, *et al.* (1982) randomly allocated women to treatment conditions where they were either able to see the scan themselves or were simply given verbal explanations. These were compared to the routine treatment being used at the time of the tests, which allowed for no vision of the scan or feedback. They found that where women were able to see their scans this resulted in more positive attitudes to the pregnancy and subsequently enhanced compliance with advice about smoking and drinking during pregnancy.

Women who were scanned with raised serum alpha fetoprotein

(Hunter, *et al.* 1987) showed greater anxiety and concerns for the baby's health prior to the procedure and benefited from reassurance.

Amniocentesis

There can be anxiety about the procedure itself, as well as anxiety about the possible outcome and diagnosis of abnormality. The decision to abort in the face of abnormality is not automatic and the procedure should be available irrespective of women's commitment to abort.

Alpha fetoprotein (AFP) screening

Hunter, *et al.* (1987) examined the longer term psychological impact of ultrasound scanning on women who had a raised serum alpha fetoprotein (AFP) and compared these with 30 control women with normal pregnancies receiving routine scanning. Subjects with raised AFP had significantly higher anxiety levels and obvious concerns for their baby's health, compared to the controls. Scanning procedures also served to improve attitudes and reduce anxiety as a result of reassurance. Farrant (1980) examined AFP tests and differentiated between those who were at risk for problems and those who were not. For the former group, the procedure was reassuring, but for the latter, the procedure raised anxiety and they were not reassured, even after results were provided. These studies highlight the need for ongoing communication for women whose worst fears (possible abnormalities in their baby) have been raised, whether or not these fears have been proved to be groundless.

Fetal alcohol screening

Fetal alcohol problems can be a cause of much suffering. There is much debate as to whether women should be asked to report their alcohol use, or whether toxicologic testing of urine samples should be used to reveal more accurate levels (Lurio, *et al.* 1991).

This problem is largely unrecognized. This can be accounted for by a number of failures: failure to acknowledge the problem, failure to elicit the information, failure to talk to the women, or failure to gain the trust of the women to report accurately. Often it is not the women's failure to report, but the obstetrician's failure to ask the relevant questions, or to gain the trust of their patients. Donovan (1991) studied a group of 58 obstetricians and reported that they did not routinely enquire about alcohol consumption because of the following:

- Bias due to their own abuse.

- Lack of training.
- Low or inadequate awareness of the problem.
- Poor awareness of the effects.
- Denial that fetal alcohol syndrome occurs in their type of practice.
- Practical problems such as lack of time.
- Disinterest.
- Reluctance to offend the patient.
- Belief that patients would lie.

This study has clear implications for potential training intervention to include such data gathering into routine care, and to alert carers to the widespread nature of the problem. It should also alert them to examine some of their own personal attitudes to alcohol to ensure sufficient time for comprehensive care, thus promoting interest and motivation in what is normally a routine, humdrum and perhaps tedious task. Carers also may benefit from greater insight and dialogue with their patient group in order to understand whether indeed patients are offended or do lie, and if so why, under what circumstances, and how they can be persuaded to do otherwise.

Jacobson, *et al.* (1991) certainly found that retrospective recall allowed for higher levels of alcohol consumption to be reported. This was endorsed by Morrow Tlucak, *et al.* (1989) who questioned subjects five years after the pregnancy, and found that positive reports increased by twenty times more than previous levels of recording.

Drugs use

Condie, *et al.* (1989) screened 600 antenatal women for amphetamines, barbiturates, cocaine metabolites, methadone and opiates, when they attended booking clinics. They found low rates of positive tests but reported a worrying finding of a high degree of false positive tests which must be a factor limiting the usefulness of such tests if they are not carried out in conjunction (and specifically with the knowledge and consent) of the women. The harmful effects of presuming a women to have used drugs when a toxicological test was a false positive must be examined. Such outcomes may affect other procedures that the woman is invited to discuss, as it may affect staff attitudes and care.

Toxoplasmosis

Toxoplasmosis screening brings with it particular problems. There is a difficulty in determining whether fetal damage has occurred and there is also a necessary delay in waiting for confirmation of fetal infection which, if the result is positive, may lead to a late termination of pregnancy. This has its own problems. Given British legislation limiting terminations up to 24 weeks, this option may not be available to women unless the infection is associated with severe fetal damage. In addition to the psychological consequences of late abortion there are also significant risks of maternal death.

Non-directive counselling is a process whereby women can assess the costs and benefits, risks and hazards of a condition prior to making a decision. Such counselling is deemed a necessary component of this procedure, given that there are possible adverse psychological sequelae of toxoplasmosis screening and the risk of a substantial number of unnecessary terminations. In order to obtain informed consent to participate in the programme, careful counselling would be necessary for all women before the initial test. It would also be needed for those in whom infection was diagnosed and for those who undergo termination of pregnancy. The basis of all such counselling must be clear and accurate information. This poses a double challenge. Firstly, those who carry out the counselling (GP, midwife, counsellor or other hospital staff) need to be fully informed and thus need training. In addition, and perhaps more fundamentally, information is lacking on the transmission risk and risk of severe fetal damage in relation to gestational age.

Unlike other screening tests, toxoplasmosis testing would need to be carried out at regular intervals for those who initially test negative. This would require multiple, rather than one off, counselling, especially if a woman subsequently tests positive. All this is compounded by uncertainties and possible hazards of some of the interventions on the pregnancy itself (Royal College of Obstetrics and Gynaecology, 1991), with possible drug reactions, side effects, and additional monitoring which may become necessary. Compliance with any treatment regimen may also need monitoring.

Background prevalence may be a factor in considering whether testing should be taken up, whether it should be offered routinely or selectively, or at all. For example Jeannel (1990) noted the variation in Europe of toxoplasmosis, with prevalence of 75 per cent in Paris, 23 per cent in London, 56 per cent in Padua, and 36 per cent in Stuttgart.

HIV testing

The problems of HIV and AIDS should not be divorced or viewed in isolation of the general antenatal screening debate. The majority of worldwide HIV infections (71 per cent) are heterosexual in origin (Mann, 1992). Maternal–child vertical transmission is well established (Peckham, 1990), despite uncertainty about the mechanisms and rate. Studies show a varying rate from 12.9 per cent in Europe, to 33 per cent in Africa. Such variation may be accounted for by background health status, virus strain, length of exposure to the virus, host factors or even couple factors, although the latter is rarely studied. There is a current increase in het-erosexual spread of HIV (Novello, 1991; CDR, 1992) and the growing rate of female HIV infection focuses the issues of reproduction (Johnson, 1992; Padian, *et al.* 1990) and paediatric infection.

Widespread antenatal HIV testing programmes (Larrson, *et al.* 1990; Moatti, *et al.* 1990; Barbacci, *et al.* 1991) mean that HIV is placed on the agenda of a broad range of women, and this invariably occurs when they first appear at antenatal clinics for routine checks. Different units have adopted programmes ranging from whole population screening, to selective screening (Barbacci, *et al.* 1991). Few studies report on pre-test counselling, although clear evidence has been gathered that HIV testing is a potentially stressful procedure for pregnant women (Stevens, *et al.*, 1989). HIV testing decisions can be more greatly influenced by the views of the carer than the views of the client or her risk behaviours (Meadows, *et al.*, 1990).

Many women are first identified as HIV positive during antenatal care (Sherr, *et al.* 1993; Beavor & Catalan, 1993). Yet Tappin, *et al.* (1991) show that with the passage of time this is less so in communities where the risk factors are clear. Johnstone, *et al.* (1989) reported little change over time of the number of pregnant women in Scotland tested, but a decline in those first knowing of HIV from such a test, with a simultaneous increase in those referred already knowing they were HIV positive was noted. Peckham & Newell (1990) reported that when comparisons were made between HIV identification in anonymous screening of Phenylketonurea (PKU) samples and known HIV infections from the obstetric/paediatric surveys in London, only 20 per cent of actual HIV cases were identified. Thus in London at least, 80 per cent of HIV positive pregnancies are currently unidentified as such during antenatal care.

HIV testing should never be undertaken without due thought and consideration and testing during pregnancy is no exception.

HIV test limitations
The test itself is limited in that it can tell whether a person has been exposed to the virus and made antibodies, but it cannot tell how the person was exposed, when they contracted HIV, the stage of illness they are now experiencing, whether they will become ill, what kind of opportunistic infections they will get, whether they will pass it on to their baby or any predictions about survival. Newly acquired infection could be missed as it takes up to 12 weeks on average for sufficient antibodies to be present for a positive test to register. This is particularly problematic during pregnancy, as many women continue to have sexual intercourse, which is rarely protected by a barrier method. Newly infected women are more likely to transmit HIV infection to their babies (van de Perre, 1991) as they are viraemic during the early stages of infection. Stevens, *et al.* (1989) showed that reassurance was significantly lower for HIV tests compared to other antenatal tests.

Cost benefit analysis

The costs of the test are high, in terms of anxiety, coping demand, stigmatization and discrimination. As no cure for HIV is yet available, interventions are limited to early treatment regimes, prophylactic treatments with uncertain long term effects on morbidity, mortality and the developing fetus. Termination of pregnancy is the major option under current debate, yet many women do not or cannot terminate. Inappropriate testing may result in alienation, with women not attending or attending late. Loss of trust may occur if women are tested without knowledge or consent. Doctors who are uncertain of their ability to do pre-test counselling were more likely to refer women (whether of low or high obstetric risk) from GP antenatal care to a hospital (Sherr & Strong, 1992). Form of delivery and retroviral treatment are also factors.

Underlying reasons for screening

The rationale for HIV testing must always be to *benefit* the recipient. Some centres test for epidemiological data gathering. Some staff desire tests as a result of their personal (misdirected) fears of infection from positive patients. HIV testing is not the solution to such fears. Instead, education should be provided. When HIV testing in pregnant women is studied (e.g. Barbacci, *et al*. 1991 n = 89; Ciraru Vigneron, *et al*. 1988 n = 60; Cowan, *et al*. 1990 n = 146; Holman, *et al*. 1989 n = 27, Irion, *et al*. 1990 n = 47; Johnstone, *et al*. 1990 n = 163; Kiragu, *et al*. 1990 n = 108; Selwyn, *et al*. 1989(a) n = 64; Selwyn, *et al*. 1989(b) n = 191; Sunderland, *et al*. 1988 n = 177; Wiznia, *et al*. 1989 n = 22) outcome measures usually centre around test uptake and termination of pregnancy, with a paucity of literature on test handling, result handling, emotional consequences, behaviour change and psychological adjustment. A few (e.g. Kiragu, *et al*. 1990) look at condom use and others look at subsequent reproduction (e.g. Temmerman, *et al*. 1990; Sunderland, *et al*. 1992).

Screening protocols

Widespread antenatal testing is often reported (see Sherr (1991) for a review) with low refusal rates, but a high failure rate in returning for results. The timing of the test, if it is carried out, needs consideration. Testing at booking clinics, if prior to 12 weeks gestation, would be ineffective in identifying any women who have become infected by the same encounter at which they conceived (clearly not a protected sexual encounter) or any sexual encounters thereafter. Continuous testing may be unreasonable and impractical – but may be the only accurate way of monitoring antibody status over time. The literature clearly shows that testing can identify some women, but that others are missed.

Barbacci, *et al*. (1991) examined 2724 pregnant women in USA and compared HIV rates in those who were selectively offered screening to those who were routinely offered screening. They found that routinely offered screening was more likely to identify HIV infected women. Larrson *et al.* (1990) showed in Sweden that universally offered screening led to almost total population uptake. In other centres, the focus has been on counselling and the role of HIV infection in pregnancy and subsequently sexual behaviour, rather than simply as an identification technique. In such centres uptake tends to be lower when women consider their individual risks and their emotional preparedness to undergo testing.

Counselling

Counselling prior to antenatal HIV testing is often not available and not reported. Some centres/clinics provide information packs, while others delegate a few minutes of discussion to another health care professional. Written information is rarely a substitute for interactive counselling and should be seen as an adjunct to counselling rather than a substitute (Sherr & Hedge, 1989, 1991). Berrier, *et al.* (1991) found that educational programmes increased the level of general knowledge, but failed to lead to positive attitudes to testing or increase desire for voluntary testing. Wenstrom & Zuidema (1989) found that risk factor identification without counselling was inefficient. Many studies aim to 'promote' HIV testing and assume low uptake rates to represent 'failure' or 'poor' outcomes. Meadows *et al.* (1991) showed that midwives did not appear to be offering accurate pre-test counselling in many cases. Only one in three women were completely satisfied with the counselling they received. Those in recognized risk groups were neither counselled nor tested. Much misinformation, especially amongst ethnic minorities, was identified.

Meadows, *et al.* (1990) showed that counselling was carried out by the midwife at the booking appointment. The refusal rate was 83 per cent. Only one third were satisfied with their counselling. In a study of uptake of HIV counselling and testing at a Scottish family planning clinic over a three month period, there was a low demand for the tests, but a steady request for advice and information from male and female patients. Advertising and awareness was promoted by use of written information (posters, information bookmarks and information cards in all condom packs). There were 17 requests for counselling over a three month period; seven of these did not proceed to have a test. Of the 17, 14 were counselled and three were given information only. Planning for pre-test HIV counselling should include the phases shown in Fig. 6.1.

Ethics and rights

HIV testing in antenatal care raises complex ethical dilemmas associated with the differences between the needs of society, the needs of the individual, and the competing needs of mother and infant. Testing of infant or cord blood also raises problems as it reflects maternal status.

Opinions of the pregnant women

The voices of the pregnant women themselves should be heard. Specific factors may account for varied uptake on offer, such as institution bias

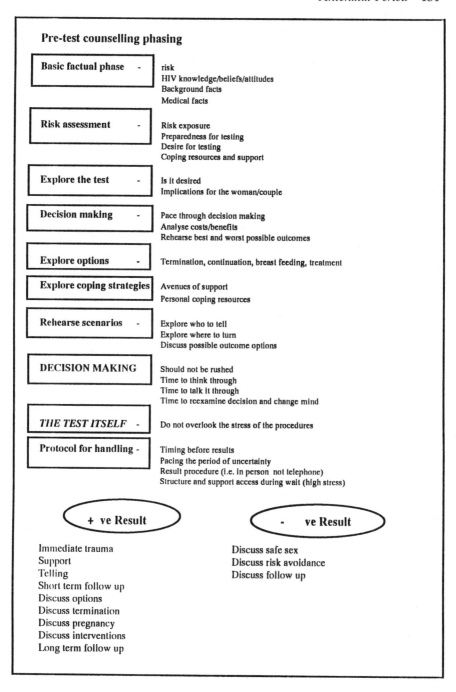

Pre-test counselling phasing

| Basic factual phase | - | risk
HIV knowledge/beliefs/attitudes
Background facts
Medical facts |

| Risk assessment | - | Risk exposure
Preparedness for testing
Desire for testing
Coping resources and support |

| Explore the test | - | Is it desired
Implications for the woman/couple |

| Decision making | - | Pace through decision making
Analyse costs/benefits
Rehearse best and worst possible outcomes |

| Explore options | - | Termination, continuation, breast feeding, treatment |

| Explore coping strategies | | Avenues of support
Personal coping resources |

| Rehearse scenarios | - | Explore who to tell
Explore where to turn
Discuss possible outcome options |

| DECISION MAKING | | Should not be rushed
Time to think through
Time to talk it through
Time to reexamine decision and change mind |

| *THE TEST ITSELF* | - | Do not overlook the stress of the procedures |

| Protocol for handling | - | Timing before results
Pacing the period of uncertainty
Result procedure (i.e. in person not telephone)
Structure and support access during wait (high stress) |

+ ve Result

Immediate trauma
Support
Telling
Short term follow up
Discuss options
Discuss termination
Discuss pregnancy
Discuss interventions
Long term follow up

- ve Result

Discuss safe sex
Discuss risk avoidance
Discuss follow up

Fig. 6.1 Planning for pre-test HIV counselling.

(Meadows, *et al.* 1991), national policy (Larrson, *et al.*, 1990), fear of identification (Barbacci, *et al.*, 1991), or limited choice (Sherr, 1993a). Generally, the majority of studies show that pregnant women endorse the offer of HIV testing, but are uncertain about personal uptake (Stevens, *et al.*, 1989). Where informed counselling has preceded testing, the uptake is low. When counselling is not reported, large percentages 'accept' testing but the return for results is low.

Testing in context of general antenatal care

HIV testing cannot simply be added to the battery of antenatal testing without examining current views on the extent to which HIV testing is similar or different to these procedures. HIV testing reflects possible life threatening illness to the baby, mother (and possibly father and other siblings). The procedures and processes of the batteries of antenatal tests often pose psychological trauma for pregnant women. Tests are often not explained, consent is lacking, informed choice is limited, feedback results are haphazard, and decision making around test outcome is fraught (Sherr, 1989).

Women attending antenatal clinics, especially on their first visit, may be exceptionally vulnerable (Oakley, 1980). The environment is strange, the experience may be new, the woman may be subjected to many confusing and humiliating procedures (Cartwright, 1979), she is concerned for the well-being of herself and her baby (Kumar & Robson, 1978) and may have little say in the process of care (Garcia, 1982). Making a choice may therefore be difficult. Truly informed choice is reliant upon comprehensive and correct knowledge and the ability to be assertive with one's decisions. Fear of imposition of HIV testing may turn women away. Some women have primary risk factors for HIV (such as drug use, poverty, prostitution) which may in themselves be barriers to early and regular antenatal care.

HIV testing and risky behaviour

One reason put forward for testing and/or counselling is to address risky behaviour, both for those who turn out to be HIV positive and those who are negative but at risk through their behaviour. Temmerman, *et al.* (1990) showed that HIV positive women who were tested and counselled subsequently showed a higher desire to conceive a subsequent child. Clearly, the desire for an uninfected baby was worth the risk for these women. Few studies examine sexual behaviour change in pregnant women (Higgins, *et al.* 1991). Termination of pregnancy is more often recorded than any measures of sexual behaviour change (as is usual with gay men, heterosexuals, drug users, haemophiliacs and all other groups).

HIV testing and termination of pregnancy

There appears to be no evidence in the literature to support the notion that knowledge of HIV is a predictor of patient desired termination of pregnancy (Selwyn *et al.* 1989; Sunderland, *et al.* 1992). Some women who terminate in the presence of HIV, do go on to have a subsequent baby to term (Sunderland, 1992). A consistent minority opt for termination and this needs to be available and handled well (see Chapter 3).

Sunderland *et al.* (1988) compared women who learned of their HIV sero-positive status while pregnant but early enough for a legal abortion, with a second group who conceived a subsequent pregnancy after HIV positive status had been established. Three out of the latter 18 women elected to terminate their pregnancy, with 15 continuing. Of the 11 who became pregnant after knowledge of HIV status, nine chose to continue their pregnancy. One subject avoided hospital or medical staff until after 24 weeks gestation for fear of having to discuss termination issue. Sunderland, *et al.* (1992) compared HIV negative and HIV positive for eighteen months post partum. They reported that 34 negative (31 per cent) and 32 positives (33 per cent) learned of their HIV status early enough to terminate. One of the 34 negatives (2.9 per cent) and six of 32 positive (18.8 per cent) chose abortion. During follow-up, there were no significant differences between pregnancies and live births for positive and negative women, or drug and non drug using women. HIV status correlated with decision to terminate but not with subsequent fertility. Of the HIV negative women 18.8 per cent and 23 per cent of HIV positive women had one or more live births. HIV knowledge was insufficient to prompt termination or avoid subsequent pregnancy. Behaviour change was noted in other areas, as pregnancy was shown as an incentive to stop drug taking. Disease state however did seem to be associated, as 10 women with AIDS did not conceive. Counselling protocols provided for extensive pre- and post-test counselling, with a policy of no direct recommendations.

Johnstone, *et al.* (1990) found that pregnant drug using women commonly terminated their pregnancy, irrespective of HIV status. Those who terminated in the presence of HIV often had previous histories of termination on other grounds. Decisions were rarely altered from original intention, especially when pregnancy was desired. Factors associated with continuation of pregnancy were:

- Current good health.
- Desire to have a child.
- Feelings against termination.
- Normative judgements, based on knowledge of women who had babies.

HIV prevalence among women who terminate their pregnancies is sometimes recorded as higher than those who continue their pregnancies.

HIV testing and vertical transmission
There is little evidence that infant infection is being prevented by proto-

cols of HIV testing. This may be associated with the current state of intervention or therapeutics. La Guardia (1991) cautions that many current studies primarily focus on protecting the fetus and reducing perinatal transmission, with little focus on reducing maternal morbidity and mortality.

Fetal echocardiography
Barton, *et al.* (1987) studied the effects of fetal echocardiography for high risk women compared to obstetrically normal women. The former group were more anxious before the procedure and had more negative attitudes. After a normal outcome, their attitudes and anxiety did not differ significantly from the controls. Psychological changes after the procedure were noted.

Antenatal testing in perspective

In conclusion, screening presents the following problems:

- Antenatal screening may raise anxiety.
- Feedback delay may have adverse emotional consequences.
- Poor communications during or after the procedure may result in dissatisfaction and raised anxiety.
- Anxiety may persist even in the presence of negative and positive test outcomes.
- Medics are particularly poor at identifying anxieties in individual women and the nature of their worries.
- The mass nature of any screening programme mitigates against the ability to respond to individuals and their concerns.

Time to prepare

'The widespread popularity of antenatal classes testifies to the desire of expectant parents for childbirth education. As there are benefits in terms of amount of analgesic medication used and in some aspects of satisfaction with childbirth, and as significant adverse effects have not been demonstrated, such classes should continue to be available'

(Enkin, *et al.* 1989)

The antenatal months give time to prepare for labour and a new family. Such preparation extends beyond the pregnant woman, to her partner and her family.

Preparation is a traditional psychological tool invoked for adaptive coping. Over and underpreparation are often seen as problematic and even predictive of poor outcome (Janis, 1971). Adequate preparation allows for rehearsal, realistic fear appraisal and planning a variety of coping strategies. Preparation is sometimes formalized within antenatal classes, sometimes given during clinic visits either by the midwives or doctors, or sometimes informalized by family and friends. Health care professionals are sometimes poorly prepared for information giving roles, yet often frown on lay information sources, calling them old wives' tales (Bourne, 1975). On examination, many of the old wives' tales turn out to be old doctors' tales. Women may have endorsed and accommodated as fact what their medical practitioners told them at the time of the birth of their baby and when their daughters proceeded to conceive, they passed on the information. Medical opinion inevitably changes with time but such widely held inaccuracies may still exist. Enkin (1982) notes that education not only increases information levels but may initiate consumer questioning – which is certainly no bad thing. Lack of information has direct effects on limiting informed choice, increasing dependence and engendering passivity, with implications for control, fear and a lack of cognitive preparation.

Houghton (1968) recorded that an overwhelming majority of her sub-jects (92 per cent) criticized the informational aspects of their experience. Cartwright (1979) recorded that, antenatally, 20 per cent of her sample wanted more information, with this figure increasing to a quarter after the birth. Information sources often varied as a class factor – probably representing professional biases as well as the biases of the women. Sherr (1981) found that women primarily sought information from medical sources despite a consistent reluctance to ask. Actual knowledge level assessment revealed an effect related to social class, but not to parity. It seemed from this study that experience did not equate expertise – a finding that the doctors and midwives were unaware of, as they felt that parity conferred greater knowledge.

The efficacy of preparation has been studied widely but the findings are generally problematic. Random allocation to information is unethical and self selection bias may account for subsequent findings. Content variation in different antenatal interventions may render various studies non-comparable. Furthermore, there can never be a truly 'non-informed' group. Enkin (1982) compared three groups of women who either attended classes, requested class attendance but were 'not accom-modated', or did not request. Class attenders used significantly less analgesia during labour, required less anaesthetic and operative inter-vention, and described more favourable experiences with lower depres-sion scores.

In a review of antenatal preparation, Enkin (1982) records consistent lowered uptake of analgesia in prepared women. There is no evidence however that they feel less pain. It may be that women who desire less analgesia attend classes, classes persuade women to use less analgesia, or classes inform women about possible side effects.

Satisfaction with antenatal classes is varied. Rautava, *et al.* (1990) described 1107 Finnish women who attended antenatal training. Although 75 per cent reported that the classes helped to increase their knowledge, criticisms were high. Courses were perceived by women as out of date, at times patronizing, inadequate and poorly presented. Psychological changes, such as emotional reactions to pregnancy, birth and breastfeeding, relationship issues and coping were poorly addressed, if they were addressed at all.

Reid & McIlwaine (1980) reported that just under half of first time mothers did not intend to go to classes and even less of the multiparous women intended to go. Mitchie, *et al.* (1990) recorded 20 per cent non-attendance (primigravidae) who were less positive about the benefits of classes, and more likely to focus on the costs of attending, believing that avoidance was a positive coping strategy. The best predictor of attendance was actual intention to attend, irrespective of demographic or attitude variables.

Pregnancy and psychological change

Do women change during pregnancy? If so, what accounts for this change? There are those who believe any change which occurs is dramatic and irreversible, whereas others see this change as minor and transitory. Some theories examine biological triggers, social or psychological prompts or explanations. The realities of any change are probably a complex interactions of many of these which ramify with great variation for different women.

A variety of psychological measures during pregnancy have been charted (e.g. Grimm, 1961; Gorsuch & Kay, 1974; Murai & Murai, 1975; Elliott, *et al.*, 1983; Sherr, 1989). The outcomes present a muddled picture, given that some workers report opposite or conflicting findings, others fail to control for medical factors which may trigger such emotional responses and others fail to repeat or follow up the measures. Elliott *et al.* (1983) notes that women vary considerably, whether they are pregnant or not and that any approach which tries to level the experience should be avoided. These measures are often invoked as predictors of post-natal outcomes, with varying degrees of accuracy.

Anxiety and pregnancy

Anxiety is an emotion which has long been associated with pregnancy, yet the extent of this association is unclear. Extreme anxiety has been associated with premature labour, but the consequences of mild or fluctuating anxiety are less well understood.

Anxiety is often a misunderstood emotion. It carries negative connotations and is seen as undesirable. Yet anxiety may be a protective positive emotion in many instances, as it is an appropriate emotion in the face of a stressor. However, it is a common and distressing emotion for many. Anxiety becomes problematic only when the levels of emotion are out of line with the levels of the stressors. It is unclear firstly, whether anxiety in pregnancy truly exists, secondly, whether it is out of proportion to the stresses of pregnancy and thirdly, whether anxiety reduction in pregnancy is beneficial or even desirable.

Niven (1992) advises 'those caring for women during pregnancy should therefore expect them to be anxious, to worry, to be easily upset'. Yet the vision of trembling tearful women may be a simple negative stereotype and flies in the face of many high achieving women who continue to function as well if not better than, their non trembling tearless male counterparts.

The way forward is to better understand anxiety triggers. High antenatal anxiety has been linked with previous abnormalities (Davids, 1961; Crandon, 1979). Anxiety is sometimes related with previous miscarriage, and in such cases it subsides in the last trimester of pregnancy, or after the anniversary of the miscarriage (Kumar & Robson, 1978). Emotional distance and worry has been noted in women who have previously lost a baby or delivered a handicapped baby (Niven, 1992). A modicum of anxiety has often been found to relate to better post-natal adjustment (Pitt, 1968; Breen, 1973) and antenatal anxiety has consistently not been related to labour complications (Beck, 1976; Astbury, 1980). Sherr (1989) noted that anxiety levels had a negative effect on staff reaction to the woman.

Many studies simply track anxiety levels in pregnant women. Some then proceed to make sweeping conclusions, whilst others gather together sets of predictors. Sing & Saxena (1991), for example, studied anxiety levels in 691 pregnant women and compared them to non-pregnant women. Not surprisingly, they found that anxiety levels at all stages were higher for the pregnant women and were reduced post partum. Some studies confuse tension and anxiety; others use a wide range of measures which purport to measure anxiety, but may indeed be monitoring or measuring other factors (such as the physical burden of increased body weight). In some studies, anxiety did not vary over the course of a pregnancy (Murai & Murai, 1975; Elliott, 1984) yet in others there were curvilinear effects over time (with the lowest levels recorded in mid-pregnancy) or a linear relationship with time (Grimm, 1961). Elliott (1984) explains that specific labour related worries at term may account for increased anxiety at this time, but Lubin, *et al.* (1975) recorded a drop in anxiety at term.

Barclay & Barclay (1976) found that increased knowledge did not lead to reduced anxiety and found that non-pregnant women expected greater depression levels in pregnancy than were monitored in pregnant women themselves. Astbury (1980) compared knowledge and anxiety in women with antenatal preparation and those without. Prepared women were more knowledgeable but displayed no difference in anxiety levels.

Studies have generally shown that anxiety intervention has beneficial effects (Ridgeway & Matthews, 1981; Wallace, 1984). Anxiety intervention can take many forms:

(1) Preparation for anxiety.
     anticipation
     education
     knowledge
     strategy
(2) Reduction of anxiety.
     psychological
     physical
     environmental
     biological
(3) Control of anxiety.
     coping strategies
     approach
(4) Removal of the stressor.
     avoidance
     re-examination of procedures and protocols
(5) Removal of the perception.
     drug treatments
     relaxation
     distraction

At the individual level, anxiety can be detrimental. Cohen, *et al.* (1989) reported on a woman with panic attack associated placental abruption and urged for treatment.

Reading (1983) reviewed studies on the impact of maternal anxiety during pregnancy on a variety of outcomes. In these studies, factors which could attenuate the effect of anxiety included:

- Trait anxiety.
- Attitudes towards the pregnancy.
- Appraisal of the stress.
- Psychosocial support.
- Coping strategies.

Interventions are clearly possible for some of these factors. Continued stress may prompt or enhance contraindicated behaviours such as alcohol consumption or smoking.

Depression and pregnancy

Most studies on depression focus on post partum depression, or measure antenatal depression as an attempt to predict post partum depression. Studies often confuse low mood with clinical levels of depression. Post partum depression is discussed in Chapter 8. Lubin *et al.*, (1975), Murai & Murai (1975) and Elliott (1984) all record that depression scores did not vary significantly over the course of pregnancy.

Practical implications

There are specific issues associated with the quality of antenatal care, its emotional impact and the opportunity it affords for beneficial input. Screening during pregnancy, for genetic, infectious or other disorders, is a central issue. In practice, all tests should be handled with care and consideration. No test is too trivial to be overlooked or not considered for any woman. As we enter the technological age which allows for multiple and expanding repertoires of antenatal testing, very careful consideration needs to be given to each particular test. This should be examined in terms of the interventions or treatments available for the condition under scrutiny, the accuracy and predictiveness of the test itself, the costs and benefits of the procedures and the time and facilities available to emotionally prepare women for the procedures.

This plethora of tests should not completely overshadow the ante-natal period which is also one marked with wide ranging change, a variety of practical, physical and emotional needs. This time is a space for the woman and her partner to prepare for labour, delivery and parenthood.

References

Astbury, J. (1980) Labour pain – the role of childbirth education information expectation. In: *Problems in Pain*, (Eds. C. Peck and M. Wallace) Pergamon Press, Oxford.

Barbacci, M., Repke, J. & Chaisson, R. (1991) Routine pre natal screening for HIV infection. *The Lancet*, 337, 709–11.

Barclay, R.L. & Barclay, M.D. (1976) Aspects of the normal psychology of pregnancy Midtrimester *American Jnl of Obstetrics and Gynecology*, 125, 207–11.

Barton, T., Harris, R., Weinman, J. & Allan, L. (1987) Psychological effects of pre natal diagnosis: the example of fetal echocardiography. *Current Psychological Rsrch. and Reviews*, 6,(1) 57–68.

Beck, A.T. (1976) *Cognitive Therapy and Emotional Disorders*. International University Press, New York.

Beevor, A. & Catalan, J. (1993) Women's experience of HIV testing and the views of HIV positive and HIV negative women. *AIDS Care*, 5(2) 177–86.

Berrier, *et al.* (1991) HIV/AIDS Education in a prenatal clinic: an assessment. *AIDS Education and Prevention*. 3(2), 100–17.

Blanche, S., Rouzioux, C., Guihard Moscato, M.L. *et al.* A prospective study of infants born to women seropositive for HIV type 1. *New Eng. Jnl. Med.*, 89,(320) 1643–8.

Bourne, G. (1975) *Pregnancy*. Pan Books, London.

Breen, D. (1973) *The Birth of a First Child*. Tavistock Publications, London.

Campbell, S., Reading, A. & Cox, O. (1982) Ultrasound scanning in pregnancy – the short term psychological effects of early real time scans. *Jnl of Psychosomatic Obstetrics and Gynecology*, 1, 57–61.

Cartwright, A. (1979) *The Dignity of Labour*. Tavistock, London.

CDR (1992) Heterosexually acquired HIV 1: infection cases reported in England, Wales and Northern Ireland 1985–1991. *CDR Review Communicable Disease Report*, vol 2, review 5, 24 April 92.

Centers for Disease Control (CDSC) (1991) *MMWR Communicable Disease Report*.

Chrystie, I., Palmer, S., Kenney, A. & Banatvala, J. HIV seroprevalence among women attending antenatal clinics in London. *The Lancet*, **339**,(8) 364.

Ciraru Vigneron, N., Nguyen TanLung, R. & Bercau, G. (1988) Prospective study for HIV infection among high risk pregnant women: follow up of 60 women, 37 children and 30 families. *IV Int. AIDS Conference*, Stockholm, Sweden.

Cohen, L., Rosenbaum, J. & Heller, V. (1989) Panic attack associated placental abruption. A case report. *Journal of Clinical Psychiatry*, **50**,(7) 266–7.

Condie, R., Brown, S., Akhter, M. & Sheehan, T. (1989) Antenatal urinary screening for drugs of addiction. Usefulness of sideroom testing. *British Journal of Addiction*, **84**,(12) 1543–5.

Condon, J.T. (1987) Psychological and physical symptoms during pregnancy – a comparison of male and female expectant parents. *Journal of Reprod. Infant Psychology*, 5, 207–13.

Coons, S., Churchill, L. & Brinkman, M. (1990) The use of pregnancy test kits by college students. *Journal of American College Health*, **38**,(4) 171–5.

Cowan, J., Kotloff, K., Alger, L., Watkins, C. & Johnson, J. (1990) Reproductive choices of women at risk of HIV infection. *VI Int. AIDS Conference*, San Francisco.

Crandon, A.J. (1979) Maternal anxiety and obstetric complications. *Journal of Psychosomatic Research*, 23, 109–11.

Davids, A. (1961) Anxiety, pregnancy and childbirth abnormalities. *Jnl. of Consulting Psychology*, 25, 76–7.

Donovan, C. (1991) Factors predisposing, enabling and reinforcing routine screening of patients for preventing fetal alcohol syndrome. A survey of New Jersey physicians. *Jnl of Drug Education*, **21**,(1) 35–42.

Dunn, D., Newell, M., Ades, A. & Peckham, C. Risk of HIV type 1 transmission through breastfeeding. *The Lancet*, 340, 585–8.

Elliott, S.A. (1984) Pregnancy and after. In: *Contributions to Medical Psychology Vol 3* (Ed. S. Rachman), Pergamon Press, Oxford.

Elliott, S.A., Rugg, A.J., Watson, J.P. & Brough, D.I. (1983) Mood change during pregnancy and after the birth of a child. *B. Jnl. of Clinical Psychology*, 22, 295–308.

Enkin, M. (1982) Antenatal classes. In *Effectiveness and Satisfaction in Antenatal Care*. (Eds. M. Enkin & I. Chalmers). Spastics International Medical Publications.

Enkin, M., Keirse, M., Chalmers, I. (1989) *A Guide to Effective Care in Pregnancy and Childbirth*, Oxford University Press, Oxford.

Farrant, W. (1980) Stress after amniocentesis for high serum alphafetoprotein concentrations. *BMJ*, 2, 452.

Fearn, J., Hibbard, B., Laurence, K. (1982) Screening for neural tube defects and maternal anxiety. *B.J. Obstet. Gynec.*, 89, 218–21.

Field, T., Sandberg, D., Garcia, R., Nitze, V., Goldstein, S. & Guy, L. (1985) Pregnancy problems postpartum depression and early mother infant interacting. *Developmental Psychology*, 21, 1151–6.

Garcia, J. (1982) Women's Views of antenatal care. In *Effectiveness and Satisfaction in Antenatal Care* (Ed. M. Enkin & I. Chalmers) 81–92. Spastic's International Medical Publications/Heineman Medical Books, London.

Garcia, J. (1985) Mothers' views of continuous electronic fetal heart monitoring and intermittent ausculation in a randomized controlled trial. *Birth*, 12, 79–85.

Garcia, J., Kilpatrick, R. & Richards, M. (1990) *The Politics of Maternity Care*, Oxford University Press, Oxford.

Goldberg, D., MacKinnon, H., Smith, R. *et al.* (1992) Prevalence of HIV among childbearing women and women having termination of pregnancy multi steering group study. *BMJ*, **304**, 1082–5.

Gorsuch, R.L. & Kay, M.K. (1974) Abnormalities of pregnancy as a function of life stress. *Psychosomatic Medicine*, 36, 352–62.

Green, J. (1990) Is the baby all right and other worries. *J. Reproductive and Infant Psychology*, 8, 225–6.

Grimm, E.R. (1961) Psychological tension in pregnancy. *Psychosomatic Medicine*, 23, 520–7.

Hall, M. & Chng, P.K. (1982) Antenatal care in practice. In: *Effectiveness and satisfaction in antenatal care*. (Eds M. Enkin & I. Chalmers). Spastics International Medical Books, London.

Hall, M., MacIntyre, S. & Porter, M. (1985) *Antenatal Care Assessed*. Aberdeen University Press, Aberdeen.

Higgins, D., Gallavotti, C.O., O'Reilly, K. *et al* (1991) Evidence for the effects of HIV antibody counseling and testing on risk behavior. *JAMA*, **266**,(17) 2419–29.

Holman, S., Berthaud, M. Sunderland, A. (1989) Women infected with HIV: Counseling and testing during pregnancy. *Semin. Perinatal*, 13, 7–15.

Houghton, M. (1968) Problems in hospital communication. In *Problems and Progress in Medical Care* (Ed. G. McLachlan) Oxford University Press, Oxford.

Hunter, M., Tsoi, M., Pearce, M. & Chudleigh, P. (1987) Ultrasound scanning in women with raised serum alpha fetoprotein long-term psychological effects. *Jnl. of Psychosomatic Obstet. & Gynec.*, **6**,(1), 25–31.

Hytten, F. (1980) *Clinical Physiology in Obstetrics*, Blackwell Science, Oxford.

Irion, O., Rapin, R., Taban, F. & Beguin, F. (1990) Voluntary screening of HIV infection in all pregnant women. *VI Int. AIDS Conference*, San Francisco.

Jacobson, S., Jacobson, J., Sokol, R. & Martier, S. (1991) Maternal recall of alcohol cocaine and marijuana use during pregnancy. *Neurotoxicology and Teratology Letter*, **13**,(5) 535–40.

Janis, I. (1971) *Stress and Frustration*. Harcourt Brace Jovanovich, New York.

Jeannel (1990) Letter, *Lancet* 11 Aug.

Johnson, A. (1992) Home grown heterosexually acquired HIV infection *BMJ*, 304, 1125–6.

Johnstone, F., McCallum, L., Brettle, R., Burns, S. & Peutherer, J. (1989) Testing for HIV in pregnancy: 3 years experience in Edinburgh city. *Scottish Medical Jnl.*, 34, 561–3.

Johnstone, F., Brettle, R., MacCallum, L., Mok, J., Peutherer, J. & Burns, S. (1990) Women's knowledge of their HIV antibody status its effect on their decision wether to continue pregnancy. *BMJ*, 300, 23–4.

Kiragu, D., Temmerman, M., Wamola, I., Plummer, F.A. & Piot, P. (1990) Paper presented at the VI Int. AIDS Conference, San Francisco.

Kolker, A. & Burke, B. (1987) Amniocentesis and the social construction of pregnancy. *Marriage and Family Review*, **11**, 304, 95–116.

Kumar, R. & Robson, K. (1978) Neurotic Disturbance during Pregnancy. In *Mental Illness in Pregnancy and Puerperium*. Sandler Medical Publications, Oxford.

La Guardia, K. (1991) AIDS and reproductive health, women's perspectives in *AIDS and Women's Reproductive Health* (Ed. L. Chen, J.S. Amor & S.J. Segal). Plenum Press, New York.

Larsson, G., Spangberg, L., Lindgren, S. & Bohlin, A.B. (1990) Screening for HIV in pregnant women. A study of maternal opinion. *AIDS Care*, 2,(3) 223–8.

Lubin, B., Gardener, S.H. & Roth, A. (1975) Mood and somatic symptoms during pregnancy. *Psychosomatic Medicine*, 37, 136–46.

Lurio, J., Younge, R. & Selwyn, P. (1991) Underdetection of substance abuse *New Engl. Jnl. Med.* **325**,(14) 1045.

Mann, J. (1992) *Plenary Address*. 8th International AIDS Conference Amsterdam, Netherlands.

Marteau, T. (1989) Psychological costs of screening. *BMJ*, **299**, 527.

Marteau, T., Johnston, M., Plenicar, M. & Shaw, R. (1988) Development of a self administered questionnaire to measure women's knowledge of prenatal screening and diagnostic tests. *Journal of Psychosomatic Research*, **32** (4–5), 403–8.

Marteau, T., Johnston, M., Shaw, R. & Michie, S. (1989) The impact of prenatal screening and diagnostic testing upon the cognitions, emotions and behaviour of pregnant women. *Jnl. of Psychosomatic Research*, **33**,(1) 7–16.

Marteau, T., Johnston, M., Kidd, J. & Michie, S. (1992) Psychological models in predicting uptake of prenatal screening. *Psychology and Health*, **6**,(102) 13–22.

Matthews, A. & Ridgeway, V. (1981) Personality and surgical recovery – a review. *BJ of Clinical Psychology*, 20, 243–60.

McIntyre, S. (1977) The management of childbirth: a review of sociological issues. *Soc. Sci. and Med.*, 11, 477–84.

Meadows, J., Catalan, J. & Gazzard, B. (1991) Maternal HIV infection. *Lancet*, 338, 386.

Meadows, J., Jenkinson, S., Catalan, J. & Gazzard, B. (1990) Voluntary HIV testing in the antenatal clinic. Differing uptake rates for individual counselling midwives. *AIDS Care*, **2**(3) 229–33.

Michelacci, L., Fava, G., Grandi, S. & Bovicelli, L. (1988) Psychological reactions to ultrasound examination during pregnancy. *Psychotherapy and Psychosomatics*, **50**,(1) 1–4.

Minkoff, H. (1989) AIDS in pregnancy. *Current Probl. Obstet. Gynec. Fertil.* November/December, 206–27.

Mitchie, S., Marteau, T.M., Kidd, J. (1990) Antenatal classes knowingly undersold. *Jnl. Reprod. Infant Psychology*, 8, 248.

Moatti, J.P., Gales, C., Seror, V., Papiernik, E. & Henrion, R. (1990) Social acceptability of HIV screening among pregnant women. *AIDS Care*, **2**,(3) 213–22.

Morrow Tlucak, M., Ernhart, C., Sokol, R. & Martier, S. (1989) Under reporting of alcohol use in pregnancy. Relationship to alcohol problem history. *Alcoholism Clinical and Experimental Research*, **13**,(3) 399–401.

Murai, N. & Murai, M. (1975) A study of moods in pregnant women. *Tohoku Psychologia Folia*, 34, 10–16.

Nielsen, C. (1981) An encounter with modern medical technology. Women's Experiences with Amniocentesis *Women and Health*, 6, 109–24.

Niven, C. (1992) *Psychological Care for Families Before, During and after Birth*. Butterworth Heinemann, Oxford.

Novello, A.C. (1991) Women and HIV infection. *JAMA*, 265, 1805.

Oakley, A. (1979) *Becoming a Mother*, Martin Robertson, Oxford.

Oakley, A. (1980) *Women Confined*. Martin Robertson, Oxford.

Oakley, A. (1984) *The Captured Womb*. Blackwell, Oxford.

O'Brien, M. & Smith, C. (1981) Women's views and experiences of antenatal care. *Practitioner*, 225, 123–5.

Padian, N., Shilboski, S. & Jewell, N. (1990) The effect of number of exposures on the risk of heterosexual HIV transmission. *Jnl. of Infect. Disease*, **90**,(161) 883–7.

Peckham, C. & Newell, M.L. (1990) HIV-1 Infection in Mothers And Babies. *AIDS Care*, **2**,(3) 205–12.

Pitt, B. (1968) Atypical depression following childbirth. *British Journal of Psychiatry*, 114, 132–43.

Porter, M., McIntyre, S. (1989) Psychosocial Effectiveness of Antenatal and Postnatal Care in *Midwives Research and Childbirth*, Vol 1 (Ed. S. Robinson & A. Tomson). Chapman and Hall, London.

Rautava, P., Erkkola, R., Sillanpaa, A. (1990) The Finnish family competence study, *Health Education Research* **5**,(3) 353–9.

Reading, A. (1982) The management of fear related to vaginal examination. *Journal of Psychosomatic Obstetrics and Gynaecology*, **1**,(3/4) 99–102.

Reading, A. (1983) The influence of maternal anxiety on the course and outcome of pregnancy. A review. *Health Psychology* **2**,(2), 187–202.

Reid, M.E. & McIlwaine, G.M. (1980) Consumer opinion of a hospital antenatal clinic. *Social Science and Medicine*, 14, 363–8.

Richards, M.P. (1989) Social and ethical problems of fetal diagnosis and screening, *Journal of Reproductive and Infant Psychology*. **7**,(3) 171– 85.

Ridgeway, V. & Matthews, A. (1982) Psychological preparation for surgery A comparison of methods *B. Jnl. of Clinical Psychology*, 21, 271–80.

Robinson, J., Hibbard, b. & Lawrence, K. (1984) Anxiety during a crisis: emotional effects of screening for neural tube defects. *J. Psychosomatic Research*, 28, 163–9.

Royal College of Obstetrics and Gynecology (1991) *Report of the Working Party on Toxoplasmosis*. Peckham, London.

Selwyn, P.A., Carter, R.J., Schoenbaum, E.E., *et al.* (1989a) Knowledge of HIV antibody status and decision to continue or terminate pregnancy among intravenous drug users. *JAMA*, 261, 3567–71.

Selwyn, P.A., Schoenbaum, E.E., Davenny, L, *et al.* (1989b) Prospective study of HIV infection and pregnancy outcomes in intravenous drug users. *JAMA*, **261**,(9) 1289–94.

Sherr, L. (1987) The impact of AIDS in obstetrics on obstetric staff. *Journal of Reproductive and Infant Psychology*, 5, 87–96.

Sherr, L. (1988) *AIDS in Obstetrics*. Paper presented to the International Conference on AIDS, Stockholm, Sweden.

Sherr, L. (1991) *HIV and AIDS in Mothers and Babies*. Blackwell Science, Oxford.

Sherr, L. (1993a) Ante-natal HIV Testing. Chapter in *AIDS Women and Psychology* (Ed. C. Squire). Sage Publications, London.

Sherr, L. (1993b) Counselling issues for women of reproductive age. In *AIDS and Women* (Ed. M. Johnson & F. Johnstone). Churchill Livingstone.

Sherr, L. & Hedge, B. (1989) *On becoming a mother: counselling implications for mothers and fathers.* Paper presented at the WHO Conference on AIDS and Mothers and Babies, Paris.

Sherr, L. & Hedge, B. (1991) The impact and use of written leaflets as a counselling alternative in mass antenatal HIV screening. *AIDS Care,* **2,**(3) 235–46.

Sherr, L. & Strong, C. (1992) Safe sex and women. *Genito-urinary Medicine,* 68, 1.

Sherr, L., Petrak, J., Melvin, D., Glover, L. & Hedge, B. (1993) Psychological trauma in female HIV infection. *Counselling Psychology Quarterly,* **6,**(2) 99–108.

Short Report (1981) Maternity Services. HMSO Publications, London.

Sing, U. & Saxena, M. (1991) Anxiety during pregnancy and after childbirth. *Psychological Studies,* **36,**(2) 108–11.

Stevens, A., Victor, C., Sherr, L. & Beard, (1989) HIV testing in antenatal clinics. *AIDS Care,* **1,**(2) 165–72.

Sunderland, A., Moroso, G., Bethaud, M. *et al.* (1988) Influence of HIV infection on pregnancy decisions. *IV Int. AIDS Conference,* Stockholm, Sweden.

Sunderland, A., Minkoff, H., Handte, J., Moroso, G. & Landesman, S. (1992) The impact of HIV serostatus on reproductive decisions of women. *Obstetrics and Gynecology,* **79,**(6) 1027–31.

Tappin, D., Girdwood, R., Follett, E., Kennedy, R., *et al.* (1991) Prevalence of maternal HIV infection in Scotland based on unlinked anonymous testing of newborn babies. *The Lancet,* 337, 1565–7.

Temmerman, M., Moses, S., Kiragu, D., Fusallah, S., Wamola, I. & Piot, P. (1990) Impact of single session post partum counselling of HIV infected women on their subsequent reproductive behaviour. *AIDS Care,* **2,**(3) 247–52.

Ussher, J. (1989) *The Psychology of the Female Body.* Routledge, London.

van de Perre, P., Simonon, A., Msellati, P. *et al.* (1991) Postnatal transmission of HIV type 1 from mother to infant: a prospective cohort study in Kigali, Rwanda. *New. Eng. Jnl. Med.,* 325, 593–8.

van de Perre, P., Hitimana, D., Simonson, A., *et al.* (1992) Postnatal transmission of HIV 1 associated with breast abscess. *The Lancet,* 339, 1490–1.

Varma, T. (1984) Maternal weight gain in pregnancy and obstetric outcome. *Jnl. of Gynec. & Obstet.,* 22, 161–6.

Wallace, L. (1984) *Psychology and Gynaecological Problems* (Ed. A. Broome and L. Wallace). Tavistock Publications, London.

Wenstrom, K. & Zuidema, L. (1989) Determination of the seroprevalence of HIV infection in gravidas by non anonymous versus anonymous testing. *Obs and Gyne,* **74,**(4) 558–61.

Wiznia, A., Beuti, C., Douglas, C., Cabat, T. & Rubinstein, A. (1989) Factors influencing maternal decision making regarding pregnancy outcome in HIV infected women. *V Int. AIDS Conference,* Montreal.

Wolkind, S. & Zajicek, E. (1981) *Pregnancy. A Psychological and Social Study.* Academic Press, London.

Chapter 7

Special Circumstances

There is a wide range of special circumstances which may prevail during a pregnancy. Some are rare, and some are common but not documented or overlooked. All these circumstances need special attention.

Abuse during pregnancy

Abuse in pregnancy is an all too common experience. Abuse refers to any physical, psychological or sexual assault on a woman that can cause pain, trauma, damage and which can have an impact for considerable time beyond the incident. True prevalence and description has not been fully established. Some studies in the USA put the prevalence as high as 7–11 per cent of the pregnant population (Helton, *et al.*, 1987; Hilliard, 1985). In Norway, similar findings were reported (Schei & Bakketeig, 1989). Such levels of abuse cannot be simply seen as a function of overall abuse, as an American study found an increased incidence of abusive violence of 60.6 per cent when comparisons were made between pregnant and non-pregnant women (Gelles, 1988). Some age factors may also be prevalent where younger women are more likely to be abused and more likely to be pregnant.

Abuse can be divided into physical and sexual abuse. Clearly, it is important to understand the implications for the psychological well being of the mother, both short- and long-term, as well as the effects and risks on the unborn baby.

Women are often reluctant to report abuse, but are more willing to divulge it if questioned in a sensitive way by their carers. McFarlane, *et al.* (1992) found that 8 per cent of their sample voluntarily reported abuse with no prompting; the figure rose to 29 per cent when questions from their medical staff addressed the issue.

The research studies currently available on abuse pose numerous methodological problems. Many concentrated solely on populations in the USA and it is therefore difficult to know to what extent these findings translate to other countries and other socio-cultural settings. In addition, many of the studies focus on small samples and it is consequently difficult to differentiate minor and major levels of abuse. Forms of abuse vary widely and may be key factors in determining outcome on an unborn infant. It is also unclear to what extent treatment for the abuse can ameliorate subsequent damage to the mother or baby. No studies give clear correlations relating to factors underlying the abuse (such as poor nutrition, or a poor emotional state) and few differentiate between single instances of abuse and multiple or continuous abuse.

Bullock & McFarlane (1989) found a higher prevalence of low birth weight where mothers had suffered abuse during pregnancy. McFarlane *et al.* (1992), in a study of 691 American subjects, found that one in six women in this prospective study had been abused, with 60 per cent of this group reporting at least two occasions of abuse. Abuse was most common around the head. The perpetrator was almost always someone known to the pregnant woman – 78 per cent had been abused by their husband or boyfriend. Particular risks were apparent in the cases of teenagers who reported multiple abuse (often by both their boyfriend and their parents). McFarlane noted that abused women were highly likely to be late attenders for antenatal care and highlighted the need to keep any avenues of dialogue on the subject open, as some women who were not abused during early pregnancy reported incidents occurring later in the course of their pregnancy.

Stewart (1992) studied a sample of 548 women in Canada and identified abuse in 36 subjects during their current pregnancy (89 per cent of the women's pregnancies were unplanned). In addition to the physical abuse, the women recorded mental abuse, threats, forced sex and fear of their partner. Yet the majority were still in the relationship, despite requiring medical treatment for the abuse. For 62 per cent, the abuse increased during pregnancy, for 30 per cent the level remained constant; only in 7 per cent did pregnancy mark a decrease in abuse. Only 2.5 per cent told the antenatal staff of the abuse. In this study, the majority of abuse was targeted at the abdomen (64 per cent) with the remainder aimed at the buttocks, head and neck or extremities. Comparisons between the abused and the non-abused pregnant women revealed the abused to be younger, more likely to be unmarried, poorly educated, unemployed and to experience emotional distress (including suicide attempts) prior to pregnancy (which was likely to be unplanned). The abused women also tended to have an unhealthy diet and an increased usage of cigarettes and alcohol, as well as prescribed and unprescribed medication and illicit drugs – this may well reflect a diminished control or a coping mechanism.

Abuse of the pregnant woman can lead to direct and indirect effects on both mother and baby. There is a direct risk of trauma and physical damage to the mother. There is a similar risk to the baby, in the case of severe violence to the abdomen, which may cause conditions such as abruptio placentae, fetal fractures, ruptures and haemorrhage (Sammons, 1981). Indirectly, the abuse may lead to emotional reactions, increased anxiety, depression, or the exacerbation of any illnesses. If a woman turns to over use of items such as alcohol, tobacco, medication or illicit drugs to help her cope with the trauma, these will have documented deleterious effects on any developing fetus (Harlap & Shiono, 1980; Kline, *et al.* 1980; Simpson, 1957; Zuckerman, *et al.* 1989) as well as on the health of the mother. If such a mother chooses to leave an abusive relationship, she may then suffer financial hardship which can directly affect her nutritional status, her likelihood to seek antenatal care and the extent to which she cares for herself adequately during pregnancy.

Women who are the subject of abuse often display a range of common reactions, often referred to as the 'battered women syndrome' (Walker, 1984). Some studies have typified such women as those who suffer from 'learned helplessness', yet other studies (Gondolf & Fisher, 1988) have shown a high degree of behavioural adaptation and resourcefulness in the victims of abuse. However, all abused women run the risk of social isolation, of detachment from social support, of shame and guilt and they may simultaneously suffer from lowered self-esteem.

There is no literature which directly links child abuse with the abuse of pregnant women, but this cannot be ruled out. In general, when working with pregnant women, one can assume:

- There is an increase in teenage abuse from parents and partners (sometimes both).
- Following abuse, there is a subsequent increase in miscarriages, low birth weight and still birth.
- Abuse is largely not recognized or identified by health care staff.
- There is a possible association between abuse and possible suicide attempts.
- The prevalence of abuse to pregnant women is increasing.

Suicide and pregnancy

Suicide during pregnancy is rare (Kleiner & Greston, 1984). The bulk of investigations are presented in the literature as case studies. While it is difficult to make generalizations from these, there essentially are two ways of addressing suicide and pregnancy. The first is to examine the occurrence and predictors of suicide during pregnancy; the second is to examine suicides and observe any pregnancy related triggers which may have contributed to the decision to commit suicide. Although suicide invariably refers to the loss of life, there is also a need to incorporate an understanding of suicide attempts and suicide ideation.

The case studies reveal underlying themes which revolve around the social pressures and supports which women experience in their pregnancies and pregnancy decisions, as well as the availability of options open to them. Over the last thirty years, case reports from Westernized industrialized countries have substantially disappeared and such low incidence can probably be directly linked to improved contraception and the availability of termination of pregnancy. This is enhanced by a more accommodating societal attitude. Data emerging from the East still reports individual cases of death during pregnancy.

Suicide in pregnancy is probably under-reported. In early pregnancy it may be missed. Kleiner & Greston (1984) reviewed the literature (spanning the period time between 1900 to 1947) on female suicides and of the 1766 reported, found that 222 (or 12.6 per cent) were pregnant. A similar review of current studies (from 1958 to 1963) revealed that 119 women (or 1.8 per cent) were pregnant out of 6454 women studies. This sevenfold decrease could almost entirely be accommodated by an understanding of social health and welfare change. In larger urban centres (e.g. New York), 2437 female suicides (from 1961 to 1980) revealed six women or 0.25 per cent to be pregnant. More recent studies (Resnik & Wittlin, 1971) found only one pregnant woman out of 202 female suicides (0.5 per cent). In the UK, the figures are also difficult to ascertain. Kleiner & Greston (1984) estimate that 1.7 per cent of maternal deaths are due to suicide. Lester & Frank (1987) examined data from the 1980 US census and found no significant relationship between suicide rates and illegitimate pregnancies.

Attempted suicides may give greater insight into the emotional suffering that some women experience. Many studies are dated, but the recorded rate is 6.6 per cent (which is still a figure nearly five times greater than the global estimated completed suicides). It is, however, unclear from the data whether these women clearly wanted to kill themselves and failed, or whether they intended to attempt and thus succeeded.

Suicide attempts and completions are disproportionately related to parity and marital status. Primiparous women are over-represented as are single women. In the 1990s, teenage pregnancy has been associated with increased suicide vulnerability. However, in other age groups, pregnancy may be a protective factor against suicide. Indeed, when Lindesay (1989) examined the relationship between suicide rates at different ages within male and female groups from 1921 to 1980, it was found that between the ages of 35–44, female suicide rates were significantly reduced.

Bayatpour, *et al.* (1992) examined the interactions between drug use in pregnancy and suicide ideation. They reported relationships between abuse, drug use and suicidal ideation. HIV infection and drug use were also correlated with increased attempts (James, *et al.* 1991).

Pennbridge *et al.* (1991) studied risk profiles of homeless pregnant adolescents and young people and found them more likely to be depressed and to have attempted suicide than those of the same age living at home.

Pregnancy in older women

Pregnancy in the over-forties is becoming more common and the mean age of first pregnancy in the West is increasing. There are considerable differences between first pregnancy in an older woman and a younger woman, as well as subsequent pregnancies in the older woman. There is also a disproportionate focus on the age of the woman rather than on the man. Pregnancies in older women therefore create a range of problems and benefits which need to be considered.

Firstly, we need to understand why an older woman is conceiving a child. In addition to the reasons that any younger woman may be conceiving, an older woman may be particularly focusing on issues such as:

(1) Difficulty in conceiving earlier in their life.
(2) A new partner can often bring about a sudden and new need to cement, enhance or even salvage a relationship. Some older women with younger partners may wish to have a baby to 'keep the relationship going'.
(3) Change of decision or a last minute rethink on whether or not to have children.
(4) Active decision to postpone conception until their career or relationship has been established.
(5) A final hurdle – often women who have reached the peak of their career find that having a baby is the one thing they have not done and wish to rectify this.
(6) Changing trends. In the 1970s women were still forced to choose between a career and a family. Now those who chose to concentrate on their careers find themselves challenged by younger women who are doing both and wish to follow their achievements.
(7) A welcome challenge. Some women fight to the top of their profession and find this a challenge in another guise. It may present an opportunity to show or prove capability.
(8) A search for permanencies.
(9) A search for meaning.
(10) A resolution to mid-life crisis.
(11) Pursuit of youth.

The interpretation by the available literature of age in pregnancy must be considered in relation to the norms of age in pregnancy; over 90 per cent of women in the UK give birth under the age of 35 years (Berryman, 1991). Perhaps because of this, age is invariably discussed in terms of disadvantages and problems rather than advantages, which certainly do exist (Berryman, 1991). Problems are probably highlighted for this age group, because any woman experiencing long-term problems, will, by the mere passage of time, find herself within the older age group still trying to conceive. There is, however, general agreement that fertility and the ability to conceive decline with age (Llewellyn Jones, 1986). Some studies have found increased problems in older women, whereas others have failed to document this systematically, especially if the women had had a child already. Down's syndrome is the most common age related problem, documented as an increase from 1.1 per 1000 (live) births at 30 years, to 9.2 per 1000 (live) births at 40 years (Mansfield, 1988). Few studies have examined the contribution of older fathers to such genetic difficulties. Clearly the impact of a Down's syndrome baby and other congenital problems in a baby, will have long-term psychological ramifications on the mother, her partner and family (see Chapter 13).

Given the age related concerns of abnormality, older women are more likely to be offered, even encouraged, to undergo screening procedures (most notably amniocentesis) to check for possible problems. The consequent apparent focus on a search for abnormalities rather than normality is often a strain for such women.

Older women are more likely to be psychologically prepared for pregnancy. They were found to be more likely to express or display the following:

- Satisfaction with maternal role (Ragozin, *et al.*, 1982).
- Feeling prepared for pregnancy (Alment, 1970).
- Higher levels of knowledge (McCaulay, 1976).
- Compliance with antenatal care and attendance.
- The ability to make conscious decisions affecting the pregnancy (Frankel & Wise 1982; Welles Nystrom & De Chateau, 1987).
- Higher career levels and thus increased socio-economic status (Ragozin, *et al.*, 1982; Wilkie, 1981).
- Greater tolerance in childrearing (Eicholz & Offerman Zuckenberg, 1980).
- Children exhibit higher intellectual development (Ragozin, *et al.* 1982).
- Longer periods of breastfeeding (Berryman, 1991).

Robinson, *et al.* (1988) compared primiparous women aged 35 years and over, with those aged younger than 31. They found some interesting differences; the older group had more autonomous styles of personality, returned to full-time work more often and displayed 'good levels' of adjustment during pregnancy and motherhood.

Teenage pregnancy

Teenage pregnancies are common. Despite the notion that such pregnancies may present difficulties, Phoenix (1991) has reported on a growing body of studies in which both the mother and child do well. In contrast to an older mother, a younger mother may be caught in social, economic and personal circumstances which throw obstacles in her path to a successful pregnancy and birth. It may be these, rather than purely age, which interact with the progress and outcome of the pregnancy. As with older mothers, one needs a clear understanding of why younger women conceive. Understanding of teenagers cannot automatically be generalized to pregnant teenagers. Those who become pregnant may differ systematically from those who do not. Studies also tend to concentrate on pregnant teenage females, with a limited understanding of their male teenage partners.

In addition to the reasons why any woman would conceive, special consideration in younger women may be given to:

(1) Accidental conception (Simms & Smith, 1986).
(2) Engineering of welfare income (i.e. becoming pregnant in order to claim state benefits). Phoenix (1991) records little support for this contention and indeed draws the contrast between wilful engineering for benefits and the high level of accidental conceptions at this age.
(3) Desire for a child.
(4) Establishing a role.
(5) Relationship factors.
(6) A wish to imitate a sibling who is also a pregnant or childbearing adolescent (East & Felice, 1992).

When considering whether younger women are adequately psychologically prepared for pregnancy, many of the problems that are encountered cannot be disentangled from employment, economic, and social factors. Yet the fact such problems exist, highlights the needs for special consideration and input for teenage mothers in order to ameliorate their position and therefore facilitate their passage through childbirth, rather than providing (unhelpful) judgements as to their suitability for parenthood. Studies on this subject tend to focus on the negative aspects of such pregnancies, showing that younger mothers:

(1) Benefit from good quality assistance. Some teenagers may be able to attend special schools for the pregnant (Geber & Resnick, 1988), whether they eventually keep their babies or place them for adoption. Such assistance as they may experience in the schools is not only positive, but has been associated with greater pleasure in pregnancy for such women (Giblin, *et al.* 1987) and may affect the decision whether to terminate or carry the babies (Ortiz & Nuttall, 1987).
(2) Benefit from social support. Satisfaction with their decision to abort or carry may be strongly associated with support from the woman's family and friends. Pregnant women were more sensitive to family influence by their mothers than their fathers (Ortiz & Nuttall, 1987).
(3) Younger mothers may have lowered knowledge on child-rearing and child-development issues (Fry, 1985). In such cases, it is more beneficial for health care professionals to supply such women with the information they lack, rather than 'blame' them for their lack of experience. This would be of direct help to them and indirect help to their children.

(4) Younger women are at greater risk of abusing their children (Butler, *et al.*, 1981). Often such risk recordings compound the problem in that they prompt scrutiny and stress for the younger mother, rather than any more positive preventive input.
(5) Younger women have increased risks of childbirth and post-partum complications (Butler, *et al.*, 1981).
(6) Younger women may have interrupted educational, career and economic progress (Edelman & Johnson Pittman, 1986).

Phoenix (1991) points out that many of the social, educational and economic factors experienced by young women may in fact predate the pregnancy and thus cannot be linked in a causative way. Positive aspects of younger motherhood are yet to be systematically recorded (Phoenix, 1991). They would include closer age links with the child, equal ability to provide love and a nurturing environment. The challenge for the caring professions in such cases is to provide adequately for the woman's special needs, facilitating positive images and adaptive behaviours rather than adopting any judgements. De Anda, *et al.* (1990) showed beneficial effects of a five week stress management course for pregnant adolescents: proof that when special care is taken, very positive effects may occur.

Women who have been raped

Rape is a devastating crime which occurs with growing frequency. Rape refers to forceful sexual intercourse, either with a known or unknown individual. The victim of such an assault may have to face pregnancy, in addition to the multiple psychological burdens of the physical and mental trauma from the rape. Under such circumstances, some women may choose to terminate their pregnancy but others will go ahead. Those involved in caring for such women need to give special consideration to the psychological needs which they may have (Kreuger, 1988).

Women who have been raped may well be experiencing a 'wrong' pregnancy (Raphael Lef, 1990) and may thus be particularly in need of special support (Burgess & Holstrom, 1974) and psychological assistance, both during and after the pregnancy. Termination of pregnancy is often seen as the only outcome in such cases; indeed pressure groups who generally condemn termination are often willing to see such situations as exceptional (Moore & Stief, 1991). However, legislation surrounding termination may interact with a woman's ability or readiness to seek it, especially when a termination may be difficult to attain or fund (Kreuger, 1988).

Women's perceptions of rape are varied. While most young women fear rape (Hall, 1987), they may not be very knowledgeable about the range of psychological trauma that may be felt during and after such an experience. Studies of young people show a belief that, following rape:

- They will experience more positive reactions from their friends than from their parents.
- They will experience more positive reactions if the rape was committed by a stranger rather than by somebody they know, no matter how well.
- Rapists are mentally ill.

Professional help should take these beliefs on board, facilitate support channels and dialogue between parents and their children, and be particularly helpful in cases where date rape resulted in the pregnancy.

Any woman who has been sexually assaulted (McGregor, 1985) needs to receive:

- Full assessment and care for any physical injuries.
- Psychological assistance in coping with the trauma of the rape.
- Full and accurate documentation for later forensic evidence (which can be difficult, painful, emotionally harrowing and seem easy to overlook at the time, but will be crucial at a later stage).
- Full assessment for a range of sexually transmitted diseases.

Rape can have long term severe sequelae. Long-term problems include dysfunctional sexual relations (Ellis, *et al.*, 1981), fears and avoidance of any activity or place which may trigger memories associated with the event. If pregnancy results from the rape, it poses systematic dilemmas. These may provoke or affect the following emotions:

- Want–*vs*–rejection. Here the baby may be wanted but the incident unwanted.
- Hate. This is a deep emotion which may surround the entire pregnancy. The mother may be unable to disentangle her hate of the incident with her emotions towards either the pregnancy or the child.
- Incident recall. The pregnancy and the child may trigger perpetual recall of the incident. The reality of the child and the acceptance that the child is 'half hers' may ameliorate this but at times of stress or difficulty the opposite may overwhelm the mother.

If the woman proceeds with the pregnancy, there are particular factors during labour and delivery which need careful handling. During pain or at the moment of labour when the baby seems a reality, the women may experience violent recollections of the rape. Some women submerge such memories, but they may resurface at such a time when their defences are down and the pain of labour becomes blurred with the pain and outrage of the rape.

A woman who has been raped may regress during confinement and have particularly need of attention. Such a woman should never be left alone during labour, and continuity of care with an informed midwife is vital. The woman should be given an opportunity to talk about the rape and this should not be simply ignored because it is inconvenient or awkward for the midwife or doctor to discuss. Staff who are uncomfortable should simply not be attending such a woman, as her needs are greater than theirs at this time. When the baby is born, she may feel ambivalence or acceptance towards the child. It is important that she realizes that love is something that grows with time and that most mothers do not feel instant burning love for the babies at the moment of delivery. Acceptance of the child and of the rape are two separate issues and should not be blurred. There may also be countless social problems which she will have to face, such as legal registration, social enquiries and even sympathy.

An increasing amount of research has been carried out on women who are raped during war situations (Swiss & Giller, 1993). Such women face the triple burden of war scarring, rape and, potentially, a pregnancy: rape and its psychological trauma occur in addition to death, devastation and destruction. Swiss & Giller, (1993) draw attention to the use of physical symptoms, as well as psychological ones to express pain. Raped women can suffer from cultural alienation in addition to their own feelings of loss of control, which may be paralysing.

Women tend to turn to medical sources if there are concerns about trauma, such as situations in which rape was associated with harm, fear of sexually transmitted diseases (especially HIV) and termination/pregnancy assistance. Medics are thus well placed to provide care. Women who experienced rape in the Bosnian conflict have been described as reacting with denial, depression or neglect of themselves and others (United Nations, 1993).

Unplanned pregnancy

Unwanted pregnancy may affect the mental health of both the mother and father. Najman, *et al.*, (1991) studied a comprehensive sample of pregnant women and found that when the pregnancy was unwanted, there were notable increases in anxiety and depression in both parents. These differences, however diminished over time. Despite early notably raised levels in mental health variables, they found that very few subjects giving birth to a baby as the result of an initially unwanted pregnancy suffered from subsequent mental health problems.

Multiple births

Multiple births occurs with increasing frequency, exacerbated by the new reproductive technologies. Twinning is quite common in the population, but more evidence of triplets, quads and quins is now emerging (Price,

Table 7.1 Growth of multiple births

Year	Triplets	Quads	Quins
1989	183	11	1
1982	70	6	–

1992), as shown in Table 7.1. Some of the figures in Table 7.1 are directly attributable to fertility drugs or multiple egg and embryo transfer.

The arrival of multiple children brings with it additional strains, some of which vary dramatically from singleton births, and some of which vary because of their sheer size rather than because of the nature of the births. These include:

Economic (Mugford, 1990) The expense of multiple births can be burdensome on many families.

Prematurity (Price, 1991) The higher the number of babies born, the more significant the risk that such births will be premature. They bring with them the accompanying problems associated with low birth weight, special care baby unit admission and may also herald longer term developmental challenges (McFarlane, *et al.*, 1990).

Parental impact (Price, 1992) This comprehensive study examined all the triplets and higher order births in the UK. They found that attribution of responsibility was a key factor and differentiated between natural and artificial causes. This study summarizes, comprehensively the obstacles faced which included:

- *Death and disability* Stillbirth, disability and death in the first year was considerably higher than for singleton comparisons. Prematurity (birth before 32 weeks) was prevalent in almost 50 per cent of the cases.
- *Demanding child care* Multiple carers are required for multiple births. Logistic factors may result in exhaustion, isolation and lack of respite for the main carers (usually mother and father). Price reported that individual attention was difficult to provide, for each baby, with consequent strain on language and personality evolvement.
- *Novelty* Multiple births are always a source of novelty and curiosity. This can be thrilling at times for the parents, but at others it can be not only burdensome, but interfering and demeaning, as they become the objects of gaze and attention.

Price also discussed the controversial and emotionally harrowing practice of 'selective feticide' where one of the fetuses is selectively aborted, either on grounds of developmental abnormality or, more recently, on the grounds of number alone. The ethical, emotional and long-term ramifications of this procedure is one for urgent debate.

Women who have experienced a previous neo-natal death

There is some speculation that the emotional state and adjustment of both mothers and fathers who are undergoing a pregnancy after a previous loss would differ systematically from those with no such history. Theut, *et al.* (1989) compared such groups and found differences between the emotional states of the mothers, compared to the fathers, with more specific anxiety increases in the mothers but no differences in either general anxieties for the mothers or any anxieties for the fathers.

Women with psychiatric history

Psychological sequelae surrounding childbirth are discussed in detail in Chapter 8. There are, however, some special circumstances which may require attention. Pregnant women with anorexia nervosa may experience problems as their body shape inevitably changes. Rand, *et al.* (1987) presented two case reports of such women and recorded anxieties and fears of obesity which peaked during the first trimester and the second post partum month. They noted that disturbed eating behaviours diminished during the pregnancy but resumed after delivery. Support and dietary counselling were beneficial.

Lemberg *et al.* (1992) examined the impact of pregnancy on 43 primiparous anorexic and bulimic women. It was found that symptoms of these conditions were reduced, but regression was noted after the birth. In this study there were no birth complications or effects on the newborn. From a psychological point of view, most women experienced anxiety about loss of control over their weight and size as pregnancy inevitably progressed. Unlike abuse, nearly half the sample had divulged their eating disorder to their obstetrician, yet the other half had been undetected.

Women who use drugs and are pregnant

Green & Gossop, (1988) evaluated 12 opiate dependent pregnant women; of these they found 1 stillbirth, 1 neonatal death, 7 *SCBU* (Special Care Baby Unit) and 3 requiring medical treatment. Poor antenatal attendance was noted and 9 of the 10 surviving babies were placed on at risk registers. Better channels of communication were needed between the treatment facilities.

Most studies are concentrated on illicit drug use by women and its various ramifications. However, Gutterman, *et al.* (1987) catalogue the other side of the coin where long-term distress was monitored, sub-sequent to pregnancy drug administration, for women with in utero diethylstilboestrol exposed daughters.

Women who were refused an abortion

There are few studies presently available examining pregnancy in women who were refused abortions (Zolese & Blacker, 1992). Very often upon refusal, such women seek illegal abortions or abortions obtained at a different site. Some women give up their children to adoption and fostering (Visram, 1972; Pare & Raven, 1970). A review of the area (Watters, 1980) concluded that unwanted parenthood had a high pro-pensity for negative effects, with allied requirements for support; either medical, social, economic, psychological or psychiatric. Stress and strain is worse if there are additional children.

The children themselves may face emotional difficulties (Matejcek, *et al.*, 1978). This study details resultant problems such as delayed devel-opment, underachievement, family problems and lowered maternal involvement. It is unclear whether these are directly a result of being a 'refused abortion' or 'unplanned/unwanted baby' or consequent upon the factors which prompted the termination request in the first place.

Women who smoke during pregnancy

There is considerable medical literature on the hazards of smoking generally and the particular hazards to the newborn of smoking during pregnancy. Many women spontaneously adjust their smoking behaviour prior to, or during pregnancy (Ihlen, *et al.* 1990). The behaviour of other people in the home and workplace of smoking pregnant women can have considerable effect on the predictors of smoking, yet few campaigns tar-get these individuals who could contribute to the reduction of smoking during pregnancy indirectly by adjusting their smoking behaviour. Studies show that partners often smoke and that their continued smoking is often the most predictive factor in relapse for the pregnant woman, either later on in pregnancy or post-partum (Cnattingius, 1989; Lodewijck & de Groof, 1990).

Instead, studies invariably examine active smoking of the pregnant mother and there is little detailed conclusive data on the impact of passive smoking, where the pregnant woman is surrounded by a smoking environment even if she herself does not smoke. A series of studies examine a variety of psychological variables in the children of smoking and non-smoking mothers. Yet their conclusions are difficult to interpret and the causal link between smoking during pregnancy and the resulting outcome is limited. The findings are further confounded by the fact that smoking may be related to low birth weight and neonatal intervention and it may be these factors, rather than the smoking, which may affect the developing child. For example Makin, *et al.* (1991) administered a battery of tests to 6–9 year old children of active smoking mothers, passive smoking mothers and non-smoking mothers. Although they found that the children of non-smoking mothers performed better on variables of speech, language, intelligence, visual/spatial abilities and behaviour, it is unclear whether these can be attributed directly to the variable under examination. The children of smoking mothers would themselves have been passive smokers all their lives. Furthermore, the reasons which prompted the mother to smoke in the first place may account for the variance, rather than the smoking itself. However, they did find that the children of mothers exposed to passive smoking had intermediate results, but such children may be exposed to another family member who smokes during their early years. Similar findings were reported by Kristjansson, *et al.* (1989).

A large study in Sweden (Cnattingius & Thorslund, 1990) showed that in over 3500 pregnant women, 32 per cent smoked daily at conception and 23 per cent had given up smoking with the onset of pregnancy. Women who smoked generally had a lower educational level than those who did not, did not live with the father of the baby, and were regularly exposed to a smoking environment (at home or at work). Subjects who continued to smoke during pregnancy were more likely to have had a previous baby (thus providing feedback which challenges the merit of fear arousing health education), or to be those who commenced smoking younger and those who smoked heavily. However, despite the fact that there is much literature on the hazards of smoking, knowledge of such hazards can still not accurately predict smoking behaviour.

Reading & Cox (1982) found that comprehensive feedback to pregnant women during routine ultrasound examinations increased the likelihood of women giving up smoking and also of adhering to other health advice during pregnancy. Other women may spontaneously quit smoking during pregnancy. Relapse rates are high, as this is often very difficult. Quinn, *et al.* (1991) studied 266 pregnant women who smoked and examined the characteristics of 41 per cent of these who spontaneously stopped smoking prior to conception. Variables associated with spontaneous quitting were:

- Absence of another smoker in the family.
- Belief in the harmful effects of smoking.
- Fewer previous miscarriages.
- Earlier initiation of antenatal care.

Those who maintained this abstinence throughout pregnancy were more likely to endorse self-efficacy for this maintenance and had a stronger belief in the harmful effects of maternal smoking. In addition, they were more likely to have experienced nausea associated with their pregnancy.

However, 1 in 5 of the spontaneous quitters relapsed prior to delivery. To attempt to aid and examine such cases, Price *et al.* (1991) gave short-term smoking intervention programmes to pregnant urban women. They were randomly allocated to an educational videotape group, a self-help booklet or received medical advice from their doctor. Of the 109 subjects, 43 per cent reduced the number of cigarettes they smoked and 6 per cent gave up smoking altogether. However, there were no differences shown in the results between the three types of treatment interventions. Burling, *et al.* (1991) randomly allocated women to regular care or to a minimal intervention condition comprising a letter giving expired air carbon monoxide rates and recommendations to cease smoking. Although the intervention group were significantly more likely to have given up smoking at the subsequent clinic visit compared to the controls, the difference dissipated closer to delivery.

A relapse back into smoking is common and it can result in a smoking environment for young babies, the effects of which may also be detrimental. McBride & Pirie, (1990) studied 567 smokers 5–9 months after delivery. Roughly 50 per cent of those who gave up smoking during pregnancy had relapsed by the first post partum month, irrespective of intentions reported during pregnancy. The company of other smokers was a strong trigger for relapse.

There is often a link between smoking and alcohol consumption. Outcome data may thus be confounded. Intervention studies have also found that it is more difficult for women to address smoking behaviour than alcohol consumption (Waterson, *et al.*, 1989). Thus the two behaviours ought to be treated separately and may have different requirements with regard to intervention and assistance.

Alcohol use during pregnancy

There is a comprehensive data set on harm caused by excessive alcohol consumption during pregnancy (Hatfield, 1985), yet there is a lack of clarity about the effect of comparatively small amounts of alcohol. Indeed, this study suggests that prevention should be aimed at chronic high consumers rather than blanket warnings for total abstinence, which may serve little purpose other than to instill unnecessary fear, anxiety and guilt.

Many women continue to drink during pregnancy. Safe levels and investigations by clinicians, let alone dialogue on this point, are often sparse. Smith, *et al.* (1987) found that subjects who continued drinking and those who stopped were very similar demographically. Predictors for continued drinking included length of drinking history, personal reported alcohol tolerance, the presence of alcohol linked illness and drinking in the family (especially siblings).

Pregnancy and transsexuals

Lothstein (1988) reported on 11 female to male transsexuals, aged between 19 and 31 years who had both experienced a pregnancy or at times raised their children. She found that the majority of her subjects felt coerced into pregnancy and were subsequently opposed to termination. They tended to carry their children to term. The high level of rape among this group ($n = 3$) was of note, especially since two had been raped by their blood fathers. Despite a variety of maternal responses, these individuals experienced many difficulties with parenting. These were related in part to their own psychological difficulties, and in part to their chaotic lifestyles.

Obstetric accidents

Ennis & Vincent (1990) have provided a comprehensive overview of the type and nature of obstetric accidents, which may have far reaching implications. They studied case reports from accidents which had reached litigation and found three common themes. These were:

- Inadequate fetal heart monitoring.
- Mismanagement of forceps.
- Inadequate supervision by senior staff.

They caution that such accidents which come to litigation, represent only the pinnacle of the problem which can result in neo-natal death, brain damage or stillbirth. Care standards were problematic in some of these studies; a small group of patients were not visited at all by doctors. Also of note was the fact that human error was most often implicated.

Parental hostage taking

An unusual phenomenon, but one which is documented at case level (Kennedy & Dyer, 1992). They incorporate a notion of primary victims (i.e. the infant taken) and secondary victims (the person who is subject to the demands made by the hostage-taker (Scott, 1978)). Little is known of the ramifications on the child and the family relations subsequent to the resolution of the hostage situation. Kennedy & Dyer point out that intervention took the form of addressing underlying family problems which attracted more importance and family attention than the incident of hostage taking itself.

Women with HIV infection and AIDS

HIV and AIDS cases due to heterosexual transmission are increasing (Downs, Ancelle Park & Brunet, 1990; Chin, 1991). Reproduction and

AIDS poses many dilemmas for women surrounding the impact of pregnancy on disease progression, the possibility and chances of vertical transmission and the options open to them. HIV infection in women closely parallels infection in children. Over 80 per cent of infant infections can be traced to transplacental spread (Peckham, 1991). However, the ramifications of HIV in women has lagged behind in documentation and understanding (Minkoff & Dehovitz, 1991). Problems such as AIDS often serve to highlight existing difficulties and societal barriers, as well as bringing new problems to the fore.

As the maternal antibody crosses the placenta, women are placed in the unique position where their antibodies are subject to scrutiny via the testing of their infants. Indeed, antibody screening of young infants can only indicate maternal HIV status with certainty. Infant infection can take up to 15 months to be established (Barlow & Mok 1993), as it is only by this age that a child will shed the maternal antibody. Newer tests (polymerase chain reaction tests or PCR) show promise in helping to identify virus earlier in neonates.

HIV testing and pregnancy

The first obstacle to be overcome relates to the problems of HIV testing in pregnancy (see Chapter 5 for discussion). Some women will be identified as HIV positive for the first time during pregnancy. Others will commence a pregnancy with known HIV infection. Others will progress through pregnancy in the presence of HIV unknown to themselves or their carers. Until opportunistic infections have been diagnosed, there is no way of telling if a woman has been infected, other than by using laboratory tests. Thus, the infection control measures needed to address this virus, should be integrated into routine antenatal and labour care in order to protect women and staff alike.

Termination of pregnancy in the presence of HIV infection

Some women may terminate their pregnancy – most will not (see Chapter 5 for discussion). Some women may have previously terminated a pregnancy in the presence of HIV, but are now experiencing subsequent pregnancy they hope to carry to term. The pregnant woman is under time pressure and termination counselling should be available if she desires it (Sherr, 1991). The essential ingredients of such counselling include:

(1) Discussion of the pregnancy.
(2) Exploration of the options.
(3) Examination of HIV and its implications.
(4) Social support.

(5) Exploring the impact on the woman and her partner.
(6) Practical implications.
(7) Future.
(8) Regrets.
(9) Allowing the woman time to think.
(10) Giving the woman support, both through the decision and afterwards.

The basis of good counselling should always be adequate factual information and the skill to impart this to the woman in an unbiased fashion.

HIV disease progression in the presence of pregnancy

Initially, it was thought that as pregnancy itself is an immune compromising state, a pregnancy could jeopardize the health of a woman in the presence of HIV and could bring on illness quicker. However, there seems to be little support for this contention and it appears that earlier studies confounded the passage of time effects (Berrebi, 1990) However, given that the mechanisms of disease progression are still only poorly understood, studies are still examining the impact of pregnancy on disease progression and updating is constantly necessary. It has been established that disease state in the mother may affect the chances of vertical transmission. Ill or viraemic (newly infected) mothers are more likely to transmit HIV than those who are HIV positive and well (Van de Pere *et al.*, 1991).

Vertical transmission

The rates of vertical transmission are only now being understood. Early studies overestimated the rates. Good prospective studies (e.g. European Collaborative Study, 1991, 1992) have shown that when large numbers of women who are well but HIV positive are followed up over a 2 year period (until true infant infection levels can be established), the vertical transmission level appears to be in the region of 13 per cent. World wide figures (Sherr, 1991) show some variation with African and South American studies which consistently report higher rates (closer to 30 per cent). This could be explained by a variety of factors, such as the virus strain, background health status and health care, length of infection, multiple exposures, host factors or other factors. This means that between 70 per cent and 87 per cent of children will not be infected. Long-term follow up of these children (and their subsequent children) has not been carried out yet, because of the newness of this infection.

Factual information

Besides HIV testing and counselling (see Chapter 5), there is a considerable input required for women who are known to be HIV positive and continue with their pregnancy. Intensive input may be required and counselling should be available for all who desire it. Good care and counselling is dependent on updated factual information on the disease which informs both the health care workers and the woman in turn. The process is hampered by the rapidly changing information base and the wide areas of uncertainty.

Current information suggests that HIV has been isolated in vaginal and cervical secretions, menstrual blood, semen, seminal fluid and it can be transmitted from men to women and women to men. Male to female transmission is greater than female to male (Van de Wijgert *et al.* 1993). Transmission can occur on a single exposure (sexual, artificial insemination, needle sharing, transplant/transfusion) yet may not occur despite repeated exposure (Sherr, 1993).

It is unknown when HIV infection of the infant occurs. It could be before, during or after delivery as virus has been isolated in fetal tissue as early as 8 weeks, in amniotic fluid and in breast milk. In twin studies, discordant twins have been identified where the first born twin is more likely to be infected than the second born.

Early studies indicated that there may be a need to carry out caesarean section in the presence of HIV, but no advantage in reduced transmission has been documented in later studies. This is still under study (European Collaborative Study, 1994).

- If a mother is symptomatic, the vertical transmission rate is increased.
- A mother who has given birth to a child previously who developed AIDS, is more likely to have a subsequent baby with HIV.
- Many women infected with HIV in the west are linked directly or indirectly to drug use. This in itself has specific implications. Drugs themselves may act as co-factors in disease expression or maternal/ fetal well being. There is no study to date which has examined the effect of withdrawal from drugs with HIV status, on an infant. Furthermore, the drug user's lifestyle may have particular elements such as nutrition, housing, social support, access to medical care, future caretaking of the child and so on, which will affect the child.
- Disease progression and the mean survival time from diagnosis to death is worse for infants than adults.
- There is no cure for HIV infection and on current knowledge, infection is life long.
- Prophylactic measures are emerging for some of the opportunistic infections and antivirals are now under investigation for use in pregnancy and children. The picture is certainly not clear and advice must be tentative, taking into account new findings as and when they emerge.

- Breast feeding is an issue currently under debate. The virus has been isolated in breast milk and breast feeding has been implicated in the spread of the disease in some cases (Dunn, *et al.*, 1992). Random allocation is obviously unethical and the protection of breast feeding for an immune compromised baby should never be dismissed lightly. The preferences of the mother should also weigh dramatically in the decision, as well as the availability of clean safe alternatives.
- Early data emerging from AZT (zidovudine) trials on pregnant women point to a possible diminishing of vertical transmission for those receiving retroviral therapy. Clearly, as the data emerges from these studies, many points will require clarification. Although vertical transmission seems to be reduced with treatment, it is not avoided. There is little data on the timing and dosage effects and whether there is a need to utilize AZT during pregnancy alone or for the infant after birth. The problems of AZT for the uninfected baby are also unknown.

Emotional trauma experienced by HIV positive women

In addition to the medical scenario, there is an overwhelming psychosocial impact of HIV and AIDS and front line workers may well have to provide disproportionate amounts of counselling or advice, given the secrecy which surrounds this condition and the reluctance many women express about turning to wider family. Emotional factors include those described below:

- Bereavement and loss, both in terms of the mother's own health, her partner's possible infection and the problems that may well surround the birth of her baby. Even if the baby is uninfected, her own illness may limit her ability to plan and enjoy long-term parenting.
- Anxiety, depression, thoughts of suicide, panic and emotional upheaval are not uncommon experiences for people with HIV infection or AIDS. The emotional burdens of pregnancy may increase these. Positive emotional states are also present and should not be overlooked. The arrival of a baby may provide many roles and reality demands for a mother and mark a new era in her life. Some women feel guilt about the possible infection of their baby, the source of their own infection and the possible infection of other loved ones.
- The dilemma of pregnancy in the first place, considering her HIV status.
- Labour and delivery problems which can compounded by infection control procedures.
- Increased medical attention and resultant interventions.
- Myriad of worries about the baby's health.
- There are additional and unique issues which only *women* infected with

HIV face, including concerns about abandonment (Worth, 1990; Kamenga, *et al.* 1991), marital breakdown, violence and divorce.

- In addition, women who are alone see HIV as a barrier to any future relationship (Worth, 1990) and children may play a key role in rooting them into the present and future, giving meaning and purpose to their lives as well as companionship, whatever the HIV status.
- Unlike other life threatening disease, HIV and AIDS still conjure up fear and secrecy (Miller & Bor, 1989).
- Social support is often a key element in adjustment to trauma, yet for women with HIV it is often difficult. Women are often the providers of social support rather than the recipients. Worth (1990) reports that male injecting drug users who lose a partner because of their own serostatus may turn to an infected woman as a last resort, rather than face being alone.

Concerns centring around the infant

Infants will either be infected or affected. Multiple illness may pose particular counselling challenges. Their mother, and perhaps their father, may be ill with HIV and the possibility of transplacental infection may herald many months of uncertainty coupled with tests and worry. For example, of the 288 children born to HIV infected mothers in the European Cohort Study (as at 31 March 1991), 83 have infection, 125 have indeterminate HIV status and 80 are not infected (Peckham, 1991). Living with uncertainty is traumatic for the family and may continue for the first 2 years of a child's life or until diagnosis can be ascertained.

AIDS in an infant is more severe than in an adult. Children who are diagnosed under 1 year of age fare less well than those who are diagnosed after 1 year. Infection often accompanies loss of developmental milestones which can be particularly distressing for parents to witness.

The current lack of totally effective treatments results in a range of psychological trauma. This can be concentrated around the stresses of long-term uncertainty, the illness of a child alongside family illness, the wider effects of HIV on siblings and grandparents, constant hospitalization, medicalization and unpleasant medical procedures.

The issue of AIDS orphans and the future care of the children on parental death, whether the children are HIV positive or not, is a further challenge.

Comprehensive management guidelines ought to be available in all maternity units (Minkof & Dehovitz, 1991). Ongoing monitoring is vital for comprehensive understanding of the unfolding patterns of vertical transmission and its correlates. Subsequent fertility is often unaffected by HIV infection in the mother (Ryder, *et al.*, 1991).

As yet, no data exists on fathers, as no testing of male partners has been reported, even though in many instances, studies show the woman's only risk behaviour is the sexual behaviour of her male partner. There is no knowledge of comparative transmission rates and prognosis for children born to families where dual infection is present, compared to only maternal infection.

Women whose babies are accidentally swapped

There is much media coverage of the tragic situations which occur, however rarely, within hospital settings where a baby is thought or known to have been accidentally swapped. It causes life long emotional devastation and can interact, though not necessarily compromise, parental-child interactions for many years.

When such situations come to light, there are a number of stages which need to be examined:

- Informing the parents.
- Dialogue with the staff.
- Record appraisal and keeping.
- Blame/guilt and culpability.
- Waiting for verification.
- Outcome.
- Reuniting parents with children.
- Short-term sequelae.
- Long-term sequelae.

Women whose first health care contact is during labour

Women who arrive in labour or who attend late for antenatal care are all too frequent. Young, *et al.* (1989) studied 201 women who only attended care in the third trimester of pregnancy. They accounted for this finding in terms of psychological and social factors, including low self-esteem, poor communication patterns with parents and partner and some psychological problems such as depressed mood.

Women from different cultures

Staff need to maintain a vigilant awareness for the nuances and special needs for women of other cultures. In cosmopolitan centres, it is all too easy to base procedure and policy on the dominant groups and to treat other groups at a distance or with awe. Currer (1986) examined the particular needs of Pathan women who had emigrated from Pakistan to the UK. Their birth experiences were affected by their exposure to male medics and multiple practices which were difficult for them to accommodate because of religious or cultural norms. Woolet & Dosanjih Matwala (1990) examined paternal presence in labour for couples from ethnic minorities. They found a discrepancy between antenatal desires and actual presence.

Pregnancy after long-term infertility (male or female)

Burns (1990) studied 20 infertility treated families and recorded memories of infertility experience and perceptions of parenting. Perceptions of parenting were compared with those of families with no such history. She found that within families where infertility treatment had occurred, self rated parenting styles were observed such as overprotection, becoming more centred around the child, but also tending to be abusive or neglectful. Examination of retrospective recall of infertility experiences was uniformly negative. Pregnancy improved marital satisfaction. They recorded an increased incidence of psychosocial problems among the infertility treated groups.

Bronham, *et al.* (1989) compared a variety of groups of patients from infertility programmes who had subsequently conceived and either lost or delivered a baby. Findings revealed marked differences, suggesting the beneficial effects of pregnancy but also describing detrimental effects of childbirth among couples successfully treated for infertility.

Phantom pregnancies

Phantom pregnancy (also known as pseudocyesis) is a rare condition (Whelan & Stewart, 1990). The condition arises when a woman believes she is pregnant when in fact she is not. Over the last few decades the incidence has decreased. The decrease can be accounted for by a number of sociological and cultural reasons, such as medical factors and the availability of reliable tests and interventions. Common features described in case reports of phantom pregnancy (Whelan & Stewart, 1990) include:

- Recent pregnancy loss.
- Recent infertility.
- Medical and psychological naïvety.
- Severe social isolation.
- Recent losses or bereavements.
- Women who hold childbearing as an all-important role.

These authors stress the interplay between mind and body, where psychological factors, endocrine factors and sociocultural factors interact.

Women who experience surgery/medical conditions and pregnancy

Schover, *et al.* (1990) studied fertility and sexual functioning in men and women after successful renal transplants. Comparisons between post transplant and pre transplant sexual desire showed significant increases for a few, but a significant proportion (about 25 per cent) remained dysfunctional. Infertility was a major concern for a small group of subjects. Regular menstruation was recorded for two thirds of the women under 50 years. Three men fathered children and two women had successful pregnancies post transplant.

Hubner (1989) examined the impact of a cancer diagnosis and the possibility of iatrogenic (caused by medical staff or medical procedures) infertility consequent upon treatments. They found high levels of life crisis in oncology patients during reproductive years. This study raised some of the important ethical and emotional dilemmas care givers must confront when approaching treatment regimes.

Willmuth (1987) provides a comprehensive review of sexuality after spinal cord injury. Cella & Najavits, (1986) examined awareness and attitudes towards infertility and procreation desires in successfully treated Hodgkin's disease males. They comment that 80–90 per cent were rendered infertile by treatment and therefore urge medics to explore pathways such as sperm banking prior to treatment.

Multiple sclerosis (MS) is a condition which engenders much debate (see Segal, 1991). Weinshenker (1989) reports that longer term MS does not seem to be affected by birth. Many doctors warn women against pregnancy in the presence of MS. Segal recounts that many women were encouraged to have a termination of pregnancy and felt emotional suffering later on.

Diabetes remains a major threat to pregnant women, contributing to congenital anomalies in 4–12 per cent of infants born to mothers with overt diabetes (Kitzmiller, *et al*, 1991). As anomalies are formed early in pregnancy (Mills, *et al.*, 1979), intensive and adequate management may dramatically affect the course of problems (Pedersen, 1977; Kitzmiller, *et al.*, 1991). Education and intensive management for glycemic control prior to pregnancy and in the early phases may play a key role in preventing excessive rates of congenital anomalies in infants.

A few fetal diseases are currently treated before birth (Longaker, *et al.*, 1991). Pre term labour has been associated with such procedures, but no effects on future fertility were found.

Semen donors and their offspring

Daniels (1989) studied 22 semen donors in Australia. Reasons for donating included a desire to help infertile couples, to evaluate fertility and financial incentives. All donors expressed an interest in the outcome of their donations and spent time thinking and musing over their potential offspring. The majority (86 per cent) would have been happy to provide information to identify themselves to the child. They were not deterred from donating if children could trace them at times in the future. Daniels describes this tenuous psychological bond and its relative importance to these individuals.

Maternal death during childbirth

Maternal death during childbirth is rare. Much of the progress in health care, nutrition, social welfare and wellbeing has contributed to the dramatic decrease in maternal mortality. But however rare the event, when it does occur, it is as dramatic as any other loss, extenuated by the circumstances and the possibility of surviving infants.

In the event of such a death during childbirth, input is needed for the partner and surviving children of the mother. Staff will also need support, debriefing and an opportunity for comprehensive dialogue and mourning. There may be possible guilt and feelings of recrimination from all those involved in the care of the mother.

The death of a mother at the very time when a child is anticipated has enormous emotional consequences, for the surviving partner, any other children and the wider family. A better understanding of the reactions of bereaved children may help staff deal with their behaviour rather than excluding them from the wards. The age of the child often has implications for the input which is needed and the coping strategies involved. However, rigid age divisions are unrealistic as individual children differ greatly. The baby, if it survives, will lose mothering, as will the siblings. Although the tasks of mothering can be replaced by many people it is important to bear in mind that the child's needs extend beyond gratification and feeding. A key and consistent individual should take over mothering of the infant and other children. Ideally, such an individual should be someone who can have sustained input over considerable time, so that the children do not have repeated experiences of loss of mothering.

With young babies it is difficult to understand their responses and reactions and interpret them as bereavement reactions – distress may be as a result of a lost reaction to their needs or to a lost individual. The longer term effects of bereavement on very young children are unknown. Studies which have attempted to examine them often have many methodological flaws which render them useless. Retrospective studies reveal little concrete data and are most useful in steering subsequent research. Prospective studies suffer from flaws where it is impossible to tease out the incidental effects of a loss (such as changed socio-economic circumstances, changed psychological mood and state of a care-giver, changed responses of children to needs) from the absence of the key mothering figure. The overwhelming message from the literature focuses on the quality of subsequent mothering as an important key factor in life adjustment. As such, when young babies are faced with a loss this ought to be a primary goal in care planning and resource input.

For older children, the level of meaning will vary. This will depend on family factors, the developmental and cognitive abilities of the individual child and the details of both the present and future circumstances of the family. The loss may be typified by a pining and despair reaction. The hardest part for the child to deal with is the fact that there will be no return of its mother. Again, irrespective of the age of the child, it seems that the level of care offered in its place is crucial in determining psychological and life adjustment.

Family adaptation to the loss determines the level of discussion, understanding, explanation and help that a children can receive. Lansdown (1990) describes how children as young as 4 can hold a meaningful discourse on death and have some concept of the notions involved. Bereavement may affect children in a variety of ways and these should be anticipated. They include:

- Anti-social behaviour (Newman & Denman, 1971; Douglas, 1970)
- General symptomatology, psychological and somatic (Van Eerdewegh, *et al.* 1982)
- Behavioural symptoms (Raphael, 1977).
- Physical problems (Morillo & Gardener, 1980; Herioch, Batson & Baum, 1978).
- Adjustment disorders after bereavement.

Future psychological problems have been tracked (Felner, *et al.*, 1981) such as school problems, school refusal and disinterest (Black, 1974 and Van Eerdewegh, *et al.*, 1982) and these have often led to more severe problems such as psychiatric disorder, depression, disrupted or difficult relationship patterns, increased sensitivity to losses and increased trauma at anniversary times (similarly to adults). This may result in individual life crises occurring at the age-anniversary point of the experienced loss.

At the point of the bereavement, these problems should be anticipated as they relate to future decisions (see Chapter 11).

The older a child grows, the closer their ideas about death correspond with adults. Perceptions of death are closely allied to perceptions of illness. In order to understand what children know and do not know about death, the following notions should be considered, as a child may express them. (See Chapter 11 for full discussion.)

- Understanding permanence (Reilly, *et al.*, 1983).
- Increasing insight with age (Kane 1979).

The age of a child and the level of support surrounding it are the two key elements in pacing. Children may have much clear insight, but their sense of time may have an individual focus. This means that a child is better able to deal with events in the more immediate future and may find events in the distant future harder to grasp. Silence, denial and pretence are three factors that can result from the family or the doctors. This can be helped by the following:

- Informing and question answering which is kept simplistic and jargon free.
- Planning for future care and management.
- Meaningful items (Kuykendall, 1989) help with the creation and retention of memories.
- Farewells are important – either overtly or symbolically; these can be easily facilitated.
- The trappings of hospital can create barriers to grief and mourning. Staff should not hide behind rules and protocols but should go out of their way to be open and supportive.

Staff who are involved in a delivery where maternal death is experienced may find their subsequent work patterns and deliveries very difficult. They may have a crisis of confidence, feel very uncertain and traumatized and may need to reappraise their entire job. This must be treated with understanding, encouragement and patience. Dialogue should always take precedence over silence.

In the instances where there were any errors, doubt or other items of question, it may well be that there will be involvement of a wider area of society, as there may be legal consequences or employment implications.

Other problems

There are a host of other problems which emerge from time to time. Such issues include:

- Women who give their children up for adoption.
- Women whose partners have died during the pregnancy.
- Women with visual or hearing impairment who may have special needs and requirements during all aspects of their care.
- Women who give birth while unconscious.
- Women who find communication in the language of the hospital very difficult.

Staff need to be constantly aware of these and to gather information for future learning.

Implications for practice

Much of antenatal care is set up as a preventive measure – to identify the small proportion of problems that may arise. Although this may generally lean towards obstetrically defined problems, this chapter is an attempt to focus on this small proportion from a psychological point of view. The lessons learned from some of the situations can often be generalized.

Essentially, there is no substitute for good grounding and knowledge of the problem areas. Empirical research must constantly supplement clinical interventions and feed the knowledge base. Such knowledge will serve to highlight the range and extent of such problems and alert workers to potentially problematic situations. Without good rapport, trust and skill, workers may be so busy delivering routine care that the women they are trying to identify may receive insufficient input.

For the more difficult psychological challenges, professionals should not only attain a good working understanding of the problem, but set up useful referral links with psychological care sources so that referral and joint working can be mobilized whenever necessary.

As pregnancy care evolves, other such situations may well come to light. Planning, policy and continuity of care are some of the fundamental tools which will ensure these problems receive adequate and prompt attention and hopefully reduce pain and suffering.

References

Adam, K.S. (1982) Loss suicide and attachment in the place of attachment. In *Human Behavior.* (ed C.M. Parkes & J. Stevenson Hinde), Basic Books, New York.

Alment, E. (1970) The elderly primigravida. *The Practitioner*, 204, 371–6.

Barlow, K.M. & Mok, J.Y. (1993) The challenge of AIDS in children. In *AIDS and the Heterosexual Population* (Ed. L. Sherr), Harwood Academic Press, Chur, Switzerland.

Bayatpour, M., Wells, R. & Holford, S. (1992) Physical and sexual abuse as predictors of substance use and suicide among pregnant teenagers. *Jnl. of Adolescent Health*, **13**,(2) 128–32.

Berrebi, A. (1990) Paper presented at *VI Int. Conference on AIDS*, San Francisco.

Berryman, J. (1991) Perspectives on later motherhood. In *Motherhood* (Ed. A. Phoenix, A. Woollett & E. Lloyd) Sage, London.

Black, D. (1974) What happens to bereaved children? *Proceedings of Meeting of Royal Soc. of Medicine*, 69, 38–40.

Birtchnell, J. (1971) Early parent death in relation to size and constitution of sibship. In *Psychiatric Patients and General Population Controls: Acta Psychiatrica Scandinavica*, 47, 250–70.

Bronham, D., Bryce, F., Balmer, B. & Wright, S. (1989) Psychometric evaluation of infertile couples. *Jnl. of Reproductive and Infant Psychology*, 7, 4, 195–202.

Bullock, L. & McFarlane, J. (1989) The birthweight/battering connection. *Am. Jnl. Nursing*, 1153–55.

Burgess, A. & Holstrom, L. (1974) Rape trauma syndrome. *Am. Jnl. Psy.*, 131, 981–6.

Burling, T., Bigelow, G., Robinson, J. & Mead, A. (1991) Smoking during pregnancy. Reduction via objective assessment and directive advice. *Behavior Therapy*, **22**,(1) 31–40.

Burns, L. (1990) An exploratory study of perceptions of parenting after infertility. *Family Systems Medicine*, **8**,(2) 177–89.

Butler, N., Ineichen, B., Taylor, B. & Wadsworth, J. (1981) *Teenage Mothering Report to DHSS*. University of Bristol, Bristol.

Cella, D. & Najavits, L. (1986) Denial of infertility in patients with Hodgkin's disease. *Psychosomatics*, **27**,(1) 71.

Chin, J. (1991) Current and future dimensions of the HIV/AIDS pandemic in women and children. *The Lancet*, 336, 221–224.

Cnattingius, S. (1989) Smoking habits in early pregnancy. *Addictive Behaviors*, **14**,(4) 453–57.

Cnattingius, S. & Thorslund, M. (1990) Smoking behavior among pregnant women prior to antenatal care registration. *Social Science and Medicine*, **31**,(11) 1271–5.

Currer, C. (1986) *Health Concepts and Illness Behaviour. The Care of Pathan mothers in Britain*. PhD Thesis, Warwick University.

Daniels, K. (1989) Semen donors: their motivations and attitudes to their offspring. *Jnl. of Reproductive and Infant Psychology*, **7**,(2) 121–7.

de Anda, D., Darroch, P., Davidson, M. & Gilly, J. (1990) Stress management for pregnant adolescents and adolescent mothers. *Child and Adolescent Social Work Journal*, **7**,(1), 53–67.

Douglas, J.W.B. (1970) Broken families and child behaviour. *Jnl. Royal Coll of Psych. of London*, 8, 203–210.

Downs, A., Ancelle Park, R. & Brunet, J. (1990) Surveillance of AIDS in the European Community. Recent Trends and Predictions to 1991. *AIDS*, **4**,(11) 1117–24.

Dunn, D., Newell, M., Ades, A. & Peckham, C. (1992) Risk of HIV type 1 transmission through breastfeeding. *The Lancet*, 340, 585–8.

East, P. & Felice, M. (1992) Pregnancy risk among the younger sisters of pregnant and childbearing adolescents. *Jnl of Dev. and Behavioral Pediatrics*, **13**,(2) 128–36.

Edelman, M. & Johnson Pittman, K. (1986) Adolescent pregnancy black and white *Journal of Community Health*, 11, 63–9.

Eicholz, A. & Offerman Zuckenberg, J. (1980) Later pregnancy. In *Psychological Aspects of Pregnancy Birthing and Bonding*, (Ed. Blum) Human Sciences Press, New York.

Ellis, E., Atkeson, B. & Calhoun, A. (1981) An assessment of long-term reactions to rape. *J. Abnorm. Psych.*, 90, 263–66.

Ennis, M. & Vincent, C. (1990) Obstetric accidents: a review of 64 cases. *BMJ*, 300.

European Collaborative Study (1991) Children born to women with HIV 1: infection, natural history and risk of transmission. *The Lancet*, **337**, (8736) 253–60.

European Collaborative Study (1992) Risk factors for mother to child transmission of HIV 1. *The Lancet*, **92**,(339) 1007–12.

Felner, R.D., Genter, M.A., Bocke, M.F. & Cowen, E.L. (1981) Parental death or divorce and the school adjustment of young children. *Am. Jnl. of Com. Psy.*, **9**,(2) 181–91.

Frankel, S. & Wise, M. (1982) A view of delayed parenting: some implications of a new trend. *Psychiatry* 45, 220–5.

Fry, P. (1985) Relations between teenagers' age, knowledge, expectations and maternal behaviour. *B. Jnl. of Dev. Psychology*, **3**,(1) 47–56.

Geber, G. & Resnick, M. (1988) Family functioning of adolescents who parent and place for adoption. *Adolescence*, **23** (90) 417–28.

Gelles, R. (1988) Violence and pregnancy: are pregnant women at greater risk of abuse? *J. Marriage and Family*, August, 841–47.

Giblin, P., Poland, M. & Sachs, B. (1987) Effects of social supports on attitudes and health behaviors of pregnant adolescents. *Journal of Adolescent Health Care*, **8**,(3) 273–9.

Gondolf, E. & Fisher, E. (1988) *Battered Women as Survivors: An alternative to treating learned helplessness.* Lexington Books, Lexington, Massachusetts.

Green, L. & Gossop, M. (1988) The management of pregnancy in opiate addicts. *Jnl. of Reproductive and Infant Psychology*, **6**,(1) 51–7.

Gutterman, E., Ehrhardt, A. & Markowitz, J. (1987) Long-term distress subsequent to pregnancy: drug administration women with in utero diethylstilbestrol exposed daughters. *Jnl of Psychosomatic Obstet. and Gynec.*, **5**,(1) 51–63.

Hall, E. (1987) Adolescents perceptions of sexual assault. *Jnl. of Sex Education and Therapy*, **13**,(1) 37–42.

Harlap, S. & Shiono, P. (1980) Alcohol smoking and incidence of spontaneous abortions in the first and second trimester. *The Lancet*, 2, 173–6.

Hatfield, D. (1985) Is social drinking during pregnancy harmless? *Advances in Alcohol and Substance Abuse*, **5**,(1–2) 221–26.

Helton, A., McFarlane, J. & Anderson, E. (1987) Battered and pregnant: a prevalence study. *Am. J. Public Health*, 77, 1337–9.

Hilliard, P. (1985) Physical abuse in pregnancy. *Obstet Gynecol*, 66, 185–90.

Herioch, M., Batson, J.W. & Baum, J. (1978) Psychosocial factors in juvenile rheumatoid arthritis. *Arthritis and Rheumatism*, **21**,(2) 229–37.

Hubner, M. (1989) Cancer and infertility: longing for life. *Jnl. of Psychosocial Oncology*, **7**,(4) 1–19.

Ihlen, B., Amundsen, A., Sande, H. & Baae, L. (1990) Changes in the use of intoxicants after onset of pregnancy. *B. J. Addiction*, **85**,(12) 1627–31.

James, M., Rubin, C. & Willis, S. (1991) Drug abuse and psychiatric findings in HIV seropositive pregnant patients. *Gen. Hospital Psychiatry*, **13**,(1) 4–8.

Kamenga, M., Ryder, R., Jingu, M. *et al.* (1991) Evidence of marked sexual behaviour change associated with low HIV 1 seroconversion in 149 married couples with discordant HIV 1 serostatus – experience at an HIV counselling center in Zaire. *AIDS*, 1991, 5, 61–7.

Kane, B. (1979) Children's concepts of death. *Jnl. of Genetic Psy.*, **134**,(11) 53.

Kennedy, H. & Dyer, D. (1992) Parental hostage takers. *B. J. Psychiatry*, 160, 410–12.

Kitzmiller, J., Gavin, L., Gin, G., *et al.* (1991) Preconception care of diabetes. *JAMA*, **265**,(6) 731–6.

Kleiner, G. & Greston, W. (1984) *Suicide in pregnancy.* John Wright, Boston.

Kline, J., Shrout, P., Stein, Z., Susser, M. & Warburton, D. (1980) Drinking during pregnancy and spontaneous abortion. *The Lancet*, 2, 176–80.

Kristjansson, E., Fried, P. & Watkinson, B. (1989) Maternal smoking during pregnancy affects children's vigilance and performance. *Drug and Alcohol Dependence*, **24**,(1) 11–19.

Krueger, M. (1988) Pregnancy as a result of rape. *Journal of Sex Education and Therapy*, **14**,(1) 23–7.

Kuykendall, J. (1989) Death of a Child. In *Death, Dying and Bereavement*, (Ed. L. Sherr). Blackwell Science, Oxford.

Lansdown, R. (1990) Paper presented at the Institute of Child Health Conference, London.

Lester, D. & Frank, M. (1987) Youth suicide and illegitimacy rates. *Psychological Reports* **61**,(3) 954.

Lemberg, R., Phillips, J. & Fischer, J. (1992) The obstetric experience in primigravida anorexic and bulimic women. *British Review of Bulimia and Anorexia Nervosa*, **6**,(1) 31–8.

Llewellyn Jones, D. (1986) *Fundamentals of Obstetrics and Gynaecology, Vol II Gynaecology*. Faber and Faber, London.

Lodewijck, E. & de Groof, V. (1990) Smoking and alcohol consumption by Flemish pregnant women 1966–83. *Jnl. of Biosocial Science*, **22**,(1) 43–51.

Longaker, M., Golbus, M., Filly, R., Rosen, M., Chang, S. & Harrison, M. (1991) Maternal outcome after open fetal surgery. *JAMA*, **265**,(6) 737–41.

Lothstein, L.M. (1988) Female to male transsexuals who have delivered and reared their children. *Annals of Sex Research*, **1**,(1) 151–66.

Matejcek, Z., Dytrych, Z. & Schuller, R. (1978) Children from unwanted pregnancies. *Acta Psychiatrica Scandinavica*, 57, 67–90.

McBride, C. & Pirie, P. (1990) Postpartum smoking relapse. *Addictive Behaviors*, **15**,(2) 165–68.

McCaulay, C. (1976) *Pregnancy after Thirty Five*. Dutton, New York.

MacFarlane, A., Johnson, A. & Bower, P. (1990) Disabilities and health problems in childhood. In *Three, four and more: a study of triplets and higher order births*, (Ed. B. Botting, A. MacFarlane & F. Price). HMSO, London.

McFarlane, J., Parker, B., Soeken, K. & Bullock, L. (1992) Assessing for abuse during pregnancy. *JAMA*, **267**,(23) 3176–8.

McGregor, J. (1985) Risk of STD in female victims of sexual assault. *Medical Aspects of Human Sexuality*, **19**,(8) 30–42.

Makin, J., Fried, P. & Watkinson, B. (1991) A comparison of active and passive smoking during pregnancy. Long-term effects. *Neurotoxicology and Teratology*, **13**,(1) 5–12.

Mansfield, P. (1988) Midlife childbearing strategies for informed decision making. *Psychology of Women Quarterly*, 12, 445–60.

Miller, R. & Bor, R. (1989) *AIDS – A Guide to Clinical Counselling*. Science Press, London.

Mills, J., Baker, L. & Goldman, A. (1979) Malformations in infants of diabetic mothers occur before the seventh gestational week: implications for treatment. *Diabetes*, 28, 292–3.

Minkoff, H.L. & Dehovitz, J.A. (1991) Care of women infected with the human immunodeficiency virus. *JAMA*, **266**,(16) 2253–8.

Moore, K. & Stief, T. (1991) Changes in marriage and fertility behavior. Behavior versus attitudes of young adults. *Youth and Society*, **22**,(3) 362–86.

Morillo, E.W. & Gardner, L.I. (1980) Activation of latent Graves disease in children. *Clinical Paediatrics*, **19**,(3) 16–63.

Mugford, M. (1990) The cost of multiple birth. In *Three, four and more: a study of triplets and higher order births*, (Ed. B. Botting, A. MacFarlane & F. Price). HMSO, London.

Najman, J., Morrison, J., Williams, G. & Andersen, M. (1991) The mental health of women 6 months after they give birth to an unwanted baby. A longitudinal study. *Social Science and Medicine*, **32**,(3) 241–7.

Newman, G. & Denman, S.B. (1971) Felony and paternal deprivation; a socio psychiatric view. *Int. Jnl. of Soc. Psy.*, **17**,(1) 65–71.

Ortiz, C. & Nuttall, E. (1987) Adolescent pregnancy. Effects of family support, education and religion on the decision to carry or terminate among Peurto Rican teenagers. *Adolescence*, **22**,(88) 897–917.

Pare, C. & Raven, H. (1970) Follow up of patients referred for termination. *The Lancet*, 1, 635–8.

Peckham, C. (1991) *AIDS and Children*. Paper presented at the AIDS and Children Conference, London.

Pedersen, J. (1977) *The Pregnant Diabetic and her Newborn*. 2nd ed, Williams and Wilkins, Baltimore.

Pennbridge, J., Mackenzie, R. & Swofford, A. (1991) Risk profile of homeless pregnant adolescents and youth. *Jnl. of Adolescent Health*, **12**,(7) 534–38.

Perakyla, A. & Bor, R. (1990) Interactional problems of addressing dreaded issues in HIV counselling. *AIDS Care*, **2**,(4) 325–38.

Phoenix, A. (1991) Mothers under Twenty. Outsider and insider views. In: *Motherhood*. (Ed. A. Phoenix, A. Wollitt & E. Lloyd), Sage, London.

Price, F. (1991) Isn't she coping well? In *Women's Health Matters*, (Ed. H. Roberts), Routledge, London.

Price, F. (1992) Having triplets, quads or quins: who bears the responsibility? In *Changing Human Reproduction*, (Ed. M. Stacey), Sage, London.

Price, J., Krol, R., Desmond, S. & Losh, D. (1991) Comparison of three anti-smoking interventions among pregnant women in an urban setting. A randomized trial. *Psychological Reports*, **68**,(2) 595–604.

Quinn, V., Mullen, P. & Ershoff, D. (1991) Women who stop smoking spontaneously prior to prenatal care and predictors of relapse before delivery. *Addictive Behaviours*, **16**,(1–2) 29–40.

Ragozin, A., Basham, R., Crnic, K., Greenberg, M. & Robinson, N. (1982) Effects of maternal age on parenting role. *Dev. Psychology*, 18, 627–34.

Rand, C., Willis, D. & Kuldau, J. (1987) Pregnancy after anorexia nervosa. *Int. Journal of Eating Disorders*, **6**,(5) 671–74.

Raphael, B. (1977) *The Anatomy of Bereavement; a handbook for the caring profession*, Unwin Hyman, Boston.

Raphael Leff, J. (1990) Psychotherapy and pregnancy. *Journal of Reproductive and Infant Psychology*, **8**,(2) 119–35.

Reading, A. & Cox, D. (1982) The effects of ultrasound examination on maternal anxiety levels. *Journal of Behavioural Medicine*, 5, 237–47.

Reilly, *et al.* (1983) Children's conception of death and personal mortality. *Journal of Paed. Psy.*, 8, 21–51.

Reinharz, S. (1988) What's missing in miscarriage? *Journal of Community Psychology* vol **16**,(1) 84–103.

Resnik, H.L.P. & Wittlin, B. (1971) Abortion and suicidal behaviors – observations on the concept of endangering the mental health of the mother. *Mental Hygiene*, 55, 10–20.

Robinson, G., Erlick Olmsted, M., Garner, D. & Gare, D. (1988) Transition to parenthood in elderly primiparas. *Jnl. of Psychosomatic Obstet. and Gynec.*, **9**,(2) 89–101.

Ryder, B., Batter, V., Nsuami, M., Badi, N., Mundele, L., Matela, B., Utshudi, M. & Heyward, W. (1991) Fertility rates in 238 HIV 1 seropositive women in Zaire followed for 3 years post partum. *AIDS*, 5, 1521–7.

Sammons, M. (1981) Battered and pregnant. *Am. J. Maternal and Child Nrs*, 6, 246–50.

Schei, B. & Bakketeig, L.S. (1989) Gynaecological impact of sexual and physical abuse by spouse; a study of a random sample of Norwegian Women. *Br. J. Obstet. Gynae.*, 96, 1379–83.

Schover, L., Novick, A., Steinmuller, D. & Goormastic, M. (1990) Sexuality, fertility and renal transplantation. A survey of survivors. *Jnl. of Sex and Marital Therapy*, **16**,(1) 3–13.

Scott, P. (1978) The Psychiatry of kidnapping and hostage taking. In *Current Themes in Psychiatry* (Ed. R. Gaind & B. Hudson), Macmillian Press, London.

Segal, J. (1991) Counselling in multiple sclerosis. In *Counselling and Communication in Health Care* (Ed. Davis and Fallowfield) John Wiley, Chichester.

Sherr, L. (1991) *HIV and AIDS in Mothers and Babies*. Blackwell Scientific Publications, Oxford.

Sherr, L. (1993) *AIDS in the Heterosexual Population*, Harwood Academic Press, Chur, Switzerland.

Simms, M. & Smith, C. (1986) *Teenage Mothers and their Partners*. HMSO, London.

Simpson, W.J. (1957) A preliminary report of cigarette smoking and the incidence of prematurity. *Am. J. Obstet. Gynec.*, 73, 808–15.

Smith, I., Lancaster, J., Moss Wells, S. & Coles, C. (1987) Identifying high risk pregnant drinkers. Biological and behavioural correlates of continuous heavy drinking during pregnancy. *Journal of Studies on Alcohol*, **48**,(4) 304–9.

Stewart, C. (1992) Abuse in Pregnancy. *Canadian Study Paper*, presented at the Annual SRIP Conference, Glasgow.

Swiss, S. & Giller, J. (1993) Rape as a crime of war. *JAMA*, **270**,(5) 612–15.

Theut, S., Zaslow, M., Rabinovich, B. & Bartko, J. (1989) Resolution of parental bereavement after a perinatal loss. *Jnl. of the American Academy of Child and Adolescent Psychiatry.* **29**,(4) 521–5.

United Nations (1993) Report on the situation of Human Rights in the Territory of the Former Yugoslavia. *United Nations Document E CN A/1993/50.*

Van de Pere, P., Simonson, A. & Msellati, P. (1991) Post natal transmission of HIV type 1 from mother to infant: a prospective cohort study in Kigali, Rwanda. *New England Journal of Medicine*, **91**,(325) 593–8.

Van de Wijgert, J.H.H.M. & Padian, N. (1993) Heterosexual transmission in HIV. In *AIDS in the Heterosexual Population*, (Ed. L. Sherr) Harwood Academic Press, Chur, Switzerland.

Van Eerdewegh, M.M. Bieri, M.D., Parilla, R.H. & Clayton, P.J. (1982) The bereaved child. *B.J. Psychiatry*, 14, 23–29.

Visram, S. (1972) A follow up study of 95 women who were refused abortion on psychiatric grounds. *Psychosomatic Medicine in Obstet. and Gynec.* 3rd Congress, Basel Karger.

Walker, L. (1984) *The Battered Woman Syndrome*. Springer Publishing Co Inc, New York.

Waterson, E. & Murray Lyon, I. (1989) Drinking and smoking pattern amongst women attending an antenatal clinic before pregnancy. *Alcohol and Alcoholism* **24**,(2) 153–62.

Watters, W. (1980) Mental health consequences of abortion and refused abortion. *Canadian Jnl. of Psychiatry*, 25, 68–73.

Weinshenker, B. (1989) The influence of pregnancy on disability from MS. A population based study in Middlesex County Ontario. *Neurology*, 39, 1438–40.

Welles Nystrom, B.L. & De Chateau, P. (1987) Maternal age and transition to motherhood. *Acta Psychiatrica Scandinavia*, **76**,(6) 719–25.

Whelan, C. & Stewart, D. (1990) Pseudocyesis. A review and report of six cases. *International Jnl. of Psychiatry in Medicine,* **20,**(1) 97–108.

Wilkie, J. (1981) The trend towards delayed parenthood. *Jnl. of Marriage and the Family,* **43,** (3) 583–91.

Willmuth, M. (1987) Sexuality after spinal cord injury. A critical Review. *Clinical Psychology Review,* **7,**(4) 389–412.

Woolet, A. & Dosanijh Matwala, N. (1990) The reactions of East London Women to medical intervention in childbirth. *Jnl. of Reproductive & Infant Psychology,* **1,** 37–46.

Worth, D. (1990) Women at high risk of HIV infection. In: *Behavioral Aspects of AIDS* (Ed. D.G. Ostrow), Plenum Medical Books, New York.

Young, C., McMahon, J., Bowman, V. & Thomson, D. (1989) Maternal reasons for delayed prenatal care. *Nursing Research,* **38,**(4) 242–3.

Zolese, G. & Blacker, V. (1992) The psychological complications of therapeutic abortion. *B. J. Psychiatry,* 160, 742–9.

Zuckerman, B., Frank, D. & Hingson, R. (1989) Effects of maternal marijuana and cocaine use on fetal growth. *N. Eng. J. Med.,* 320, 762–8.

Chapter 8

Childbirth

The ultimate moment in every pregnancy arrives with the onset of labour and the birth of the baby. Drew, *et al.* (1989) questioned post partum mothers to identify important features of labour and postnatal care. They showed that midwives and obstetricians ranked items similarly, thus demonstrating a global appreciation of the issues which matter to women. However, Johnston (1982) has shown that although medical staff are good at itemizing which type of general worries most patients may have, they are very poor at identifying individual patients and their particular worries. Thus they may misdirect input. Drew, *et al.* (1989) summarize the key needs for mothers in childbirth, many of which are endorsed by other studies:

- Explanations of procedures (Kirke, 1980).
- Involvement of the mothers in administering or choosing such procedures.
- Presence of partner.
- Presence (with good rapport) of qualified hospital staff (Stevenson, 1981; Woollett, *et al.*, 1983).
- Physical comfort of the postnatal ward.

Zweig, *et al.* (1986) studied patient satisfaction with obstetric care (n = 255) and concluded that satisfied subjects were more likely to have had continuity of care and to have attended classes. Perceived doctor concern was also an important component of satisfaction.

Medical interventions: 20th century innovations

Medical interventions cover a variety of procedures which are undertaken for a multitude of reasons. The literature expresses criticism when the implementation of the procedures is unnecessary or of questionable use (Chalmers & Richards, 1977; Chard & Richards, 1977; Chalmers *et al.* 1989). Concern is also expressed in situations where the individual assessment of particular patient circumstances is overlooked and when the procedure is carried out for excellent medical need but in such a way as to minimize patient accommodation and adjustment, let alone understanding and satisfaction.

The overall cost of marginally necessary procedures is inevitably borne by the mother who is rarely apprised of the benefits and hazards prior to the procedure. Chalmers (1982) concludes that some procedures are necessary (indeed life saving) for a few mothers but are ill advised as general routine policy for all.

Most medical innovations take on a standard pattern. They evolve to redress a realistic problem. If they do this with success they are fostered often unquestioningly, until routine application becomes questionable. A mixture of consumer query and medical challenge often leads to a more rational policy of utilization with selective use. However, on the road to such a balance, the women are seldom consulted. Such intervention patterns can be observed with episiotomy, inductions, various forms of analgesia, pubic hair shaving, position in labour and suturing.

Labour and delivery

This area marks the focus of many studies. The analysis available examines the way delivery is handled, by whom, with what roles and practices and how these affect the participants. It includes a dialogue about the place of delivery (home or hospital), the attendants at delivery (medical, midwifery, family), the social norms and procedures governing delivery and how all of these factors affect subsequent behaviour.

There are many routines associated with delivery, which all move in and out of vogue. These change as a result of necessity, insight, fashion, convenience, 'science' or consumer desire. For example, routines such as the immediate removal of a baby after birth from the mother and father were once standard practices, but have been abandoned (and indeed are now frowned upon) as society sways in its attitudes (Klaus & Kennel, 1976). Scientific findings and studies are responsible for the re-establishment of parental role in the labour ward.

Pain management

> 'A young doctor came in to see me. And I was doing, I was counting away, thumping the bench [NCT relaxation technique] and he thought I was saying the last rites or something and he said "never mind dear, I will get you something for the pain" and I said "no, I don't want anything."'

> 'Anyway they gave me some drugs and I was on, I think ... I can't remember – they didn't tell me what it was.'

Pain and pain relief are the most common themes when discussing childbirth. Despite the fact that psychology has much to contribute to the area of pain, pain experience and pain management, surprisingly little has been adopted. The psychological impact of different pharmacological pain management regimes (such as pethidine, epidural, entonox) may contribute greatly to their efficacy and to subsequent rates of satisfaction.

Pain perception varies among individual women, even if the pain stimuli is similar. Lowe (1989) examined predictor variables for pain. Confidence in the ability to handle labour was the most significant predictor of all components of pain during active labour. Pain is a poorly understood concept with many intervening variables and contributing factors. Fridh, *et al.* (1988) found a number of psychological and social variables contributed additionally to pain experience, including the partner's feelings towards the pregnancy, previous termination history and personal emotional feelings and expectations.

Long-term recall for pain has been reported as exceedingly accurate by Niven (1988) who followed up 33 women three to four years after the birth. The study noted that simply recalling the pain had resulted in negative effects in a few subjects, but the majority were acknowledged to have experienced some positive consequences. The stability of pain reporting over time was endorsed by Cogan & Spinnato (1988), yet Norvell, *et al.* (1987) suggest that subjects tended to deflate the intensity of their labour pain and therefore cautioned workers against studies which rely on retrospective assessments of labour pain.

Pain management of labour has reached a pinnacle: as far back as 1970, (British Births Survey) only 3 per cent of women were recorded to have received no drugs for pain in labour. Concerns about pain and its management invariably relate to the matching of tolerance with pain experience and analgesia use, the role of expectations about pain and particularly the role of explanations from staff about the effects, sensations and options available.

Some pain management strategies are endorsed, yet have unpleasant side effects. For example, Morgan, *et al.* (1982) showed that of 1000 women, 536 were given epidural analgesia. Despite greater reported pain relief than pethidine, longer labours and higher assisted deliveries were noted for 51 per cent of these women, compared to 6 per cent who received pethidine. Even when satisfaction with pain management is good (Light, *et al.*, 1976), lowered satisfaction is recorded with explanations of medications used.

Pain management also involves sensitive communication and good rapport. Copstick, *et al.* (1986a) examined the relationship between partner support, use of pain control techniques and epidural anaesthesia in 80 primiparous women. They found that psychological pain control techniques did not reduce the intensity of labour pain, nor did their use allow subjects to endure labour without epidural anaesthetic. However, the use of the techniques was correlated with a reduction in frequency of anaesthesia usage, especially when subjects were supported and encouraged throughout their labour, and where the labour was short.

Pain experience is often unrelated to fulfilment or feelings of satisfaction and achievement reported by women (Salmon, *et al.* 1990). Yet these feelings do seem to be related to intensity and pattern of uterine contractions as measured in a study by Corli, *et al.* (1986).

Psychological findings are rarely incorporated into pain management schedules in the labour ward, despite their obvious utility. Possible uses for such factors include:

Distraction

This is known to increase tolerance and is a technique taught by the National Childbirth Trust. Simply placing a woman in a sensory reduced environment (delivery room) and keeping her there for extended time can mitigate against distraction and decrease her tolerance levels. Mobility, change of position and environment can all help distract, which in turn can affect pain perception, pain coping and tolerance.

Personal control of pain

Self control has been well documented as a factor in pain tolerance and management. It is also useful in any crisis situation which labour may well accommodate. Robinson, *et al.*, (1979) utilized self control with the administration of pethidine. Subjects who self administered were compared with those receiving a standard dose. Self administering subjects reported equal pain but used less pethidine. The obvious benefits were associated with superior condition of their babies at birth in terms of APGAR scores (a standard measure on a 10 point scale of the baby's condition at birth).

Control may be linked in with maternal confidence. Lowe (1989) examined the relationships between perception of pain and a variety of variables. With regression techniques to examine the variance in the subscales of the pain rating inventories, confidence in ability to handle labour was the most significant predictor of all components of pain.

Leventhal, *et al.* (1989) reported that directed coping provided the best account for the decline in pain and distress during active labour. Accurate expectations also contributed to adjustment.

Brewin & Bradley (1982) caution workers not to assume that personal control is the only important kind of expectation. They compared women who had not attended classes with women who had. They found that class attenders were characterized by the belief that both they and the medical staff had great control over the process of childbirth compared to those who did not attend classes. Personal control over duration was significantly predictive of reported discomfort among attenders but not among non attenders. Perceived staff control was significantly predictive of discomfort in non attenders but not in attenders.

Body position

There is much of interest written about body position during labour. Its efficacy may be physiological, but additional psychological factors may also be prevalent. Upright individuals are better able to engage in eye contact and therefore better able to verbalize their wants, needs, demands and questions. They are also more likely to receive such interactions. Mobility would also enter into this analysis; a mobile person can choose where they want to be; the stationary person has less choice. Indeed, many women are strapped down (by machinery, but strapped none-theless) which enhances their passivity and focuses their attention on pain rather than on coping.

Choice

Coping is often enhanced by the personal choice of the women concerned and respect thereof by staff.

Biofeedback

There are many psychological interventions based on this notion, in which feedback from bodily processes is given to individuals, either verbally or mechanically. This facilitates their ability to monitor and adjust conscious control to bodily functions. Duchene (1989) examined the effects of biofeedback on childbirth pain with 40 primiparous women who were randomly assigned to biofeedback or a control group. Subjects using biofeedback reported significantly lower pain from admission to labour and delivery, as well as at delivery and 24 hours post partum. In addition, such labours were on average two hours shorter and medications were reduced by 30 per cent. These provide exciting preliminary data although few units utilize biofeedback.

The impact of pain management on the baby must also be taken into consideration. Muhlen, *et al.* (1986) found that the elective use of medication in childbirth for 109 infants was noticeable. They studied firstborn babies at birth and followed them up on their first, fifth and twenty-eighth day of life. Poor scores were recorded even where anaesthesia was minimal.

It should be noted that one form of pain management does not neces-sarily exclude another and multiple forms could be collated to improve efficacy. However, women's experiences of pain and pain management during labour can be varied. This is typified by the woman who stated:

'They just gave me the injection. They said, "We will give you an injection to help you to sleep, help you rest." But it had a really bad effect on me and I really regret having it.

There are few comprehensive studies of drug free labour. Indeed, in many studies these are conflated with women who have short periods of inhalation analgesia. One woman stated:

'I was in control nearly the whole time and I didn't take any pethidine, although that was one thing that the nurses tried to persuade me to have'.

Pethidine

'The pethidine must have lowered down my consciousness quite a bit. When the baby was finally born he did not breathe; I did not even care, I did not even know, I did not even notice.'

All medication must be considered not only in terms of its primary effect but also in its subsequent indirect effects on the mother and baby. Some workers are loathe to admit to such effects. Rosenblatt, *et al.*, (1980) showed that absorption rates of the drug were important indicators of after effects, with high absorption related to reduced alertness and poorer auditory and visual responses. Higher doses of pethidine related to decreased maternal interaction with the infant immediately after delivery.

Infants of mothers who have received pethidine have been shown to exhibit depressed sound localization (MacFarlane & Turner, 1978), respiration (Rosen, *et al.*, 1960; Chamberlain, *et al.*, 1975) and depressed feeding (Kron, *et al.* 1966, Dubignon, *et al.*, 1969).

Epidural

Wuitchik, *et al.* (1990) examined the relationships between pain, cognitive activity and epidural analgesia during labour. They found that epidural anaesthesia significantly reduced subjective pain behaviour but did not seem to affect coping or distress related cognitive activity during active labour. Barbour (1990) studied epidural anaesthesia and relative levels of client satisfaction in a large cohort of women. Satisfaction was not optimum. Problems surround the speed and availability of the procedure on request, as well as problems associated with administration of the procedure and pain experience despite the procedure. After effects have also been recorded. Some are short-term, e.g. headaches. Others can be related to epidural accidents which can cause longer term problems. Indirect effects may also relate to the reason the epidural was used in the first place (such as problem labours). Some studies have documented an increased use of forceps and episiotomies in the presence of an epidural. The effects of the analgesia often mean that women are unable to either receive or perceive the pushing sensation. The procedure is now being developed to ensure that timing can minimize this effect and thereby reduce the occurrence of instrumental deliveries.

Morgan, *et al.* (1982) recorded low satisfaction in a large comprehensive study of women receiving epidural analgesia during labour. This may be accounted for by the increased need for assisted deliveries, the logistics associated with epidural provision, the problems associated with instances partial or total failure of the epidural (Melzack, 1984).

Holding the baby

In 1979, Cartwright found that over 60 per cent of women in her study were not allowed to hold their baby immediately after delivery. Emotional support for the mother during labour is now emerging as paramount and women who are left alone represent an abhorrent scenario. Controlled trials to evaluate the impact of such support have shown tangible benefits (such as reduced labour length, lowered augmentation of labour, fewer fetal problems). Such findings have focused attention on the needs of the labouring woman which marks a welcome improvement in maternity care.

Support

Cogan & Spinnato (1988) studied the effects of social support during premature labour. A group of women were allocated a supportive companion supplied by the hospital. Compared to a group who had no such support, the supported group had fewer abnormally long labours, used medication less frequently and reported improved neonatal well-being, as judged by APGAR scores.

Hodnett & Osborn, (1989) evaluated the physical and psychological impact of continuous one to one support on childbirth outcomes for 103 low risk women. They found that three major variables were predictive of perceived control during childbirth. These were expectations of control, the presence of the continuous professional caregiver and pain medication usage. The importance of the supportive professional input was therefore emphasized.

Thune & Moller (1988) found that post partum emotional disturbance was related to unmet needs reported by women. These were mostly omissions by the midwife during delivery.

Niven (1985) studied the effect of husband presence on the experience of pain during birth. No differences in the intensity of pain were reported. However, differences did emerge when subjects were categorized according to the helpfulness of the partner (rather than simply their presence).

Kennell, *et al*. (1991) studied the impact of a 'doula' or supportive birth companion on labours in a randomly allocated trial. Here 212 women received continuous support, another 200 were observed and a control group was generated (with neither observation nor support). It was found that support was related to significantly reduced caesarean section rate and forceps deliveries. Epidural anaesthesia was utilized by 7.8 per cent supported women, compared to 22.6 per cent (observed) and 55.3 per cent for controls. In addition, oxytocin use, duration of labour, prolonged infant hospitalization and maternal fever showed the same pattern. This study makes an excellent case for the role of a psycho/social supporter in the labour ward.

Such a study should mark a cornerstone in policy. It would be of interest to understand why these findings occurred. They describe some interesting comparisons between the supportive attender and the partners, where the former touched the labouring women 95 per cent of the time, compared to 20 per cent by male partners. This is a surprising finding and may reflect social constraints and 'job description' rather than ineffectual actions by the male partners. It may well be that partners should be trained to touch and help in labour rather than simple observe or accompany the women. It may well be that the doula affects the mother's behaviour but also affects the staff behaviour who feel they are under scrutiny or see, by way of example, how one can interact and gain the sympathy and trust of the woman in labour. The notion of 'continuous' support receives little attention in this paper and it would be of interest to know if the doula was the only continuous supporter in a ward of changing staff.

Other factors affecting labour experience

Time of day
Copstick, *et al.* (1986b) examined the relation between time of day to outcome factors in 147 women. They found that primiparous mothers who noted first contractions at night had shorter labours than those commencing during the day. This was explained by either mothers sleeping through early contractions or increased utilization of epidural and augmentation during daylight time when staff were more likely to be available. Night shifts seemed to contribute to interventions in this study. Harkness & Gijsberg (1989) studied 29 women and confirmed that pain and stress associated with labour were lower for women who started their second stage at night. This study examines the ethological implications of nocturnal birth.

Artificial rupture of the membranes
The procedure has been studied both in terms of its appraisal by women and its impact on their experience of labour. Niven (1992) found a relationship between the procedure and increased pain reporting. This could be due to the nature of the labour after the procedure, or the suddenness of the contractions. Cartwright (1979) noted dissatisfaction with the procedure.

Cultural factors
Many cultural variations have been noted, including the expression and the experience of pain, labour behaviour and partner attendance (Woollett & Dosanijh Matawala, 1990).

Doctors and power

'I thought – well, you just believe them because they are the medical profession. You just think what they say is gospel truth'.

The notion of power and role has been described in detail in psychological theories (see Chapter 1). Power is certainly a theme permeating the childbirth arena. The medical profession holds high status and, by default, power. There are many contributions to the power imbalance which are striking in childbirth.

Whilst it is women who give birth, very often their doctors will be men. Gender roles feed into power imbalance. The trappings of the environment feed subtly into the power equation. Women are the strangers, or 'guests', the professionals are their hosts within the hospital and all allied behaviour about guests become relevant. Homebirths can dramatically reverse this factor. Power artefacts are also added. These range from the series of complex mechanical 'toys' (which only the doctor can 'play' with), the sophisticated measurement and outputs of such machinery (which only the medics can read, understand and interpret) and uniforms which imply power. Dress and accoutrements all identify roles. Doctors wear stethoscopes, white coats, pens and scissors. Midwives wear uniforms, hats, colour codes (and even name labels). In contrast, women have their clothes taken from them. Pyjamas, slippers or even bare feet also play a role in denoting power and can be a potent determinant of a woman's behaviour.

Freedom to move can determine or confer power. Medics can navigate the entire environment without question. Women cannot. Their partners are even more tentative and can only enter 'with permission' or on 'invitation' – to be excluded at the whim of anyone.

'I kept calling for my husband: "In a minute, in a minute" she kept saying'.

Body position can also affect power relationships. Women giving birth are sitting, lying or crouching. Doctors and midwives are standing, bending or leaning. At times they may perch on the bed – many messages can be contained therein.

Knowledge is power, as are choice, control and decision making. Many women will make total sacrifices of all their power status in the bargain which gives them 'a live baby'. Currer (1986) describes how women can be prepared even to breach fundamental religious beliefs to reach this goal.

Many units have attempted to address some of the power issues. Tokenism is an attempt to deny these. Such acts can be seen where staff knock on a door before entering a labour ward or room. It would be interesting to note how often (if ever) they are denied entry (or indeed if they even wait for an invitation). Some staff abandon uniforms. This may be an attempt to redress power balance, but in effect may disturb some women who seek out a powerful individual to take control where they fear to tread. But it may also provide mixed messages where the women is further confused by limited information as uniforms (at least) conveyed factual information without the need for dialogue about role, status, qualifications and hygiene and even provide reassurance. ('The crisp white gown made me feel reassured – I had arrived'.)

Communication can also have many power laden components. At worst, women can be bypassed completely. Kirkham (1989) describes how staff often speak to partners, thus bypassing the women. Similar frustrations and discriminations are often reported by handicapped people (e.g. 'Does your friend take sugar?'). Content and tone both play a role. Some staff can take on parental type nuances within their speech. Censure can occur, especially related to behaviour, noise or emotional expression. This is made worse by the fact that childbirth, one of the most harrowing of human experiences is usually carried out in public, often in the presence of strangers. Free expression is, therefore, almost of necessity, hampered. Indeed, Kennell *et al.*, (1991) notes that this extends to partners who are reticent to even touch their wives during labour whereas the doula women, who are employed to do so, feel much freer to have physical contact.

Deferring to expertise

Control and expertise are specific issues in childbirth. Many women are passive, unquestioning and defer to experts without much question. Comments from women's discourse of their experience highlights this notion (Sherr, 1989).

'So I said no, I had not thought of an epidural but he said because my blood pressure had gone up again – I don't suppose they want you to be in stress. So I said if you think I should have one I will have one, but I would rather not'. [She did].

'I had to have an injection to make me sleep. And I wondered then – I don't need an injection to make me sleep ... but I don't like injections and I said "do I have to?" and they said "yes", so anyway I had the injection.'

Control

There is a reluctance experienced by women to look at or examine their own notes (Sherr, 1989). There is often collusion with the medics to enforce this by sealing envelopes, not showing files and keeping information secret or locking it up or via the use of jargon.

'They gave me my records sealed up in an envelope to take with me. I wish I had now opened them. I thought I could just undo those strings and put them in another envelope, they are not going to know – but I thought perhaps it's best not to . . .' [she did not].

Professional–patient interactions

Many women report brief interactions of poor quality. One possible explanation or dissatisfaction with communication may be the brevity of an interaction (Ley, 1977; Byrne & Long, 1976).

'Examination by the consultant lasts about 2 seconds. The doctor at the hospital sort of just comes along, does what he has got to do and is off again.'

Explanations

Cognitive coping, especially with new or frightening experiences, often hinges on the provision of comprehensive and understandable information.

'Oh no, no, they don't tell you anything. No they don't tell you why they are doing anything; they just do it.'

Moss, *et al.* (1987) studied 96 primigravidae women. The prospect of the birth for these women was a major worry during their pregnancy and many had negative expectations. On the whole, these proved justified, and bad memories of the experience predominated. Most dissatisfaction with the hospital stay centred around inadequate help, particularly with breastfeeding. This is in sharp contrast to the rationale put forward for the move to hospital deliveries where 'expert help can be on hand'. Greater dissatisfaction was particularly noted by middle class women – whose expectations were perhaps higher – and by women who experienced caesarean sections. This again is interesting given that much intervention and screening is introduced 'in case' of problems. Yet when birth is medicalized, the promised care is not delivered to the extent that it is expected.

One of the most insightful studies published to date on information giving during labour is a poignant account by Kirkham (1989). The study ought to be read in full. In summary, this insider research reports on the informational experiences from 113 observed labours (representing 90 consultant unit deliveries, 5 home confinements and 18 general practitioner unit deliveries). Observations were supplemented by interviews at 36 week gestation and post partum, as well as brief interviews with attendant midwives. This sensitive study reports great efforts to maintain academic neutrality and 'observer' status while balancing the demands of humanity and the situation. The findings form the basis for a number of themes. It is unclear whether these themes represent the total experience, or whether more sophisticated categorization and analysis would be useful. The themes which are tentatively expounded include:

Initiation
Women were reported as being initiated into subservient patient roles very effectively. There was a specific role of the admission interview which conveyed the rules to women with great efficiency. Controlling styles were reported with the effect of adjusting replies and interaction from the women.

Need to please
Kirkham reports on the intense need to please observed in the women. Such behaviour is typified by the adoption of polite, subservient behaviour, self denigration, passivity and silence.

Information needs
Kirkham noted that the women had an ardent need for information, which contrasted vividly with the inconsistent practices of information imparting. She noted a class difference in information seeking. Women of lower social class were less likely to be given information and were classified as disruptive when they sought it out.

Equilibrium
Kirkham describes with great subtlety the notion of the order of the ward and how any threatening behaviour or information demands may destabilize this order. She also describes how many of the interactions are constructed to maintain rather than destabilize this order.

Hierarchy effects
Senior staff had a direct inhibiting effect on the passage of information from junior staff. The power permeated in the presence and absence of such senior staff to the point where junior midwives, often on the front line, chose the path of least resistance, desisting from providing any information at all, with the philosophy of 'say nothing to be safe'.

Blocking styles

A number of examples are expounded in the study where pleas for information and dialogue are effectively blocked by tactics of deflection, ignoring the requests, short sharp conclusions to opening attempts at communication by women and the creation of multiple barriers. Kirkham suggests an explanation for this phenomenon may be a method of avoiding interaction, evading any reference to emotions or circumventing any deeper issues.

Reassurance

There are a number of examples of how reassurance opportunities are missed or dealt with in non optimum ways. Essentially, the study shows that midwives deflect pleas for reassurance or deny the emotional experience, rather than become drawn in to the provision of true reassurance. The process was compounded by midwives using patter, meaningless phrases, descriptive monologue or overspeaking.

In conclusion, Kirkham noted the subtle use of language and the strong influence of the medical dialogue. This study certainly raises some fundamental questions. Although the methodology could be tightened up and little theorizing is presented to account for these interactive patterns, it is one of the few applied studies which gives in depth views on current information transfer within the labour ward.

Place of birth

Place of birth raises many questions nowadays. Skibsted & Lange (1992) examined the need for pain relief in uncomplicated deliveries in an 'alternative birth centre' and compared these findings with those gathered at an obstetric delivery ward in Denmark. The alternative birth centre provided a low technology home-like environment. They studied 295 women and found that the use of pethidine for pain relief (predominantly administered to young subjects and first time mothers) was four times greater on the obstetrical ward than the alternative centre. They concluded that the attitude and behaviour of staff had a significant impact on analgesia administration.

Fleming, *et al.* (1988) compared home and hospital delivered mothers and noted the former had higher birth satisfaction, higher feelings of control and greater amount of immediate contact with the baby. Although home and hospital births may reflect a self selection bias initially this study goes on to describe the role of expectations. When subjects had negative feelings towards interventions prior to birth and then experienced these their satisfaction was reduced. Furthermore, these workers found a relation between birthing variables and affectionate behaviours towards the baby at three months follow up.

Position

Position during labour has been extensively studied. Mobile women report less pain, have more effective contractions and use correspondingly less analgesia, with consequently favourable ramifications on the baby. Melzack, *et al.* (1991) studied the effect of maternal position on pain comparing those vertical (sitting or standing) with those horizontal (side lying or supine). They found that a quarter of the subjects felt less front pain and half the subjects felt less back pain when vertical compared to horizontal.

Anticipation

Women can anticipate labour with eagerness or dread (and many emotions inbetween). Some women oscillate between emotions. Preparation for labour plays an important part in the months leading up to childbirth. There are a variety of studied comparing outcome (post birth) between prepared, non prepared or differentially prepared women (see Enkin, *et al.* 1989 for a comprehensive review). However, the entire area is confounded by the non random selection to treatment groups, the ethical problems which would be associated with so doing, and the fact that outcomes always relate to labour delivery and post partum with few investigations of how preparation helps the actual progress of pregnancy.

In general it has been found that prepared women tend to differ from unprepared women in the amount of analgesia they request or are give n and the myriad of allied factors. It is unclear whether it is the preparation that reduces pain in teaching them alternative or even stoic coping. On the other hand, those who choose to seek out a labour with reduced analgesia may be disproportionately represented among preparation class attenders.

Few studies give detailed content accounts of the courses yet alone provide appraisal by the attenders. Antenatal classes are invariably treated as a standard intervention variable, despite the fact that they can vary enormously and hence have differential impact depending on content, bias of the leaders, efficacy of the teachers, rapport, attendance, and motivation.

Care during labour

'And I said don't leave me, don't leave me'.

Care during labour has been the focus of much attention. Studies examining levels of support in labour (Kennell, *et al.*, 1991) give some insight.

Of greatest interest in this study is the description of 'usual care', which reads:

'Patients were confined to bed as soon as possible after admission to allow for electronic fetal monitoring. When admission blood work was completed, an intravenous infusion was started for each patient. Artificial rupture of membranes was done routinely after 5 cm of cervical dilatation so that internal monitoring could be obtained if needed. For the management of pain ... was utilized at the patient's request, or if, in the judgement of nursing and or medical staff, the patient was unable to deal with her pain as evidenced by vocalization restlessness or lack of cooperation between contractions.'

This report (in 1991) gives a clearer indication than any birth care books, of a 'modern' birth. Studies have examined a wide range of issues of care, including who is present, the management of pain, emotional support of the labouring woman, environment and background factors, continuity of care, doctor versus midwife care and home versus hospital care (Garcia & Garforth, 1990; Enkin, 1982).

Inductions

The induction of labour can be carried out for medical, social or pragmatic reasons. Cartwright (1979) recorded the experiences of women undergoing inductions. Preparation was low, retrospective and dissatisfaction was often noted. Advantages for the women were concentrated around the ending of tiresome waiting and the certainty of timing which facilitated planning. Disadvantages of inductions were related to the increased incidence of analgesia usage, physical constraints resulting from the paraphanalia to carry out the induction (including drips and tubes) and comments about the increased level of assisted delivery associated with inductions. These factors in turn had ramifications. Riley (1976) reported greater pain levels in just under a half of the subjects in induced births.

Accurate studies of induction are problematic, given that they may draw conclusions which result from the original reason for the induction, rather than those which result directly from the procedure. A sophisticated study was carried out by Chalmers, *et al.* (1976) to study induction systematically which found no advantages and several disadvantages of routine induction. Very often examinations used in the preparation for inductions exclude the women totally. For example, Enkin, *et al.* (1989) present a chapter called 'Preparing for induction of labour' and concentrate on preparing the cervix with no mention of preparing the women to whom the cervix belongs. When examining the effects, the same authors do include a section on the effects on the mother, but this is directly associated with medical indices (such as pyrexia, uterine hyperstimulation, retained placenta and post partum haemorrhage) rather than emotional or psychological ones.

Out, *et al.* (1986) compared women who chose elective inductive or spontaneous onset of labour and scrutinized their underlying motives. Of a group of 237 women, almost half opted for elective induction. These women had usually more complaints during pregnancy and menstrual periods, more complicated obstetric histories and displayed greater levels of anxiety about their forthcoming labour. The motives for induction were generally those which engendered feelings of safety and a desire to shorten the duration of pregnancy. The authors discuss this in the light of trust in physical reproductive functions.

Recognition of the onset of labour

It is safe to assume that recognition of the onset of labour is always best assumed in retrospect! Many women report a wide range of experiences which trigger the onset of labour. There is a wide variation in experience as evidenced by the 10 women studied in depth by Sherr (1989). They reported:

(1) 'I said I am going in, I don't feel right. You must excuse me if they send me home again if it is a false alarm.'
(2) 'I started getting pains and the doctor came and said they were just testing contraction and it was the effect of the drip wearing off. I was having these awful pains, but they told me that it was just the drip wearing off. They told me I wasn't in labour, and you believe them.' [baby delivered 3 hours later].
(3) 'I just did not realize. So I walked up to the nurse – I must have sounded really stupid – I said to her "Do you think I could have some aspirin" – she said "Yes, I will bring you some in a minute". I said I am a bit wet, I said [membranes rupturing]. I must have been in quite a daze.'
(4) 'We came downstairs and then they seemed to stop, and I said "Alright, perhaps I will go back to sleep." You know I just kept thinking that nothing was going to happen.'
(5) 'I knew it could not be labour because they didn't say that was how it started.'
(6) 'I got this awful period pain right in the bottom of my stomach and I didn't know what it was'.
(7) 'I was very uncomfortable but no pains or anything. And my husband was saying "Have you started?" and I don't know whether I had started or not. I mean, I had never had a baby before'.
(8) 'I had what were very mild contractions for quite a few hours which weren't as bad as I thought they would be so I didn't realise they were actually labour pains'.

(9) 'I think the pains were quite bad and there was never anything like you learned in the NCT, where you had first stage and second stage. There wasn't. Like you should go into slow labour and it builds up. Well it wasn't there.'

(10) 'So luckily on the Friday night I started – I take it, because I didn't really know. They said to time your contractions when they came regularly but they did not seem to.'

Episiotomies

Episiotomy, a peculiarly western procedure, is carried out on varying numbers of women. The chances of having an episiotomy seem to be related more to place of birth than any labour related factors. In 1958, one fifth of first time mothers were given an episiotomy. By 1978 this figure was closer to 91 per cent. Oakley & Richards (1990) recorded an episiotomy rate of 98 per cent in their sample. Episiotomy rates may increase if staff are inexperienced or if protocols demand. Although the medical advantages are often emphasized, the psychological disadvantages should also enter the equation.

Painful stitches and painful tears are the cause of much maternal suffering, which is often experienced silently, shrouded by embarrassment. If the pain is excruciating, it can mar the first days or weeks of the mother's experience of and input into the baby's life. There are no studies comparing the pain levels and discomfort comparing a natural tear during childbirth with an episiotomy, despite the fact that one of the oddly logical reasons given for episiotomy is to 'avoid tearing'. The longer term ramifications are also of major concern. Reading (1982) reported that pain as a result of episiotomy in recently delivered mothers was not only high, but lasted for extensively long periods of time, with over one in ten women still reporting pain three months after suturing.

Episiotomy difficulties have been graphically described by Kitzinger (1983) and Reading (1982), with results including prolonged healing, impaired or impossible sexual functioning and problems with breastfeeding due to the inability to sit down. The DHSS committee examining breastfeeding in 1978 noted that three quarters of mothers who breastfed had stitches; one fifth of these reported that the sutures interfered with feeding. When they examined differences in mothers with painful stitches, they found that 22 per cent gave up breastfeeding compared to 16 per cent of women who had non painful stitches.

The hazards of episiotomy may not only be limited to the labouring woman. In a recent study comparing HIV prevalence in midwives in a sample of hospital midwives and home birth attendants in Africa, HIV transmission to midwives was more prevalent for midwives who performed episiotomy than those who did not.

Caesarean section

The entire range of antenatal procedures are mounted 'in case something goes wrong'. Despite the fact that most births are normal, there is a small percentage that does not follow this course and caesarean deliveries may result. As a result, millions of women are now subjected to countless procedures to seek out and identify the very few who need specialized input. How does the health care system care for women when they are indeed identified?

The initial point of note is that there is very little literature on the experience, very few comprehensive protocols that balance the need for medical intervention and care with the psychological needs of childbirth and few long-term follow up studies. Those that have been done very often are cataloguing the obvious and it is surprising that such few strides have been made to accommodate the physical and psychological needs of women experiencing caesarean sections. These women, simultaneously experience all the similar effects of major abdominal surgery and those of any mother recently delivered of a new born baby and are in need of both nursing and midwifery care, as well as medical and emotional support.

Caesarean rates have recently shown a dramatic increase. In the USA it accounted for 4.5 per 100 births in 1965 and had reached 24.1 per 100 by 1986 (Localio, *et al.*, 1993). In Canada and the UK, similar increases have been noted, but not at such high levels. Of particular note is the finding that rates can vary for different institutions. This may reflect the particular populations (and their problems) who attend such institutions, the institutional approach or policy, or a complex interaction of both factors. Localio, *et al.* (1993) studied 60 490 deliveries over 31 hospitals and found a positive association between malpractice claims risk and the rate of caesarean delivery.

The psychological ramifications of caesarean sections have yet to be fully understood. Oakley & Richards (1990) point out that the very name 'section' as opposed to 'surgery' or 'operation' reflects some of the difficulties surrounding the procedure and the psychological adjustment and reaction to it. They note that after a caesarean section 'the kinds of demands that looking after a new born baby are likely to make involve activities that are probably forbidden to any patient on a surgical ward for some days (if not weeks) after abdominal surgery'.

Caesarean sections can be planned or unplanned. They can occur after an arduous labour or prior to the onset of labour. They are always (in theory anyway) associated with an obstetric concern. Any studies which examine subsequent child development in the presence of a caesarean delivery must consider the confounding effects of the procedure with the effects of the reasons which instigated the procedure in the first place. Furthermore, such medical problems may require other interventions (for example, admission to a special care baby unit) and this may ultimately interfere or interact with child development. The psychological effects and the ability to adjust and cope to these may vary according to the nature of the section (planned or unplanned) and the procedures used (general or epidural anaesthesia) (Lipson & Tilden, 1980).

Padawer, *et al.* (1988) compared the psychological adjustment and experience of women experiencing an emergency caesarean section compared to those delivering vaginally. They found that women delivered by caesarean section were significantly less satisfied with the experience, yet no differences were found in psychological adjustment. Hillan (1989) reported that 48 per cent welcomed the section, seeing it as the end of a traumatic labour. Over a quarter of the women expressed terror and fear, for the procedure, their own life and their baby. Despite antenatal attendance, few were prepared for the procedure. Most antenatal coverage had been to reassure them of the low likelihood of caesarean sections rather than informing them of the realities associated with the procedure.

Post partum support seems unable to match the needs of women after caesarean section. Nearly all the subjects examined in Hillan (1989) reported intense pain of long duration. Nearly a third of the women commented specifically on the lack of understanding, sympathy, input and care from staff on the post natal wards, who seemed unaware of their discomfort (and even failed to note this within hospital records).

One of the major problems related to caesarean sections is the link with subsequent pregnancy difficulties (Hemminki, 1987) and the consequent high rate of repeat sections. Subsequent deliveries after a caesarean section were studied by McClain (1987). One hundred subjects were interviewed in the third trimester of a pregnancy following a previous caesarean section and again after delivery. Some mothers (Hillan, 1989) find the thought of a repeat section a disincentive for a further pregnancy.

Trowell (1982) compared a group of primiparous women undergoing unplanned sections with another experiencing vaginal deliveries. She found that caesarean mothers differed in their interaction with their new born babies one month after the birth (looking more but smiling less), showed heightened negative recall of their labour experience, expressed greater levels of self doubt at parenting and were more likely to express negative moods. Some of these effects were still present one year post partum. Trowell also noted variation in the behaviours of the babies. Yet her sample was very small (16 in each group) and it is unclear whether the caesarean section itself can be seen as causative. However such a study does mark the way forward and highlights the extreme vigilance that is needed for mothers undergoing caesarean sections where particular attention should be paid to care, support and ongoing assistance.

Kendell (1981) report an association between caesarean delivery and admission to a psychiatric hospital in the first three post partum months.

Once again, many of the studies tend to concentrate on the negative impact of a procedure rather than use the research to highlight the perceived benefits or ways of minimizing harmful effects. In general the major physical and psychological effects, when they are noted, are often concentrated in the few days after delivery. Some studies fail to record systematic differences, whereas others note effects which include difficulty in breast feeding (Lipson & Tilden, 1980), reduction in self esteem (Cox & Smith 1982; Marut & Mercer, 1979), and a delay in baby naming (Marut & Mercer, 1979). There does seem to be cultural variation and some studies (Bradley, *et al.*, 1983) do not find these difficulties (if indeed they are difficulties). Many of these findings may be directly related to the pain levels, pain medication, wound effects, sutures and mobilization restrictions. This renders comparisons difficult with vaginally delivered women as the two types of birth are truly not comparable. Some of the findings can be similarly explained. For example, a woman who is less mobile as a result of her section may rely more on staff to handle her baby. This may increase her exposure to conflicting opinions, poor communications or censure and it may be these factors that adjust self esteem. On a practical level, many of the psychological consequences are linked up with post surgical demands made on a mother and with the emotional reactions to the surgery. Hillan (1989) reported that women with caesarean sections reported fewer sexual difficulties post partum and were able to resume sexual activity earlier than those vaginally delivered with painful perineum.

Ameliorating factors for negative effects of caesarean sections include:

- Paternal presence (Shearer, *et al.*, 1988; Cain, 1984).
- Use of epidural anaesthesia rather than general anaesthesia (Shearer, *et al.*, 1988).
- Availability of paternity leave (Hwang, 1987).

Post partum care

This century has seen marked changes in the nature and duration of post partum hospital care. Childbirth usually used to be accompanied by extensive stays in hospital (sometimes up to two or three weeks). Changing time, ethos, economics and appraisal has adjusted the average length of stay and the practices during the stay. Short stays are fairly common in the UK now. In addition to duration of stay, there are the important aspects of what happens during the stay, irrespective of duration.

Porter & MacIntyre (1989) question the whole content of post natal hospitalization. They examine the promises given to women (in terms of education and rest) in the light of the realities available. They conclude that there is little opportunity for quality dialogue, rest is rarely available (endorsed by Ball, 1989) and hazards include conflicting advice and contradictory information. When these workers examined antenatal and post natal women they observed that post natal women were the least likely to ask any questions (which is surprising, giving the removal of time restraints) with only 28 per cent of their sample observed asking any questions at all after delivery and the majority at the six week check up after discharge. Furthermore, the specific problems (tiredness, feeding and availability of childcare) that women experienced were rarely responded to. Embarrassing or sensitive topics (such as contraception) were handled in an unsatisfactory manner – often in public.

Feeding

Society as a whole is focused on how babies should be fed. Motivations for this concern can be well meaning, but can also be intrusive. Among the clamour, few listen to the voices of the women themselves. Breast-feeding is in vogue at the moment and is encouraged. Bottle feeding promotions in developing countries have backfired as the lack of sterile conditions may cause more problems than the nutritional aspects of formula solve. Indeed, sometimes mothers have been advised to drink the formula and then breastfeed their babies. Sherr (1989) found that women who desired to bottle feed were shunned and reported difficulties in gaining advice.

Women are often given conflicting advice on breastfeeding (which can be on demand or scheduled), such as advice to demand feed their babies four hourly! Social class also plays a role in breastfeeding (Cartwright, 1979) as well as the helpfulness of nurses. Cartwright (1979) noted that 75 per cent of mothers were not allowed to feed their babies when they wanted to do so, but had to adhere to hospital schedules, which were probably constructed for the convenience of staff rather than mothers (Fisher, 1985). Moss, *et al.* (1987) found that a major source of dissatisfaction with their hospital stay was inadequate help with breast-feeding.

Breastfeeding was studied by Jones (1986) where 1525 consecutive subjects were interviewed after delivery and 649 breastfeeding mothers followed up 12 months later. More than half were first time mothers. Attitudes were influenced by the number (or lack) of children they had had, problems encountered while establishing breastfeeding, and embarrassment.

Thomson (1989) studied factors associated with bottle feeding and breastfeeding. This study examined a number of factors which contributed to feeding decisions. These include:

- Culture.
- Emotional embarrassment.
- Sexual factors.
- Role models.
- The role of advice in feeding decisions.
- Convenience.

- Socio-economic status.
- Personal and normative attitudes.

In a small empirical study, it was noted that women come to feeding decisions very early in their pregnancy. Feeding decisions are invariably discussed, often with husbands, who can be fairly influential in the outcome. Intention to breastfeed did not necessarily result in trouble free feeding, with a sub group of women abandoning breastfeeding after initial attempts. Such cessation was examined in relation to professional support (or the lack of it), with clear implications for the potential role of helpful carers in this aspect of child care and maternal health. Help with breastfeeding is variable. Porter & McIntyre (1989) noted that little help was given to women at the six week post partum check. In addition, fathers of bottle fed babies become involved with feeding much earlier on and extend their contribution to preparation of feeds (Lewis, 1986).

Moss, *et al.* (1987) note that a large proportion of their subjects had experienced emotional upheaval or practical difficulties when first feeding their baby. Other women report physical discomfort and pain associated with nipple tenderness (Drewett, *et al.*, 1987), episiotomy pain (Reading, 1982), or exhaustion (Niven, 1992). There is some evidence that women may abandon breastfeeding because their partners are embarrassed or troubled by the practice (Thomson, 1989).

Niven (1992) discusses infant gender differences in feeding patterns and explanations given by mothers. Few workers examine the wider and longer term social context and restraints which may hinder breastfeeding. Freed (1993) notes that, with regard to breastfeeding, there is a considerable gap between what the profession teaches and what it preaches. This interesting study shows a shortfall in professional training on breastfeeding, with many obstetricians and paediatricians limited in knowledge, desirous of more information, or indeed actively recommending against breastfeeding. Even when women are encouraged to breastfeed and succeed, there are still societal barriers (*The Times*, 1993). A study by the Royal College of Midwives showed that some restaurants would not allow women to breastfeed their babies on the premises. Women report that they were instructed to 'retire to the lavatory, the office or the street' to feed their baby. This study noted much opposition from men to feeding, with over half of the sample of men opposed to women breastfeeding in public.

Maternal and paternal nutrition post partum

There is so much focus on feeding the baby that many forget the mother who may also require feeding! Women, who do not eat during labour and may well labour for hours on end, rarely receive a wholesome meal until they return home (Niven, 1992; Currer, 1986). This is almost an intolerable situation given the nutritional demands made on the mother by her new baby. Food plays a key role in factors other than nutrition. It is a ritualized and social activity which is often ignored in hospitals. It is almost unheard of for food to be provided for fathers who accompany women during the long hours of labour. Hot drinks or refreshments are rarely offered to partners or visitors, despite their social function, their low cost and the enormous token of 'emotional' caring it could display.

Pain other than labour

There is so much focus on pain during birth that few writers bother to examine pain after birth, yet alone address themselves to amelioration of such pain. There are many pains that women report, including post episiotomy pain (Kitzinger, 1987; Reading, 1982), after pains, nipple pain, piles, sutures, and, least discussed, emotional pain. One woman described the pain of hearing her infant crying while blood was taken for bilirubin counting as being 'worse than myriad contractions'. When birth has been traumatic, with forceps or caesarean section there are enormous levels of pain, made worse by the demanding schedule of a tiny infant.

Some women report that labour pain blurs the thinking of staff about any other or subsequent pain and analgesia is often simply not contemplated, despite the fact that it would be routine in other settings. Some women report that they are sutured after tearing or episiotomies without pain relief. Some report annoyance and exasperation from the staff doing the suturing as 'I was not able to keep still'. Some women report intense pain from the administration of drips, made worse by restricting bindings. Some women find artificial rupturing of membranes extremely painful. Even internal examinations in the presence of contractions can be excruciating. This is rarely mentioned, studied or even discussed.

Hospital care

'And then the midwife came and the first thing she did was took all my clothes off and put them in a plastic bag. And I thought this was an incredible cheek.'

The usual place of birth for most women (in the west) is hospital. Home deliveries are currently increasing and in some countries (such as The Netherlands) there has always been a consistent level of home deliveries. The pros and cons of such hospital deliveries and the various options available (such as general practitioner units, short stay, own midwife care) vary from centre to centre. From the psychological point of view, simply being in hospital creates a set of environmental factors which impact on the experience. A hospital is a strange social environment into which a women will enter at a time when she is least able to exert control, adjust, and accommodate change.

Rules

'You were woken up just when you felt like going to sleep'.

'Oh, I must have been changing him on the bed and I got yelled at'.

Being in hospital brings with it many rule factors which are either explicit (such as visiting hours, when to eat meals, who may be present with the woman during her labour) or implicit (such as rules about where to change the baby, who is in charge, what is permissible). The latter are rarely made explicit.

Conducive environments

'But it was a bit military. I did feel when I came out that I had been released from an army camp.'

There needs to be some analysis of the modern environment into which women, at the very moment of childbirth, are hurtled. Although the theory talks about provision of rest and care, helping and teaching new mothers, establishing breastfeeding and loving environments, the reality may be very far removed. Women find themselves in dormitory type accommodation with strange women as their roommates, attended by overworked midwives, many of whom they have never met before. There are often rules limiting their contact with people they love and need. Very little patient education is carried out on the wards and there is a high possibility of problems such as cross infection, poor quality food, a lack of privacy, being woken by other people's babies and staff noise.

Continuity of care

'You never saw the same doctor twice, and they never told you who they were and they didn't say "Hello, I am doctor ..." you just sort of thought this was the doctor. It could have been anybody really, it could have been the porter.'

One of the major consumer criticisms has been aimed at continuity of care, or the lack thereof. This has specific implications for building up therapeutic relationships, trust and familiarity. It also means that any inter-personal dialogue has to be established at every interview. As a result, care may rely on standard routines rather than one which is an understanding of an individual's needs.

Conflicting advice

One problem associated with the team approach, the hospital environment, and the division between experts and patients is the conflicting advice given to women at all levels. Women may well hold the belief that there is certainty among the professions, there is truth and there is pure knowledge. All science, however, is much more murky than this, and for every method there are many pathways.

Even the most compliant, willing woman can flounder when given conflicting advice. Conflicting advice leaves a woman unable to decide who to follow and also threatens her confidence that the system has anything to offer at all. Indeed, conflicting advice can sometimes be the first betrayal of the system to the woman. It is also very common that the most rigid advice comes from the most inexperienced professionals and flexible, adaptable advice comes from experienced practitioners. The mere provision of advice may conflict with her own views, which may be rarely explored, sought or endorsed.

In reality, women make arbitrary decisions about who to believe. They either believe the most senior person (who must know), the most junior person (who is approachable and perhaps liked), the most affable person (because that makes intuitive sense and they can identify with them), or simply the last person who spoke to them (or indeed, the first person who spoke to them). It is a brave woman who can believe in herself amongst all this.

At best the system which creates such problems can be seen as inconsistent. At worst it results in behaviours such as the abandonment of breastfeeding (Thomson, 1989), lowered mood or exasperation.

Fathers

Paternal involvement in labour and childbirth is not new. What is new is the recent attention being paid to fathers, with the evolving understanding of their role, contributions and needs and a corresponding observation of the care, treatment and handling which they receive (Barbour, 1990).

Literature on fathers in relation to childbirth encompasses their role in the relationship, in conception, during pregnancy, in the labour ward and post partum. Early writings on fathers presented a gender stereotyped father as one who provided for and sheltered the mother as she began the business of mothering (Winnicott, 1964). Fathers were often viewed as superfluous, out of focus or simply not viewed at all. For example,

Bowlby (1969) considered the relationship to be between the mother and child and consequently paid scant attention to paternal relationships, despite much anecdotal (and empirical) evidence of long lasting, fruitful or troubled relationships between children and their fathers. However, recent emergence of interest in fathers (Lamb, 1981) has now provided a focus on them as a group.

Phoenix, *et al.* (1991) caution against views which assume inter-changeability between mothers and fathers when role differentiation may still be present, even if it is not desired or desirable. Indeed, they put forward the notion that the 'New man is much more a figment of media imagination' than reality as empirical studies show higher female involvement and responsibility for children is still predominant (Lewis & O'Brien, 1987; Phoenix, *et al.*, 1991; Brannen & Moss, 1990). Indeed, books on child development published as late as the 1970s do not even have an index entry for the term 'fathers' (e.g. Konger, *et al.*, 1974).

Paternal role in an antenatal setting
Many fathers do attend antenatal clinics with their partners, but few are invited (or dare to enter) into the consultation. Barbour noted only 8 per cent doing so, a finding confirmed by Lewis (1986). Such reticence to enter consultations is certainly not as a result of negative treatment or dismissal. Fathers seem to attend ultrasound scans and amniocentesis procedures with greater frequency.

Antenatal classes are essentially geared towards women, with a slow evolving acknowledgement of the rights and needs of men. The National Childbirth Trust has long encouraged male attendance. Some obstacles to male attendance, besides lack of an invitation, include daytime scheduling, lack of childcare (where fathers may stay at home to look after siblings to allow their partner to attend; the provision of childcare would free him to attend as well), a non conducive environment (in which the attendees are mainly women) or simply a lack of relevance or focus on the needs of the couple. This is short sighted, given that many men now attend during labour and delivery and will be also faced with their new born baby.

Labour
Paternal presence during labour and delivery was frowned upon in the west as recently as 30 years ago. In some cultures, it is sometimes taboo for the father or any males to be present, whilst others accommodate or encourage such attendance. In the west there has been a marked shift with a paternal presence of 67 per cent recorded by Garcia (1985), 70 per cent by Cartwright (1979) and 90 per cent by Jacoby (1987). This movement has come about as a result of benefits recorded as a result of paternal presence (Antle May & Perrin, 1985), social or partner pressure (Barbour, 1990), personal decision (Lewis, 1986), consumer demand or societal expectation. Most mothers endorse paternal presence (90 per cent); only 5 per

cent do not want it and 5 per cent are ambivalent (Garcia & Garforth, 1990).

Within the labour ward, paternal presence is usually seen as helpful to the woman. Given this assumption, it is even more surprising that such paternal aids and helpers are not provided with adequate information, forewarning and training. The medical environment, with its high technology and complex equipment, may be alienating (Perkins, 1980) and serve to intimidate or obstruct true involvement. Indeed, this may be by design rather than by accident and certainly make clear the power imbalance between the father and the staff.

Advantages of paternal presence

Father's role
Clearly there are distinct advantages for the father himself, his partner and his baby if he desires to be present and this is respected. It means he can be part of the process, observe, experience and assist in whatever way possible rather than simply imagine or support from a distance.

Facilitator
The father may be a trusted individual who can facilitate procedures and protocols. He will probably know his partner better than the staff and can provide support at moments of trauma.

Communications mediator
Many women note that they see their partner as their 'ambassador' in the labour ward, and consequently acquaint him with their wishes and see him as supporting their needs in negotiating with staff. Staff, on the other hand, may secure his support to persuade or dissuade the woman on a variety of courses of action.

Disadvantages of paternal presence

Inhibiting maternal choice
Now that paternal presence is, for the most part, seen as desirable, Phoenix, *et al.*, (1991) reports that paternal absence is seen as aberrant or deviant by staff, frowned upon and seen as indicative of relationship, coping or cultural problems. Indeed the assumption that the father ought to be present may inhibit real choice for some women, who may prefer another companion such as a female friend, mother or sister.

Public emotional response to what is a very personal event (Barbour, 1990). Yet no one considers the same may be true for the woman.

Intrusion
Both mother and father may be under the microscopical gaze of mid-wives, who may observe (and often judge) the nature of their relationship and its interaction (Barbour, 1990).

Mediator for persuasive communications
A helpless father may play many roles in impeding or facilitating pro-cedures. For example, Sherr (1989) found that paternal presence was a factor predictive of higher pain medication during labour. Possible explanations for this finding may be that a father, watching, helpless, as his partner experiences pain, may be instrumental in persuading her to take medication. The staff may harness his support to persuade the wife. On the other hand, it may simply be that the presence of the father means that the emotional support role is assumed by him and this may interact with the midwife/mother relationship. If a true understanding is not established, there may be a greater tendency for the midwife to use pain medication.

Staff reaction to paternal presence

Barbour (1990) recorded staff as encouraging, yet noted censure if fathers did not attend. They were critical of fathers, especially when they did anything for distraction during the long hours of labour.

Policies vary according to hospitals on whether fathers are allowed to be present during instrumental and caesarean deliveries. The practice has been endorsed by study findings (Cain, 1984; May & Sollid, 1984). The role in such circumstances is usually peripheral with the father being guest/observer but still being able to provide a link for the mother in terms of dialogue, description and mediation.

Paternal involvement
Touching and holding the baby is seen as a crucial step for mothers (Klaus Kennell 1976). Yet Garcia & Garforth (1990) noted that there was often considerable delay for fathers, with 19 per cent touching the baby immediately after delivery, while the remaining 81 per cent waited between one minute and one hour to touch their baby (a mean wait of 9.8 minutes).

Hospitalization post partum is intended to provide 'rest for the mother' and 'train her in parenting skills'. In reality, it may not provide either and may also serve to ensure no rest for the father and deny him any training in such skills (Lewis, 1986).

In some countries such as Sweden, paternity leave is available. In most others, this is not the case. Many fathers plan their annual leave to coin-cide with the arrival of their new baby, but some are unable to do so and are thus restricted in their visiting, access and contribution to the care of their new baby.

Fathers whose babies were born by caesarean section are often recorded as more involved with the baby while their partners recover from surgery (Pedersen, 1981; Hwang, 1987; Oakley & Richards, 1990).

Worries about the well being of self and baby

'My main worry was, was it alright, was it normal'.

'I don't know, it seemed a long time to me, like you know when you are having a car accident; everything is happening slowly. And I looked and said "Is he alright?" And they said "Oh yes", and I looked and thought – he shouldn't be that colour and he is not making any noise.'

'When I was conscious and he said it was a baby girl I was worried then because it wasn't there, I could not see it'.

Kumar & Robson have shown that the majority of women show emotional peaking surrounding concerns for the well being of themselves and the baby.

Discharge

Discharge from hospital is a time when women can look at the care and experience they have had as they contemplate the future with their baby. Some women, especially those with little experience of or exposure to young babies, find these tasks challenging, awesome, overwhelming or pleasurable. It is rarely a single emotion but usually a catalogue of experiences which fluctuates with time and the presence or absence of crises.

Comments about overall appraisal of the experiences are mixed (Sherr, 1989) and include:

1. 'I have thoroughly enjoyed my whole pregnancy, labour and being a mother. Totally – I would recommend it.'
2. 'I think it was alright, but in the long run I have got a lot to grumble about.'
3 'What with that and everything else it just seemed awful, and I got very depressed.'
4 'So it was the stitches, the feeding and the jaundice. Everything else was fine.'

The impressions of women using maternity services

There have been a number of studies set up to examine the views of the users. There are sampling and methodological problems with data gathering, which may affect outcome and results (see Jacoby & Cart-wright, 1990). Recruitment may be non random: those with more to grumble about may be disproportionately represented in studies.; may include more middle class than working class women; refusal may exclude a silent group. There are some who argue that the vociferous are the spokeswomen of the silent.

Yet all these studies do seem to emerge with comparable themes. Generally, there is a need to set up investigations to monitor maternal responses to a variety of obstetric procedures. In the past, this was usually in reaction to the procedure. Good practice would allow for early evaluation. Ideally, consumer views should feed the process rather than battle against it. The major problems focus on the provision of information, advice, continuity of care and personalized treatment.

Implications for practice

A pendulum of focus can be clearly traced. In the early days when the overriding issue of mortality and morbidity demanded most attention, there was little focus on the emotional wellbeing of the mother, let alone her wider family. Now, with dramatic improvements to the medical wellbeing of the mother and baby, the focus has moved to the psychological experience.

This chapter has given a global overview of many aspects of labour and delivery. These need to be addressed, understood and incorporated into care packages. No practice should escape regular scrutiny. Routines that seemed vital at one time may outdate quickly. There is a usual pattern to new regimes. Often they are originally spurned, then grasped with gusto and implemented irrationally. After trial and error, they tend to settle down to a more adaptive pattern. Yet during this adjustment phase there are many casualties. They tend to be the women.

References

Antle May, K. & Perrin, S. (1985) Prelude, pregnancy and birth. In *Dimensions of Fatherhood* (Ed. S. Hanson & F. Bozett), Sage, California.

Ball, J.A. (1989) Postnatal care and adjustment to motherhood. In *Midwives Research and Childbirth* (Ed. S. Robinson & A. Thompson). Chapman and Hall, London.

Barbour, R. (1990) Fathers: the emergence of a new consumer group. In *The Politics of Maternity Care*. (Ed. J. Garcia, R. Kilpatrick & M.P.M. Richards), Oxford University Press, Oxford.

Bowlby, J. (1969) *Attachment and Loss – Vol 1 Attachment* London Hogarth Press, London.

Bradley, C., Ross, S. & Warnyca, J. (1983) A prospective study of mothers' attitudes and feelings following caesarean and vaginal births. *Birth*, 10, 79–83.

Brannen, J. & Moss, P. (1990) *Managing Mothers: Dual Earner Households after Maternity Leave*. Unwin Hyman, London.

Brewin, C. & Bradley, C. (1982) Perceived control and the experience of Childbirth. *British Jnl of Clinical Psychology*, 21, 263–9.

Byrne, J.S. & Long, B.E. (1976) *Doctors Talking to Patients*. HMSO, London.

Cain, R. (1984) Effects of the father's presence or absence during a caesarean delivery. *Birth*, 11, 10–15.

Cartwright, A. (1979) *The Dignity of Labour*, Tavistock Publications, London.

Chalmers, I. (1982) Pregnancy. In *Effectiveness and Satisfaction in Antenatal Care*, (Ed. M. Enkin & I. Chalmers). William Heinemann Medical Books, London.

Chalmers, I. & Richards, M. (1977) Intervention and causal inference in obstetric practice. In *Benefits and Hazards of the New Obstetrics* (Ed. T. Chard & M. Richards). Spastics International Medical Publications, London and Philadelphia.

Chalmers, I., Zlosnik, J.E., Johns, K.A. & Campbell, H.L. (1976) Obstetric practice and outcome of pregnancy in Cardiff residents 1965–73. *BMJ* 1, 735–8.

Chalmers, I., Enkin, M. & Keirse, M.J. (1989) *Effective Care in Pregnancy and Childbirth*. Oxford University Press, Oxford.

Chamberlain, G., Howlett, B. & Claireaux, C. (1975) *British Births* 1970. Vol 2, Obstetric Care. Heinemann Medical Books, London.

Chard, T. & Richards, M. (1977) (Eds) *Benefits and Hazards of the New Obstetrics*. Spastics International Medical Publications, London and Philadelphia.

Cogan, R. & Spinnato, J. (1988) Social support during premature labor effects on labour and the newborn. *Jnl. of Psychosomatic Obstet. and Gynec.*, 8,(3) 209–16.

Copstick, S., Taylor, K., Hayles, R. & Morris, N. (1986a) Partner support and the use of coping techniques in Labor. *Jnl. of Psychosomatic Rsrch.* 30,(4) 497–503.

Copstick, S., Taylor, K., Hayes, R. & Morris, N. (1986b) The relation of time of day to childbirth. *Journal of Reproductive and Infant Psychology*, 4,(1–2) 13–22.

Corli, O., Grossi, E., Roma, G. & Battagliarin, G. (1986) Correlation between subjective labour pain and uterine contractions. A clinical study. *Pain*, 26,(1) 53–60.

Cox, B. & Smith, E. (1982) The mother's self esteem after a casesarean delivery. *Maternal Child Nursing*, 7, 309–14.

Currer, C. (1986) Health concepts and illness behaviour: the care of Pathan mothers in Britain. Unpublished PhD Thesis, University of Warwick.

Drew, N., Salmon, P. & Webb, L. (1989) Mothers, midwives and obstetricians views on the features of obstetric care which influence satisfaction with childbirth. *Brit. Journal of Obstetrics and Gynaecology*, 96, 1084–88.

Drewett, R., Kahn, H., Parkhurst, S. & Whiltey, S. (1987) Pain during breastfeeding: the first three months post partum. *Journal of Reproductive and Infant Psychology*, 5, 183–7.

Dubignon, T., Campbell, D., Curtis, M. & Partlington, M.W. (1969) The relation between laboratory measures of sucking food intake and perinatal factors during the newborn period. *Child Development*, 40, 1107–20.

Duchene, P. (1989) Effects of biofeedback on childbirth pain. *Jnl. of Pain and Symptom Management*, 4,(3) 117–23.

Enkin, M. (1982) Effectiveness of Ante natal preparation. In *Effectiveness and Satisfaction in Antenatal Care* (Ed. M. Enkin & I. Chalmers) William Heinemann Medical Books, London.

Enkin, M., Keirse, M. & Chalmers, I. (1989) *A Guide to Effective Care in Pregnancy and Childbirth*, Oxford University Press, Oxford.

Fisher, C. (1981) Community Midwife – the gentle approach. *Nursing Focus*, **3**,(4) 562.

Fisher, M.C. (1985) How did we go wrong with breast feeding? *Midwifery*, **1**,(1) 48–51.

Fleming, A., Ruble, D., Anderson, V. & Flett, G. (1988) Place of childbirth: influences feelings of satisfaction and control in first time mothers. *Jnl. of Psychomatic Obstet. and Gynec.*, **8**,(1) 1–17.

Freed, G. (1993) Breast feeding. Time to teach what we preach. *JAMA*, **29**,(2) 243–5.

Fridh, G., Kpare, T. & Gaston Johansson, F. (1988) Factors associated with more intense labor pain. *Research in Nursing and Health*, **11**,(2) 117–24.

Garcia, J. (1985) Mothers' views of continuous electronic fetal heart monitoring and intermittent ausculation in a randomized controlled trial. *Birth*, 12, 79–85.

Garcia, J. & Garforth, S. (1990) Parents and new born babies in the labour ward. In *The Politics of Maternity Care* (Ed. J. Garcia, R. Kilpatrick and E. Richards), Clarendon Paperbacks, Oxford.

Garcia, J., Kilpatrick, R. & Richards, M. (1990) *The Politics of Maternity Care*. Clarendon Paperbacks, Oxford.

Gillot de Vries, F., Wessel, S., Busine, A. & Adler, A. (1987) Influence of a bath during labor on the experience of maternity. *Pre and Perinatal Psychology Jnl.*, **1**,(4) 297–302.

Harkness, J. & Gijsberg, K. (1989) Pain and stress during childbirth and time of day. *Ethology and Sociobiology*, **10**,(4) 255–61.

Hemminki, E. (1987) Pregnancy and Birth after Caesarean Section. A survey based on the Swedish Birth Register *Birth* 14, 12–17.

Hillan, E. (1989) Caesarean section: indications and outcomes. PhD Thesis, University of Glasgow.

Hodnett, E. & Osborn, R. (1989) Effects of continuous intrapartum professional support on childbirth outcomes. *Rsrch. in Nursing and Health*, **12**,(5) 289–97.

Hwang, C. (1987) Caesarean childbirth in Sweden. Effects on the mother and father infant relationship. *Infant Mental Health Journal*, 8, 91–99.

Jacoby, A. (1987) Womens preferences for and satisfaction with current procedures in childbirth. Findings from a National study. *Midwifery*, 3, 117–24.

Jacoby, A. & Cartwright, A. (1990) Finding out about the views and experiences of maternity service users. In *The Politics of Maternity Care* (Ed. J. Garcia, R. Kirkpatrick & M. Richards) Clarendon Paperbacks, Oxford.

Johnston, M. (1982) Recognition of patients worries by nurses and by other patients. *British Journal of Clinical Psychology*, 21, 255–61.

Jones, D. (1986) Attitudes of breast feeding mothers. A survey of 649 mothers. *Social Science and Medicine*, **23**,(11) 1151–6.

Kendell, R. (1981) The social and obstetric correlates of psychiatric admission in the puerperium. *Psychological Medicine*, 11, 341–50.

Kennell, J., Klaus, M., McGrath, S., Robertson, S. & Kinkley, C. (1991) Continuous emotional support during labor in a US Hospital. *JAMA*, **265**,(17) 2197–201.

Kirke, P. (1980) Mothers' views of obstetric care. *Br. J. Obstet Gynaecol.*, 87, 1029–33.

Kirkham, M. (1989) Midwives and information giving during labour. In *Midwives, Research and Childbirth* (Ed. S. Robinson & A. Thomson), Vol 1 Chapman and Hall, London.

Kitzinger, S. (1983) *The New Good Birth Guide*. Penguin, London.

Klaus, M.H. & Kennel, J.H. (1976) *Maternal Infant Bonding*. C.V. Mosby, St Louis.

Konger, P., Mussen, J. & Kagan, J. (1974) *Child Development and Personality*. 4th edn., Harper and Row, New York.

Kron, R.E., Stein, M. & Goddard, K.E. (1966) Newborn sucking behaviour affected by obstetric sedation. *Pediatrics*, 37, 1012–16.

Kumar, R. & Robson, K. (1978) Neurotic disturbance during pregnancy and the puerperium. In *Mental Illness in Pregnancy and the Peurperium*, (Ed M. Sandler). Oxford University Press, Oxford.

Lamb, M. (1981) *The Father's Role in Child Development*. Wiley & Sons, New York.

Leventhal, E., Leventhal, H. & Shacham, S. (1989) Active coping reduces reports of pain from childbirth. *Jnl. of Consulting and Clinical Psychology*, 57,(3) 365–71.

Lewis, C. (1986) *Becoming a Father*. Open University Press, Milton Keynes.

Lewis, C. & O'Brien, M. (1987) *Reassessing Fatherhood*, Sage, London.

Ley, P. (1977) Psychological studies of doctor patient communication In *Contributions to Medical Psychology 1*, (Ed. S. Rachman) Pergamon, Oxford.

Lipson, J. & Tilden, V. (1980) Psychological integration of the caesarean birth experience. *American Jnl. of Orthopsychiatry*, 50, 598–609.

Localio, A., Lawthers, A., Bengston, J. *et al.* (1993) Relationship between malpractice claims and caesarean delivery. *JAMA*, **269**,(3) 366–73.

Lowe, N. (1989) Explaining the pain of active labour: the importance of maternal confidence. *Research in Nursing and Health*, **12**,(4) 237–45.

MacFarlane, A. & Turner, S. (1978) Localisation of human speech by the newborn baby and the effects of pethidine (Meperidine). *Develop. Med. Child Neur.*, 20, 727–34.

McClain, C.S. (1987) Patient decision making: the case of delivery method after a previous caesarean section. *Culture, Medicine and Psychiatry*, 11,(4) 495–508.

Marut, J. & Mercer, R. (1979) Comparisons of primparas' perceptions of vaginal and caesarean births. *Nursing Research*, 28, 260–66.

May, K. & Sollid, D. (1984) Unanticipated caesarean birth from the father's perspective. *Birth*, 11, 87–95.

Melzack, R. (1984) The myth of painless childbirth. *Pain*, 19, 321–37.

Melzak, R., Belanger, E. & Lacroix, R. (1991) Labor pain: effect of maternal position on front and back pain. *Jnl. of Pain and Symptom Management*, **6**,(8) 476–80.

Morgan, B., Bulpitt, C., Clifton, P. & Lewis, P. (1982) Analgesia and satisfaction in childbirth. *The Lancet*, 2, 808–810.

Moss, P., Bolland, G., Foxman, R. & Owen, C. (1987) The hospital inpatient stay. The experience of first time parents. *Child: Care Health and Development*, **13**,(3) 153–67.

Muhlen, L., Pryke, M. & Wade, K. (1986) Effects of type of birth and anaesthetic on neonatal behavioural assessment scale scores. *Aust. Psychologist* 21,(2) 253–70.

Niven, C. (1985) How helpful is the presence of the husband at childbirth? *Jnl. Reprod. Infant Psychol.*, 3, 45–53.

Niven, C. (1988) Labour pain: long-term recall and consequences. *Jnl. of Reproductive and Infant Psychology*, **6**,(2) 83–7.

Niven, C. (1992) *Psychological Care for Families Before, During and After Birth*. Butterworth Heinemann, Oxford.

Norvell, K., Gaston Johansson, F. & Fridh, G. (1987) Remembrance of labour pain. How valid are retrospective pain measurements? *Pain*, **31**,(1) 77–86.

Oakley, A. (1989) *Women Confined: Towards a Sociology of Childbirth*, Martin Robertson, Oxford.

Oakley, A. & Richards, M. (1990) Women's experiences of caesarean delivery. In

The Politics of Maternity Care, (Ed. J. Garcia, J. Kilpatrick & M. Richards), Oxford University Press, Oxford.

Out, J., Vierhout, M., Verhage, F. & Duivenvoorden, H. (1986) Characteristics and motives of women choosing elective induction of labour. *Jnl. of Psychosomatic Rsrch.*, **39**(3) 375–80.

Padawer, J., Fagan, C. & Janoff-Bulman, R. (1988) Women's experiences of caesarean versus vaginal delivery. *Psychology of Women Quarterly*, **12**,(1) 25–34.

Pedersen, F. (1981) Cesarean childbirth: psychological implications for mothers and fathers. *Infant Mental Health Journal*, 2, 259–63.

Perkins, E.R. (1980) *Men on the Labour Ward*. Leverhulme Health Education Project Univ. of Nottingham Occasional Paper, no 22.

Phoenix, A., Woollett, A. & Lloyd, E. (1991) *Motherhood Meanings Practices and Ideologies*, Sage, London.

Porter, M. & MacIntyre, S. (1989) Psychosocial effectiveness of antenatal and postnatal care. In *Midwives, Research and Childbirth*, vol. 1 (ed. S. Robins & A.M. Thompson). Chapman and Hall, London.

Reading, A.E. (1982) How women view post episiotomy pain *BMJ*, 284, 28–9.

Reading, A. & Cox, D. (1982) The effects of ultrasound examination on maternal anxiety levels. *Journal of Behavioural Medicine*, 5, 237–47.

Riley, C. (1976) What do women want? The question of choice in the conduct of labour. In Benefits and Hazards of the New Obstetrics Clinics (T. Chard & M. Richards). In *Developmental Medicine*, No 64, 62–71. SIMP Heinemann, London Lippincott, Philadephia.

Robinson, J.O., Rosen, M. & Evans, J.M. (1979) A controlled trial comparing maternal opinion of patient administered intravenous pethidine with intramuscular pethidine for labour. *British Jnl of Anaesthetics*, 79.

Rosen, M., Mushin, W., Jones, P. & Jones, E.V. (1960) Field trial of obstetric analgesics. *BMJ*, 3, 263–7.

Rosenblatt, D.B., Redshaw, M. & Notarianni, L.J. (1980) Pain relief in childbirth and its consequences for the infant. *Trends in Pharmacological Sciences*, **1**,(13) 365–9.

Salmon, P., Miller, R. & Drew, N. (1990) Women's anticipation and experience of childbirth: the independence of fulfilment, unpleasantness and pain. *B. Jnl. of Med. Psy.*, **63**,(3) 255–59.

Shearer, E., Shiono, P. & Rhoads, G. (1988) Recent trends in family centered maternity care for caesarean birth families. *Birth*, 15, 3–7.

Sherr, L. (1989) Anxiety and Communication in Obstetrics. Unpublished PhD Thesis, Warwick University.

Skibsted, L. & Lange, A. (1992) The need for pain relief in uncomplicated deliveries in an alternative birth center compared to an obstetric delivery ward. *Pain*, **48**,(2) 183–6.

Stevenson, E. (1981) Consumer expectations. *Australas. Nurs J*, 10, 18–21.

The Times (1993) Nov 6, Pg 7 'Restaurants welcome breast feeding'.

Thomson, A. (1989) Why don't women breast feed? In *Midwives, Research and Childbirth Vol 1* (Ed. S. Robinson & A. Thomson) Chapman and Hall, London.

Thune, K. & Moller, K. (1988) Childbirth experience and post partum emotional disturbance. *Jnl. of Reproductive and Infant Psychology*, **6**,(4) 229–40.

Trowell, J. (1982) Possible effects of emergency caesarean section on mother child relationship. *Early Human Development*, 7, 41–51.

Winnicott, D. (1964) *The Child, the Family and the Outside World*. Penguin, Harmondsworth.

Woollett, A. & Dosanijh Matwala, N. (1990) Asian women's experiences of childbirth in the East End – the support of fathers and female relatives. *Jnl. of Reproductive and Infant Psychology*, 8, 11–22.

Woollett, A., Lyon, L. & White, D. (1983) The reactions of east London women to medical intervention in childbirth. *Jnl. Reproductive and Infant Psychology*, 1, 37–46.

Wuitchik, M., Bakal, D. & Lipshitz, J. (1990) Relationships between pain, cognitive activity and epidural analgesia during labour. *Pain*, **41**,(2) 125–32.

Zweig, S., Kruse, J. & Lefevre, M. (1986) Patient satisfaction with obstetric care. *Jnl. of Family Practice*, **23**,(2) 131–6.

Chapter 9

Psychological Conditions Associated with Childbirth

'And then I went home, devastation. . . .'

Although most women experience childbirth as a challenge, only a small proportion proceed to show childbirth related problems requiring psychiatric help (Dalton, 1972 a and b; Braverman & Roux, 1978). Post partum depression and psychosis are the two major areas but there are other problems which could benefit from study. It must be remembered, however, that despite the enormous changes a woman undergoes as a consequence of childbirth (especially a first birth), psychiatric disorder is rare. Complaints of pregnancy (such as nausea) are invariably not psychosomatic.

Many conditions are measured in simplistic studies, using unsophisticated theory and design to simply collate copious amounts of checklist-type inventories which are often given to women post-natally. With multiple correlations, a variety of workers seek to explain associations with little strong validity. Many of the studies fail to examine in depth factors for individuals, which may account for both mood variation and the outcome measures. For example, a woman who has a poor screening test results, has protein in her urine or is informed of placental malfunction, may indeed react with high anxiety, low mood and panic. These physical problems may then be associated with poor post partum outcome for the infant. Studies rarely examine individual factors and continue to dish out rather meaningless psychiatric inventories (Lobel, *et al.* 1992, Moore, *et al.* 1991).

Of greater concern is the use of medication in response to psychological problems. A dialogue about the relative risks and benefits of these is crucial, as there are major concerns associated with the use of antipsychotics, antidepressants, benzodiazepines and lithium carbonate in both pregnancy and the post partum period (Cohen, *et al.* 1989). If a mother breastfeeds while using such drugs, psychotropic drugs can be found in the milk and the baby therefore probably receives the same dose per kilogram as the mother.

Some views examine the whole area of psychological trauma from a feminist perspective (Phoenix, *et al.* 1991). In this study it was shown quite clearly how a view of childbirth within society is crucial if one is to understand the true extent of emotional trauma and upheaval that it forces a woman to face. It may be at the very point of childbirth that her role as a 'woman in society' is made explicit, by social norms, or even her own expectations of her role in life. This raises the question of 'disturbance' and some studies argue quite forcefully that it is society rather than the women which may be symptomatic. By labelling and treating women, the cycle is further entrenched and the disparity of justice is perpetuated.

This argument is endorsed by the crude measuring facilities currently available to catalogue and define these conditions. Some studies simply rely on individual judgement, while others use questionnaire style inventories of mood variation. It is unclear to what extent such scores relate to quality or quantity of emotional experience. If such conditions truly exist, then there is the added burden of understanding what causes them. As identification and categorization are often difficult, there mere label of a condition may differ from centre to centre (indeed from practitioner to practitioner) and studies may not include women with like experiences.

Such methodological problems have beset the area and much of the useful data lies with the qualitative description of women's experiences and the strategies which they find useful.

Ussher (1989) states that labelling is unhelpful and that unhappiness and depression are not confined to the post partum period, but may extend for years reflecting problems with the 'job' of mothering. Indeed, when men provide primary care for children, they are significantly more likely to report depression than their female partners (Jenkins, 1985).

Post partum breakdown

The rate of post partum problems is low and show variation in different cultural settings as a result of different incidence, treatment, reporting or recognition. The problems are often categorized as depressive or psychotic, either mild or severe. Mild reactions are often labelled 'post partum blues'. Explanations for these problems vary depending on the school of thought. Some see it as biological and attributable to hormone level variation (the 'raging hormone' theories), those who view women as fundamentally psychologically fragile (Ussher, 1989) and those who acknowledge the trauma and change that a newly delivered woman may have to encounter (Phoenix, *et al.* 1991) as she undergoes a labour, is plucked out of her normal environment at the very moment she may feel pain and fear, is surrounded by professionals, machinery and technology and is then forced to spend the night in an 'all girls' ward, away from her loved ones, more often than not with torn skin, sutures, and a strange little bundle to ponder.

It is reported that 1 in 100 mothers experience post partum mood fluctuation. This can be of a depressive or psychotic nature. Recognition of mild and major mood changes is important, as is the ability to deal appropriately and rapidly with these. Much psychological suffering is earmarked 'baby blues' and never receives the appropriate counselling and attention, let alone prevention.

There are considerable differences between post partum depression and psychosis (Chalmers & Chalmers, 1986). Admissions to a mother–baby unit in a psychiatric hospital showed the majority were diagnosed with major depression. The next highest proportion were diagnosed psychotic, followed by schizophrenia, bipolar disorders, anxiety and deferred diagnoses (Buest, *et al.* 1990).

Predictors of psychological morbidity following birth were catalogued by Timsit, *et al.* (1986), among primiparous women with no previous history of psychological disorder. They found socio-economic and familial factors, difficult pregnancy and birth, recent psychological trauma and persistent conflict associated with post partum anxiety and depression.

Short-term depression

Variability of mood after labour and delivery are understandable, and it is strange that this needs to be labelled in order to receive adequate attention and input. It is documented by various workers either as a psychiatric syndrome or more descriptively as a mood state (Kennerley & Gath, 1989). Psychologists would see an obvious post partum mood variation accounted for by a variety of factors including:

- Heightened emotional experience.
- The physical experience of labour.
- The arrival of the baby.
- Pain.
- Institutionalization.
- Social deprivation (removal from family and friends).
- Sleep disruption, disturbance or denial.
- Drug effects.
- Loss (privacy, pregnancy, role).
- Anxiety (associated with their health, their baby's or their family left at home).
- Exhaustion.
- Excitement.
- Fear and challenge.
- Uncertainty.

Few studies have attempted to standardize or quantify such emotional expression. Women who cry (even if they stub their toe on metal hospital beds) may be classified as suffering from post partum depression or blues. One woman reports:

'My father had arrived to see me – we had not seen each other for five years. He was brought straight from the airport to the hospital, where I was with my two day old baby. Unfortunately, he arrived in the morning when no visitors were allowed. I begged the nursing staff to let him in. They were adamant – he should return from 3 to 4. I could not believe that my father was separated from me by one wall and the frustration and anger I felt made me burst into tears. "Oh dear" they said "post-partum blues – perhaps if she saw her father she would feel better." I was then allowed to see my father – not because I was joyous at having a baby boy and exhilarated to see him, but because I was suffering from a psychological condition and he was seen as a medical cure!'

Some studies categorically attribute such mood to 'variation in hormone level' O'Hara (1987). Again, the raging hormone theory raises its head in the life experience of women. It attributes mood variation to hormone changes which are out of control, unpredictable and overwhelming.

Hapgood, *et al.* (1988) monitored mood in 66 post partum women according to visual analogue scales for 14 days. They noted that dysphoric mood was temporarily related to childbirth, but concluded that lability of mood was related to psychiatric symptoms up to 14 months post partum and was a strong predictor of later psychopathology. They also noted that maternity blues were unrelated to variables associated with labour experience.

Knight & Thirkettle (1987) report on a study of primiparous women, evaluating their expectations and experiences and then comparing these with mood after birth. Although fluctuating levels of depression and anxiety were reported, these are not necessarily equated with clinical levels of depression or anxiety. They found that subjects who rated the birth experience as being unpleasant (in the face of contrary expectations) showed high mood variation. Fear of birth and general personality anxiety predicted post partum downturned mood. Birth experience and expectations did not predict post partum depression.

Long-term depression

Post-partum depression has been recorded in 10–15% of birthing mothers (O'Hara, 1987). Dalton (1971) recorded a rate of 8 per cent for depression which was sufficient in severity to merit psychiatric input. This should be viewed in conjunction with a further 25 per cent whom she recorded exhibited mild disturbance. Martin (1977) found a rate of 13 per cent and Braverman & Roux (1978) a rate of 14 per cent. Factors which are associated with its occurrence in addition to the impact of the birth, are often recorded as stressful life events, relationship discord and individual personality attributes, or even breast feeding (Alder & Bancroft, 1988). Such depression can either be primary and secondary. Women with pre-existing depression may find this is exacerbated during and immediately after the pregnancy. Secondary problems identified only after the pregnancy are said to have a more positive prognosis. Depression generally is more amenable to input than psychotic type reactions. Women who have depressive reactions after pregnancy are often found to have similar episodes after a subsequent pregnancy.

Nicolson (1989) found that elements of depressive reactions post partum were normal and appeared to be reactive to changing situation and life circumstance. They conceptualized the depressive reactions in the form of a bereavement where reactions represented a mourning over a previous social role and identify. They emphasized the role of grief work for such women.

Boyce, *et al.* (1991) examined predictors of post-natal depression. They studied 149 non-depressed women antenatally and then studied post-natal depression at 1, 3 and 6 months post partum. They concluded that there were increased risks to post partum depression where low spouse care was present, where spouses were particularly controlling and for subjects who themselves were highly sensitive. Other predictors included low maternal care and paternal overprotection. They also noted that these various risk factors had an impact at different post partum times.

One of the problems associated with depression is not only the longer term consequences on the mother, but the consequences on her new baby. Caplan, *et al.* (1989) studied the emotional development of children when mothers had experienced depression. Childhood behavioural difficulties were associated with mothers who were concurrently depressed, as well as marital discord at the time of the pregnancy and a previous history of paternal psychiatric problems. However, these workers found that the cognitive abilities of the 4 year old children showed no clear links with the depression of the 92 women examined.

Stein, *et al.* (1991) compared 49 mothers with depressive disorders with 49 control mothers who had no psychiatric symptoms post partum. They found that the former group exhibited reduced quality of interaction (measured according to means such as sociability, sharing and parental facilitation). Where mothers had recovered from depression, some social and developmental differences were still noticed. Gotlib & Whiffen, *et al.* (1989) compared families where the mother was diagnosed with post partum depression and families where no such diagnosis existed. The former, together with their husbands, reported greater levels of marital dissatisfaction and exhibited more dysfunctional coping strategies.

Treatments vary from drug treatment to supportive interventions or environments, with varying outcomes (Jacoby Miller, 1985).

Stress

Some groups, such as teenagers, have been recorded as experiencing greater than average stressors. De Anda (1992) studied 120 pregnant adolescents and described how many experienced dysphoric affect in response to stress. Stress levels of great magnitude were often accompanied by intense anger and frustration. The study examined strategies adopted for coping with such levels of stress and found that active coping was infrequently employed. However, when coping strategies were utilized, they usually included positive attempts such as relaxation and distraction, compared to deleterious attempts such as substance abuse or aggressive outbursts. The most common source of stress for these adolescents centred around the father of the unborn baby in just under half the cases (43 per cent) signifying the need for help to be targeted to the social network rather than simply to the pregnant teenager.

Levin & DeFrank (1988) reviewed 30 years of findings on pregnancy outcomes and stress. He differentiated four categories of outcomes, namely low birth weight, prematurity and ante partum and intra partum complications. He concluded that there were systematic differences between stress and anxiety and the concepts should not be used interchangeably. Life change stress was predictive of prematurity and ante partum complications and anxiety was predictive of complications. Yet there is little evidence which separates the causes of such anxiety, which in itself may be associated with the outcome.

Psychotic breakdown

Post partum psychosis is reported with a frequency of occurrence one in every 1000 deliveries (O'Hara, 1987). Two separate groups can be distinguished:

(1) Women with an existing psychotic condition who have a baby.
(2) Women who have a psychotic episode immediately following the birth of their baby.

The prognosis for the former is poorer. Marks, *et al.* (1991) studied women with previous psychiatric disorder after childbirth, compared with those with no previous psychiatric history. It was found that 51 per cent of those with a psychiatric history relapsed. Of these 28 per cent were psychotic and 23 per cent were non psychotic. Only in the latter non psychotic group were significant life events recorded in the year preceding psychiatric illness.

Mental health characteristics of women who are pregnant and have had a previous history of psychosis have been studied (McNeil, 1988). This study followed 88 women and found that women who were actively disturbed and in contact with a psychiatrist during pregnancy were at increased risk of post partum episodes.

The most important methodology for studying these problems is to understand whether they are primary and secondary problems, i.e. did they predate the pregnancy or are they a result of the pregnancy? This will be the most direct clue to intervention targeting. There is a need for the provision of care, for systematic data gathering to understand prognosis and to provide input for subsequent pregnancies in the presence of previous breakdown.

Baby snatching

This is a distressing problem, which will have a lifelong effect both on the victims and those who carry out such behaviour. There are two types of snatching – premeditated and spontaneous. The psychology of those who snatch babies can be divided into three: *deviant*, *disturbed* and *distressed*.

Deviant	Criminal, usually covers kidnapping, want to cause pain or suffering, seeking reward, or with another vested interest in mind.
Disturbed	Suffering from an aberration: a mental state which causes them to differ from normative and societal behaviour. Such people are usually unaffected by the response of the grieved who suffer from the disappearance of their baby.
Distressed	Those who want a baby but cannot have one. They need to be loved, to parent, to make a statement. This sort of snatcher responds to the emotions of the losers.

The outcome of such a trauma can vary enormously, depending on whether the baby is found or not. Ramifications can be divided into short, medium- and long-term effects. In the short-term, the parents suffer from excessive immediate trauma of the loss, reliving the circumstances of the snatching act and are often riddled with recriminations, guilt and anger. In the medium-term, they find it very difficult to resume normal life after the event. Having previously carried out their everyday life in the constant expectation that awful things do *not* happen, when something so out of the ordinary and disturbing, like the disappearance of a baby does occur, the event affects decision-making and an entire analysis of rational existence. In the longer term, adjustment to the event may be very slow in coming. Overprotection is common and can be expected and understood. Both the parents and child will suffer.

When the baby is not found, there is a heightened grieving, emotions very similar to those described in any loss, but with the added guilt, pain and outrage tempered by the eternal hope of finding the baby. Such situations are rare, but in instances where they do occur they make for chilling reading. Some have been documented within extreme social conditions (such as war).

Suicide in pregnancy

Generally suicide in pregnancy is a rare event (Kleiner & Greston, 1984 – see Chapter 6). Trauma associated with a pregnancy or a termination is often noted as a triggering event in retrospective studies of women who commit suicide later on in life.

The studies that do exist are mostly at case level and should all be viewed in the context of underlying themes such as the availability of termination in the case of an unwanted pregnancy and social pressure and options. The low incidence in the West is probably related to legislation concerning both availability of contraception and termination together with more accommodating societal attitudes. Generally the circumstances of suicide during pregnancy are associated with:

- Societal morality and inability to support women.
- Women who are unmarried.
- Women who are deeply unhappy.
- Reactive triggers to unforeseen circumstances.
- Pregnancy which is resultant upon rape.

Munchausen's syndrome by proxy

This is a condition where parents create illness or feign symptoms in their children to gain hospital admission. Sometimes they go to great lengths and damage their children (Meadow, 1977). This problem is typified by a parent seeking out extensive and unnecessary treatment, fabricating symptoms and conditions often appearing at different medical care venues and resulting in unnecessary investigations, treatments and interventions.

There are a variety of forms of health care seeking which can be examined under this heading (Maguire, 1991). The first is an extension of anxiety where the exaggeration of existing illness (i.e. grounded in possible or probable fact) prompts an excessive search for help (Masterson, *et al.* 1988). This can result in overuse or inaccurate use of medication, and harm can result. The second form is where the parent fabricates symptoms. The third is one where the parent takes active steps to create symptoms, at times administering noxious substances to the child (Orenstein & Wasserman, 1986). The behaviour is most often attributed to the mother. Libow & Schreier (1986) describe women seeking help because of their inability to cope; women who are somehow addicted to medical care and attention and the child becomes an effective tool in meeting the need. The most dangerous form is the last where parents actually incur damage. Numerous psychological theories have been invoked to explain this behaviour, often rooted in the family function or the maternal personal needs or concerns.

Anorexia and bulimia in pregnancy

Lemberg, *et al.* (1992) studied the impact of pregnancy on 43 primiparous women with a history of anorexia and bulimia, together with data from 17 obstetricians. Symptoms were reduced during pregnancy but significant regression was noted after the birth. There were no signs of deleterious effects on the birth or the infant. They noted that the women experienced anxiety about losing control over weight during pregnancy. Women expressed concern over the health of their infant. Of note was the fact that less than half (44 per cent) confided their eating disorder to their doctor revealing the shame and secrecy which surrounds eating disorders which may impede good antenatal care (see Chapter 7).

Psychiatric disturbance

Some studies presume that pregnant women are psychologically disturbed. An examination of a group of 81 pregnant women (33–34 weeks) carried out by Hrasky & Morice (1986) typified such attitudes. Two well established inventories were completed, (the GHQ and Present State Examination). They found that, according to the questionnaire data, 30.7 per cent of the women were psychiatrically disturbed. This is a harsh label to place on women simply based on the score of a questionnaire where some of the questions may relate to the physical and emotional conditions about their pregnancy (such as tiredness, difficulty in mobility, concern over future job change, financial matters or impending labour). They conclude there is a 'high rate of psychiatric morbidity'.

Sterilization

Burnell & Norfleet (1986) examined psychological factors for 297 men and 215 women who received vasectomies and tubal ligations, 6 weeks after they had experienced the procedure. Half the group were from large families. Women were most likely to report a history of medical, gynae-cological or psychiatric problems. Half of the women had had four or more pregnancies, while a third had experienced a recent pregnancy. In addition, contraceptive experience was unsatisfactory for most. Women were more likely than men to report improved psychosocial adjustment after the procedure – despite more medical complications with the procedure.

Abuse of parents by children

Although most abuse is discussed in terms of child harm (see Chapter 10), there are also rare situations in which children can physically turn on adults. Mouren, *et al.* (1985) found 35 instances of children who abuse their parents among 6000 files in one hospital records. All social categories were represented, with a marked decrease among the severely disadvantaged social groups. Factors associated with the cases included marital discord, single motherhood and weak fathering. These authors also noted that one or both parents were exhibiting psychiatric features such as mood or personality problems. Most abusing children were boys and the majority were first born or only children. Most aggression was solely or disproportionately aimed at the mother. Situations under which abuse occurred invariably were those where parental yielding to child demands was at issue.

Implications for practice

Although severe psychological trauma is abnormal in pregnancy and childbirth, when it occurs it causes enormous amounts of confusion and suffering for all concerned. Such cases demand the dual need for good links to specialized help, while simultaneously allowing for a comprehensive understanding for the more widespread emotional fluctuations which can permeate at all levels of childbirth. Often the situation centres around the ability to cope with a problem rather than the nature of the problem itself. Some families can cope and will be able to contain great levels of upheaval, whilst others need early intervention. Prevention and pre-empting is always desirable, but when it is not possible, then staff need to be aware, sympathetic and able. It is also important for staff to acknowledge where their own limits lie.

References

Alder, E. & Bancroft, J. (1988) The relationship between breast feeding, persistence, sexuality and mood in post partum women. *Psychological Medicine*, 18, 389–96.

Boyce, P., Hickie, I. & Parker, G. (1991) Parents, partners or personality. Risk factors for post natal depression. *Jnl. of Affective Disorders*, **21** (4), 245–55.

Braverman, J. & Roux, J. (1978) Screening for the patient at risk for post partum depression. *Obstet Gynec*, 52, 731.

Buest, A., Dennerstein, L. & Burrows, G. (1990) Review of a mother–baby unit in a psychiatric hospital. *Australian and New Zealand Jnl. of Psychiatry*, **24** (1), 103–8.

Burnell, G. & Norfleet, M. (1986) Psychosocial factors influencing American men and women in their decision for sterilization. *Jnl. of Psychology*, **120**, 2, 113–19.

Caplan, H., Cogill, S., Alexandra, H. & Robson, K. (1989) Maternal depression and the emotional development of the child. *B. J. Psychiatry*, 154, 818–22.

Chalmers, B. & Chalmers, B. (1986) Post partum depression; a revised perspective. *Journal of Psychosomatic Obstet. and Gyne.*, **5**, 2, 93–105.

Cohen, L., Heller, V. & Rosenbaum, J. (1989) *Psychosomatics*, **30**, 1, 25–33.

Dalton, K. (1971a) Prospective study into puerperal depression. *B. J. Psychiatry*, 118, 689.

Dalton, K. (1971b) *Depression after childbirth*. Oxford University Press, Oxford.

de Anda, D., Darroch, P., Davidson, M. & Gilly, J. (1992) Stress and coping among pregnant adolescents. *Journal of Adolescent Research*, **7**, 1, 94–109.

Gotlib, I. & Whiffen, V. (1989) Stress coping and marital satisfaction in couples with a depressed wife. *Canadian Jnl. of Behavioural Science*, **21** (4), 401–18.

Hapgood, C., Elkind, G. & Wright, J. (1988) Maternity blues. Phenomena and relationship later post partum depression. *Australian and New Zealand Jnl. of Psychiatry*, **22** (3), 299–306.

Hrasky, M. & Morice, R. (1986) The identification of psychiatric disturbance in an obstetric and gynaecological population *Australian and New Zealand Jnl. of Psychiatry*, **20** (1), 63–69.

Jacoby Miller, E. (1985) Successful treatment of the mother–infant relationship in a mother suffering from severe post partum depression. *Infant Mental Health Jnl.*, **6** (4), 210–13.

Jenkins, R. (1985) Sex Differences in Psychiatric Morbidity. *Psychological Medicine Monograph Suppl. 7*, Cambridge University Press, Cambridge.

Kennerly, H. & Gath, D. (1989) Maternity blues. Associations with obstetric psychological and psychiatric factors. *B. J. Psychiatry*, 155, 367–79.

Kleiner, G. & Greston, W. (1984) *Suicide in Pregnancy*. John Wright, Boston.

Knight, R. & Thirkettle, J. (1987) The relationship between expectations of pregnancy and birth and transient depression in the immediate post partum period. *Jnl. of Psychosomatic Research*, **31** (3), 351–57.

Lemberg, R., Phillips, J. & Fischer, J. (1992) The obstetric experience in primigravida anorexic and bulimic women. *British Review of Bulimia and Anorexia Nervosa*, **6** (1), 31–38.

Levin, J. & Defrank, R. (1988) Maternal stress and pregnancy outcomes. A review of the psychosocial literature. *Jnl. of Psychosomatic Obstet. and Gynec.*, **9** (1), 3–16.

Libow, J. & Schreier, M. (1986) Three forms of fictitious illness in children. When is it Munchausen by Proxy? *Am. Jnl. of Orthopsychiatry*, 56, 602–611.

Lobel, M., Dunkel, S., Schetter, C. & Scrimshaw, S. (1992) Pre natal maternal stress and prematurity. A prospective study of socioeconomically disadvantaged women. *Health Psychology*, **11** (1), 32–40.

McNeil, T. (1988) A prospective study of post partum psychoses in a high risk group. *Acta Psychiatrica Scandinavica*, **77** (5), 604–10.

Maguire, J. (1991) Health illness and the family. In *The Psychology of Health* (Ed. M. Pitts & K. Phillips). Routledge, London.

Marks, M., Wieck, A., Checkley, S. & Kumar, R. (1991) Life stress and post partum psychosis. A preliminary report. *B.J. Psychiatry*, **158** (10), 45–9.

Martin, M. (1977) A maternity hospital study of psychiatric illness associated with childbirth. *Irish J. Med. Sci.*, 146, 239.

Masterson, J., Dunworth, R. & Williams, N. (1988) Extreme illness exaggeration in pediatric patients: a variant of Munchausen's by proxy? *Am. Jnl. of Orthopsychiatry*, 58, 188–95.

Meadow, R. (1977) Munchausen's syndrome by proxy: the hinterland of child abuse. *The Lancet*, ii, 343–5.

Moore, M., Meis, P., Jeffries, S. & Ernest, J. (1991) A comparison of emotional state and support in women at high and low risk for pre term birth with diabetes in pregnancy and in non pregnant professional women. *Pre and Peri Natal Psychology Journal*, **6** (2), 102–27.

Mouren, M., Halfon, O. & Dugas, M. (1985) A new form of intrafamily aggressiveness: parents beaten by their children. *Annales Medico Psychologiques*, **143** (3), 292–5.

Nicolson, P. (1989) Counselling women with post natal depression. Implications from recent qualitative research. *Counselling Psychology Quarterly*, **2** (2), 123–32.

O'Hara, M. (1987) Post partum blues, depression and psychosis. A review. *Jnl. of Psychosomatic Obstet. and Gynec.*, **7** (3), 205–27.

Orenstein, D. & Wasserman, A. (1986) Munchausen's syndrome by proxy simulating cystic fibrosis. *Pediatrics*, 78, 621–4.

Phoenix, A., Woollett, A. & Lloyd, E. (1991) *Motherhood, Meanings, Practices and Ideologies*. Sage, London.

Stein, A., Gath, D., Bucher, J. & Bond, A. (1991) The relationship between post natal depression and mother–child interaction. *B. J. Psychiatry*, 158, 46–52.

Timsit, M., Timsit, B., Manni, A. & Monnier, M. (1986) Recent maternity and anxio depressive manifestations. *Acta Psychiatrica Belgica*, **86** (4), 502–8.

Ussher, J. (1989) *The Psychology of the Female Body*. Routledge, London.

Chapter 10

The Impact of the Baby on the Family

The arrival of a baby into a family will herald many changes. The dynamics, needs, structure and roles of all family members will be dramatically and eternally changed. The new baby will create a niche for itself within the family, bringing to it a new personality, new stresses, rewards and challenges. A number of themes will be discussed, but truly comprehensive data should be gathered from detailed child development texts, such as Shaffer (1993), Bremner (1988).

Becoming a parent

Parenting may be a new role for the individual or a couple. It may be eagerly anticipated, dreaded or accepted without much fuss. The limits of this may be markedly different for new parents and existing parents who have a subsequent baby. The cumulative effects can be viewed from social, economic, or psychological standpoints, as parenting affects many areas of everyday life such as roles, marriages, sexuality, finance, housing, and life satisfaction.

As pregnancy marks impending parenthood, there is much focus on the impact this has on the mother (with less focus on the father, despite the fact that the impact of a new baby may be great on his life too). Few couple-based studies exist. This is probably due to the 'medical' focus of pregnancy which focuses disproportionately on the mother's biological parameters and fails to examine the critical social, emotional and relationship factors which mark the context and social meaning of pregnancy and parenthood.

However, social and emotional preparation for pregnancy cannot be dissociated from the major impact of the hospitalization and medicalization of childbirth. This process, to an extent, will determine social behavioural patterns, in terms of help seeking, labour planning and the abdication of control. It also determines much of the psychological experience which is controlled (willingly or unwillingly) by the health care professionals who surround the women at the time of birth. Woollett, *et al.* (1983) described social class differences in the approach to childbirth with working class women fostering greater endorsement for the 'medicalization' of childbirth than their middle class counterparts.

The fetus as a member of the family

Stainton (1985) studied 25 couples in the eighth month of pregnancy and related that parents described individualized characteristics for the unborn baby. Thus an awareness of an unborn infant as a separate person with meaningful behaviours was identified, underlying the early sense of the individual and its impact with discernible behaviour patterns, needs, wants and reactions. This confirms studies which show that the fetus hears and responds to sounds at least 24 weeks (at the latest) of pregnancy and has achieved full consciousness by 32 weeks.

The formation of new relationships

Most parents form relationships with their new baby long before birth. Studies examining feedback during ultrasound scanning (Reading, *et al.*, 1982) have shown how visual imaging of the new baby can directly effect parents' initial concepts of the infant and change their behaviour in ways which may affect the development of the infant.

Although much antenatal time is taken up following the biological parameters of the pregnancy, more women would enjoy time and effort which would allow them and their partners to foster emotional links with their baby. Simple use of feedback and explanation could contribute greatly to this process, yet few studies have examined this aspect of relationship building. Anecdotally parents gather much thrill and excitement from the movement of their baby. Few practitioners even guide mothers around their own abdomen to differentiate the fetus's body parts, with the result that women may report caution and awe at attempting to do so on their own.

Zeannah, *et al.* (1987) asked pregnant women questions about the personality of their forthcoming baby. After birth they examined interactions between the parent and child. They found that mothers who had difficulty in imagining what their child would be like were less responsive to their babies, whilst their babies looked, smiled and vocalized less than babies of mothers who had had a clear visual picture of the child.

Classic 'first meetings' between mother and child occur immediately at birth. This is probably why so much attention is focused on the behaviour and delivery position. The first feel and touch of the baby, the warmth of human skin, and the introductions all have special significance. The modern trend for such personal moments to occur in public has not been fully examined. Fathers may feel restrained and mothers may be intimidated. On the other hand, conducive atmospheres are certainly reported where first meetings are enhanced by helpers. There are a multitude of factors which could interfere or affect such vital first meetings. These are as follows:

The emotional state of the mother

This may depend on the length and arduousness of the labour, the analgesia effects (if any) and the support, pain, exhaustion or elation she may feel. The practice of episiotomy adds the unwelcome need for suturing. Not only can this procedure be painful and unpleasant for the mother, it also occurs at the very time when the mother may want to be with her baby.

The appearance of the baby

This may be affected by apparatus such as forceps, which may cause bruising. The shape of the baby's head, the colour at birth, or the need to resuscitate may all affect the mother's immediate impression. The sex of the baby may also interact with parental reaction, depending on the desired sex of the fetus, normative behaviour to different sexes, partner reaction and expectations.

The environment

The physical environment can facilitate or impede the experience and expression of emotion. It is probably because of this key factor that home and hospital births are so directly contrasted. Some hospitals attempt to integrate environmental facilitators to aid the process (such as home-looking pictures, bedding and artefacts). However, it is often the atmosphere rather than the simple physical features which differentiate the two environments; reactions as well as wallpaper may need adjustment. Hospital births may also often result in delayed handling of the baby (Garrow & Smith, 1976).

The state of the infant

An extremely ill infant with immediate problems may need sudden intervention and this may take precedence over parental contact. More subtle effects caused by analgesia have been monitored on infant state (Rosenblatt, 1984). Infants can be affected by drowsiness, breathing difficulties or sensory responses.

Those present

Classic research examines the reactions at birth of mothers only. However, not only are fathers often present but their very presence may affect maternal behaviour (Clarke-Stewart, 1978). Fathers show equal attention to their newborns as mothers, given the chance (Parke & Swain, 1980).

Although much attention is focused on these first moments, there is comprehensive psychological literature to endorse the evolving interactions in relationship formation. This allows for change and development over time, input from both the parents and the baby and adjustment and accommodation according to circumstance (Sameroff, 1975, 1978).

Following these first introductory moments, Robson & Moss (1970) then studied first time mothers in depth over the first few weeks of the life of the infant and found an evolving relationship which peaked at 12 weeks, rather than immediately after birth. Indeed these workers noted that about a third of their women reported distance and flat emotions at the time of delivery. The relationship with the baby was complex and the baby's behaviour, together with their heightened personal investment, played a role in the evolving emotional closeness.

Premature babies

With the advent of neonatology, many babies who would have died ten years ago may well survive as a result of periods spent in intensive care. The experience of intensive care, its traumas and hurdles, its anxiety filled days and often the need to pace life day by day can be traumatic for parents, siblings and staff.

Perrin, *et al.* (1989) examined the notions held by parents of the fragility of their child, in the absence of objective evidence, in which they compared premature and full-term babies. Parents of premature babies who remained healthy, perceived their children to be more vulnerable than parents of healthy full term babies, while the greatest sense of vulnerability was expressed for children with ongoing health and/or developmental problems. The authors concluded that the level of prematurity led to a greater sense of infant vulnerability than the nature of neonatal problems.

The recent improvement in the survival of very low birth weight infants has long-term implications for health and development (McCormick, *et al.* 1992). In general, such babies that survive show low rates (5 per cent to 20 per cent) of severe handicap (Aylward, *et al.* 1989; Escobar, *et al.* 1991). However, when such studies are extended to older children, higher levels of severe disability and other types of health related problems are documented (McCormick, 1989; Hunt, *et al.* 1988). There are, however, many methodological problems which hinder accurate interpretation, such as intervening factors, small sample sizes, limited outcome measures and other intervening socio economic variables. McCormick, *et al.* (1992) found that when children are studied at school age, decreasing birth weight was associated with morbidity for a series of measures, including multiple health problems. Socio economic status worsened the situation for low birth weight children, irrespective of birth weight.

Bonding and attachment

Attachment is the term utilized to describe 'the powerful emotional tie that babies develop to their mothers' (Scarr & Dunn, 1987). This theory evolved from early animal studies which showed animals imprinting their mothers; these theories were then adapted to humans. Much of the literature was embodied in the work of John Bowlby (1982) who examined childhood attachments in relation to the corresponding separation anxiety that a child may experience if such attachments are broken.

Such theories evolved at a crucial time in history when there was large scale unemployment and a need for mothers, who had a previously been running the country while the menfolk were at war, to return to the home and free up jobs for returning soldiers. Society latched on to these theories with great tenacity, despite the fact that many of the tenets of Bowlby's initial work would not stand up to severe scrutiny along methodological and theoretical grounds. Bowlby described specific behaviours which made up attachment behaviour and provided ways to measure a 'separation response', which was seen as the corollary of attachment. According to the theory, attachments needed to be formed solely with the biological mother and negative longer term outcomes in social functioning for institutionalized children were cited as evidence to back up the theory. Clearly, such negative outcomes may not simply be due to the availability of a mother, but may reflect multiple variables associated with institutionalized care or individual factors accounting for the institutionalization in the first place.

Much work has now been done to put these theories in perspective. Scarr & Dunn (1987) typify them as theories created in order to keep mothers at home. Schaffer (1976) views the theories in terms of their context and points out the implications they had on health care policy. Some of the routine practices of removing babies from their mothers immediately after birth now had a 'scientific' reason to be abandoned. In addition, any invocation of the attachment theories allowed for much needed change in the practices surrounding hospitalization of children. Parents were now welcomed instead of excluded and incorporated into care. However, the theories do raise a number of critical questions:

(1) What does attachment really mean?
(2) Is there a biological base to the concept?
(3) Are attachment figures confined solely to biological mothers?
(4) Does attachment play a role in the development of the child?
(5) Is the concept of attachment useful and helpful in understanding a child's development.

A scrutiny of the theories has led to a much more reasoned approach to infant bonds. Klaus & Kennell (1976) claimed that the early interactions between solely the mother and the infant were crucial. For this to be true, it would mean that fathers would never be capable of sustaining meaningful relationships with their children, which is clearly not the case. It therefore seems that it is 'early interaction' rather than 'mother' which forms the key to these theories. The power of such theories were that they marked a turn around of macabre labour ward practices and allowed, indeed encouraged, the parents to take control and interact freely and lovingly with their new infant. Dunn & Kendrick (1982) noted that multiple attachments were indeed positive and found that children with exclusive intense relationships with their mothers suffered more distress and negative behaviours on the arrival of a sibling than those with relationships with their father and other adults.

Maternal and paternal deprivation are other possibilities which may occur. Maternal deprivation can be examined as a short- or long-term phenomenon. Short-term deprivations range from placement in day care, to hospitalization or residential stays. Bowlby (1969) describes some of the emotional reactions of children separated from their families during stays in hospital. These include phases of acute distress and protest, misery and despair, which are eventually followed by a detached contentment. However, these emotional reactions are not universal and can also be affected by the age of the child (they will be most acute in younger children), the gender of the child, the individual temperament of the child, the pre-existing emotional ties, and experience of separation (especially if this experience had a positive outcome) (Rutter, 1982). Many studies compound the effects of separation with the effects on the child of the procedures experienced whilst separated. Thus a child experiencing painful and frightening procedures during a separation may reasonably be more affected than a child experiencing good quality day care or excitement during the separation.

Longer term deprivations are invariably due to separation, divorce or death. The impact on the developing child is again unclear as separations rarely occur in a void. For example, a divorce not only signifies a separation but may also point to much parental argument, strife and stress. Parental death may mark a changed life style, altered income and socio-economic status, and may also directly affect the mood and care taking abilities of the surviving parent. Rutter (1982) concludes that it is the quality rather than the quantity of care which is the key variable in determining healthy infant adjustment to both short- and long-term separations.

The early environment

There is much concern that the early environment plays a critical role in determining long-term infant well being. There is certainly evidence supporting and refuting the importance of the early environment. This is examined in terms of critical versus sensitive periods, quality versus quantity of social interactions and care, and sensory stimulation and environment which may interact with vision, hearing, motor development and even language. Comprehensive texts exist giving details of child developmental factors (Shaffer, 1988).

Mothering

There is a vast amount of literature examining attitudes to mothering. This extends from maternal characteristics to include subsequent child factors, which range from infant health problems, hyperactivity, restlessness, feeding problems, sleep problems, colic, birthmarks, blemishes, feeding, development, ego development, weight gain, vocalization, smiling in a seemingly never-ending list. There is little overall theory to make sense of this vast array of findings, especially when conclusions are contradictory. The area is fraught with methodological problems, where correlational evidence is often utilized to infer causation (which it cannot or should not do). The hidden agenda is the subtle meaning attached to such studies which set out to define 'perfect' mothers who can duly provide 'perfect' babies, as if by recipe.

A more helpful approach is to understand the range of individuality and the way in which a variety of experiences may have subsequent effects on any given individual. This will free the findings from judgemental and subjective descriptions and allow for an understanding of processes in context. The most comprehensive work on the subject (Rutter, 1982) concludes that mothering has a lot to offer a child, but that the concept of maternal deprivation should be treated with caution. Several attachments are good (Rutter, 1982), and the needs of children invariably show that the quality of child care (whether by mothers or others) is the most beneficial factor.

There are some practical factors associated with mothering that can directly affect infant well being.

Maternal age There is an emerging literature examining the impact of maternal age on childrearing. Studies generally record some difficulties in younger mothers and hint at an 'optimum' (i.e. younger) age for mothers. Yet Ragozin *et al.* (1982) showed high levels of interaction with older mothers. These studies need to examine factors other than age which may contribute, such as socio-economic and relationship status, as well as whether the individual is well prepared. Once again, an isolated focus on maternal age with no consideration of paternal age leaves these studies without a comprehensive look at the entire picture. If both parents are teenagers, could that differ from a situation where there is a father in his 30s or 40s and a younger mother? What happens to older women with younger men? Clearly the dynamics of the situation are complex (see Chapter 6 for further details).

Maternal smoking has been correlated (Butler & Golding, 1986) with attendance of children at hospital surgeries. There was a consistent relationship between heavy maternal smoking and other outcomes such as non attendance at dental clinics and low uptake of immunization. Passive smoking also poses a risk to children. Again, most studies examine maternal smoking habits without examining paternal habits and their ramifications (see Chapter 6). The explanation for such findings is not simple. It may be that health values of the mother are low as a result of smoking and this factor is simply reflected onwards to the baby. It may be that smoking is taken up or continued for reasons of other stressors, which in turn account for the low uptake of health care services for the baby. Of course, there may also be the fear of censure from such health personnel about the level of smoking in the presence of the baby and this may inhibit attendance.

Home accidents have been studied in terms of parental factors (Kellmer Pringle, 1980) ranging from car accidents and seat belt usage to health promotion (Mayall, 1986). Uptake and ramifications do show relationships between some parental factors. These can be best summarized (Maguire, 1991) by an emerging pattern of mirrored self care behaviour from parent to child.

Maternal employment has attracted much interest. The literature has been reviewed and the conclusion reached that employment on its own will not necessarily affect either attachments the infant has made, or any subsequent development of the child, especially as working mothers often offset their absence by high quality interactions when they are able to be present. Other factors, such as job satisfaction, improved income, and emotional well being need to be offset against maternal presence. In general, the quality of alternative care is the best predictor of infant adjustment, both in the short- and long-term (Lamb, 1981, 1987; Howes, 1990).

Fathers: is there really a 'new man'?

As fathers become a more visible 'consumer' group, studies are now trying to systematically evaluate the needs, expectations and experiences of fathers.

Literature which focuses purely on mothering may be limited as it views the parent-child interaction out of context and may negate the important impact of the father, not only on the child, but on the mother and her mothering (Phoenix *et al.*, 1991). Clarke-Stewart (1978) noted that in the presence of fathers, mothers paid significantly less attention to their children and were less responsive. Sensitivity to infant needs is often seen as heightened in the presence of a good marital relationship and when this breaks down, children may get poorer quality of attention and interest (Hetherington, *et al.* 1982).

Fathers may be often absent (Henwood, *et al.* 1987). The effects of such absences are difficult to monitor accurately, as the very absence may trigger changes in the mother in terms of her economic situation, her role, her range of responsibilities and her ability to indulge in a relationship, share and navigate feelings and practicalities (Hetherington, *et al.* 1982).

Lemmer (1987) reviewed nursing research on fathers and found that these fell into the following categories: the experience of pregnancy from the father's perspective, response to their wife's body image, somatic responses to pregnancy, the effects of anxiety, stress and support on health during pregnancy, antenatal attachment and the father's actual experiences during the birth.

Nicolson (1990) looked at women's expectations and men's promises in the light of media images of fatherhood. It was found that these did not coincide and in fact contributed to relationship stress. Despite support for the idea of parenthood, they gave unrealistic messages about the degree of active parenting support. Such unmet expectations may contribute to strain and breakdown. Another study looked at parenting (Grossman, *et al.* 1988) to find predictors of paternal parenting involvement in terms of time spent in caretaking. Both paternal and maternal characteristics related to the level of paternal involvement. Paternal involvement may vary with age (Cervera 1991), who studied 15 families where the mother was aged between 13 and 19.

Shapiro (1987) studied 227 expectant and recent fathers, who described the double bind of being encouraged to become involved but simultaneously being considered as outsiders. It was of especial note that while their presence was requested, their feelings and reactions were rarely consulted or inquired. A series of major concerns was identified, which expectant fathers felt but which were rarely addressed. These were queasiness, increased responsibility, distaste of obstetrical/gynaecological matters, uncertain status of paternity, and the potential loss of either the spouse and/or child.

Couvade is a common but poorly understood phenomenon where the father experiences somatic symptoms during pregnancy, for which there is no recognized physiological basis (Klein, 1991). Such symptoms include indigestion, appetite variation, weight gain, diarrhoea or constipation, headache and toothache. Such symptoms commonly arise in the third month of pregnancy and usually resolve with the birth of the baby. Varied interpretations have been given for the syndrome, most of which are not based in solid research. Some are conflicting and include an expression of ambivalence about impending fatherhood or, at the other extreme, a statement of paternity. Some workers attribute symptoms to 'parturition envy'. Wide individual variation is reported.

Ferketich & Mercer (1989) studied the health status of men 8 months after the birth of the child and during the pregnancy. Health perceptions were affected by negative life events, self-esteem, mastery and depression or anxiety. Richards (1983) noted that premature babies had increased involvement with their fathers. This was described in detail by Levy Shiff & Mogilner (1989), who noted that fathers carried out many direct caring routines such as feeding, holding and changing when babies were premature. This could be explained by a number of factors including the possible threat, the heightened needs, the encouragement from the unit, the commitment because of the trauma. Yet when the child was extremely sick with extensive care needs, fathers tended to recede somewhat compared to mothers. Again, this could be accounted for in terms of needs for emotional sustenance, time off work or caring challenges.

Siblings

There is evidence that different sibling positions in a family have certain characteristics: children in similar positions in other families experience similar roles.

There is no evidence that this is hereditary and it is therefore thought to be a result of treatment or circumstance (Dunn, 1983). Children often spend more time with their siblings than with their fathers. Not only do families affect children but siblings can affect each other. Siblings try to be different. If one child relates to a given parent, it is common for the second child to relate to the other parent.

If there are large gaps in age, children may take up the role of sibling caretaker (e.g. Whiting & Whiting, 1975). Concerned and helpful roles were found by Dunn & Kendrick (1982). Often children are attached to older children as they would be to a parent. Siblings as young as 3 years of age were sophisticated in adjusting their speech to accommodate the baby (Dunn & Kendrick, 1982) by utilizing exaggerated tone, simple sentences, incorporating repetition and showing high proficiency with explanations. There were some consistent differences between sibling and maternal speech. Siblings showed no motherese (facilitative language) and the goals of speech adjustment seemed to differ from adults in that they appeared to be utilized to encourage play rather than teaching.

One consistent finding in the literature is of a language advantage for the first child. This can be accounted for by different language models, shared classes with other children, diluted teaching where there is not so much one-to-one attention with parents and friends (Zajonc & Marcus, 1975). Language development in the younger child may be influenced by the presence of siblings. It may encourage language development, especially as a result of overhearing conversations or it may lead to language delay as children compete for attention and their acoustic environment is blurred by multiple speakers rather than single directed speech.

Siblings have been found to have better skills at teaching tasks to younger siblings than unrelated adults. Teaching can also benefit the first child (Tizard & Hughes, 1984). Siblings can thus form definitive social role models and this can directly affect social abilities.

Most studies examine the sources of difference by looking at age and sex. However, the evidence on sex is inconsistent. Some studies found that same sex siblings had more positive interactions, but sometimes this was not found. One male and one female were found to have greater cooperation in some studies. Dunn (1983) cautions that the issue is much more complex and feels it is related more to parental attitudes and roles.

Therefore, the situation is not static, but changes over time as the children reach different ages and different stages.

Initially the older child imitates the younger and then with time the younger child starts to imitate the older – ultimately moving to mutual imitation. Various emotions between siblings have been recorded. Cooperation with siblings and peers varies. Often it is helpful and positive. Sometimes there is antagonism, jealousy and aggression. Physical aggression is common (Parke & Salby, 1983). Often parents allow this to occur in family settings, but not in public. Shaffer (1988) comments that sibling relationships are often 'paradoxical' as they can be simultaneously close and conflictual.

Large families will have a corresponding effect on the amount and quality of individual attention any sibling may receive. Feiring & Lewis (1984) note that mothers and fathers ask fewer questions and provide less positive child feedback in larger families; correspondingly, the children ask less of the parents in larger families. Language is also affected by the arrival of a sibling, where dialogue with older children is often focused on the new baby (Phoenix *et al.*, 1991). However, this is not necessarily 'detrimental' and Dunn & Kendrick (1982) claim that this may encourage older children to develop the notion of putting events into perspective. Children without siblings ('only' children) have their own hurdles. They may struggle with peer relations, yet they can still flourish without them.

Gender issues

Gender attributes are imposed from birth either formally (such as naming) or informally (such as colour coding of APGAR cards, baby clothes and flowers).

The gender of a baby has been shown to determine maternal responses. Condry & Condry (1976) examined the responses to infants (dressed as either boys or girls) and found that reactions differed systematically according to gender perception, in preference to the eliciting behaviour.

Differences were noted in the extent of interaction (with a same gender bias) and with the type of the interaction (more boisterous with boys, more soothing with girls). Fathers talked most to baby boy first borns. Gender of the baby is often the key stimulus to which adults respond.

There are some systematic sex differences which have been recorded. It is unclear whether these are biologically determined or whether they result from societal expectations, differential handling or differential stimulation and exposure. Those which are commonly catalogued include (Shaffer, 1988):

(1) Females show more extensive verbal abilities when compared to

males. This is recorded on systematic verbal, reading and word fluency tests.

(2) Males consistently attain higher scores than females on visual and spatial tests.

(3) Mathematical reasoning skills are often more accomplished in boys than girls.

(4) Aggressive characteristics are more often recorded in males than in females.

(5) Males show a greater level of physical activity.

(6) Girls are more likely to report feelings of timidity and fear.

(7) Males are more vulnerable to developmental hazards.

It should be noted that although these traits have all been documented, there is no evidence that they are true for every individual child and they in fact may result from expectations and experience rather than as a result of innate factors. The studies therefore need to be examined in context. They evolve from historical biases, and rarely control for factors such as parental attitudes, differences, self discrimination, learning exposure or opportunities. However, there are certainly intense influences on the developing child according to sex role, sex typing and gender factors, which have powerful effects on their evolving life pattern.

Temperament

There are a wide range of differences in temperament noted in young babies. These vary according to differences in parental acceptance and expectations and to parental concepts of what constitutes the normal range of emotion and temperament. The various forms of temperament measured include notions of irritability, ease of placating, passivity and decreased attention span leading to a notion of 'easy and difficult children'. Hewson, *et al.* (1987) found that observers were able to pick out babies whose parents also described them as difficult.

Child abuse

Perhaps the most extreme problem of parenting is child abuse. This can take various forms, ranging from psychological abuse, to physical and sexual abuse. Abuse can occur as an isolated incident or as a prolonged and extended experience (the latter is thought to be more harmful).

The fine line between discipline and abuse is often difficult to draw. For example studies of child smacking show that, by the age of four, 75 per cent of 700 children in a Nottingham study (Newson & Newson, 1968) were smacked at least once a week; 3 per cent were hit with an implement.

Primary child abuse is often child specific and may commonly be present in a large family where only a single child is abused. This lends credence to theories which attempt to accommodate abusing traits in both the abuser and vulnerability traits in the child. Many studies have examined the course of events in abuse incidents. If the precipitating incidents can be understood, then the subsequent intervention can be better targeted.

In general, studies have shown that abuse occurs in families with fewer children, less contact with extended families, fewer learning opportunities, increased marital breakdown, poor housing and urbanization. However, people who abuse their children can be drawn from all walks of society, social class, cultural background, economic and educational standing. There are some claims that those who abuse were themselves subjected to abuse (Belsky, 1981). The complexities of abuse are yet to be unravelled. An understanding of the problems and forms of abuse will allow for higher quality intervention by health care professionals when it occurs, or prevention in situations which may trigger abuse.

Families: a broader context

There is clear evidence that families (mothers, fathers, siblings and wider family members) have a dynamic and changing influence on any one member which will affect different individuals in a different way, and should be viewed more in terms of a continuum than an absolute. There is little comprehensive literature on the role and impact of grandparents on development, despite countless anecdotal accounts of their profound effect. McHaffie (1990) and Niven (1992) studied grandparents in the care and support in cases of premature birth. Grandparents played a key role in the provision of emotional support. Difficulties they experienced included the lack of information and the barriers they encountered on trying to seek the necessary information.

Similarly, parenting patterns and infant development in extended families is not fully understood. Most Western studies are based on the nuclear family, despite the fact that extended families are common, as are reconstituted families. Kibbutz children are brought up with extended families and communal forms of care. Different child care styles are now subject to more rigorous examination.

The challenge for the future is to understand the impact of single parenthood, increased maternal employment, multiply reconstituted families and older parents.

Implications for practice

Although medical care separates obstetrics and paediatrics, this model does not concur with psychological experience. Evolving models of comprehensive care can no longer overlook or delegate the care and needs of the whole family when dealing with childbirth. Quality care will attempt to understand the role of the infant in the family, and the various adjustments that need to be incorporated into holistic care if this is to be fully accommodated. There is every reason to believe that a variety of practices in the early days after childbirth may set up patterns or pathways which may dramatically affect subsequent family interactions.

References

Aylward, G., Pfieffer, S., Wright, A. & Verhulst, S. (1989) Outcome studies of low birth weight infants published in the last decade: a meta analysis. *Journal of Paediatrics*, 115, 515–20.

Belsky, J. (1981) Early human experience: a family perspective. *Developmental Psychology*, 17, 3–23.

Bowlby, J. (1969) *Attachment and Loss 1* – Attachment. Hogarth Press, London.

Bowlby, J. (1982) *Attachment and Loss II – Attachment*. 2nd edn, Basic Books, New York.

Bremner, J.G. (1988) *Infancy*. Blackwell Science, Oxford.

Butler, N. & Golding, J. (1986) *From Birth to Five: a Study of the Health and Behaviour of Britain's Five Year Olds*. Pergamon, London.

Cervera, N. (1991) Unwed teenage pregnancy. Family relationships with the father of the baby. *Families in Society*, **72** (1), 29–37.

Clarke-Stewart, A. (1982) *Daycare*. Harvard University Press, Cambridge, Mass.

Clarke-Stewart, K.A. (1978) And daddy makes three: the mother–father–infant interaction. *Child Development*, 49, 466–478.

Clarke-Stewart, K.A. (1989) Infant day care. Maligned or malignant? *American Psychologist*, 44, 266–73.

Condry, J. & Condry, S. (1976) Sex differences: a study in the eye of the beholder. *Child Development*, 47, 812–819.

Dunn, J. (1983) Sibling relationships in early childhood. *Child Development*, 54, 787–811.

Dunn, J. & Kendrick, C. (1982) *Siblings*. Grant McIntyre, London.

Escobar, G., Littinberg, B. & Pettiti, D. (1991) Outcome among surviving very low birthweight infants: a meta analysis. *Arch. Dis. Child.* 66, 204–11.

Feiring, C. & Lewis, M. (1984) Changing characteristics of the US family. Implications for family networks, relationships and child development. In *Beyond the Dyad*. (Ed. M. Lewis), Plenum, New York.

Ferketich, S. & Mercer, R. (1989) Men's health status during pregnancy and early fatherhood. *Research in Nursing and Health*, **12** (3), 137–48.

Garrow, D. & Smith, D. (1976) The modern practice of separating a newborn baby from its mother. *Proceedings of the Royal Society of Medicine*, **69** (1), 22.

Grossman, F., Pollack, W. & Golding, E. (1988) Fathers and children. Predicting the quality and quantity of fathering. *Dev. Psychology*, **24** (1), 82–91.

Henwood, M., Rimmer, L. & Wicks, M. (1987) Inside the family: changing roles of men and women. London Family Policy Studies Centre, Occasional Paper, no. 6.

Hetherington, E., Cox, M. & Cox, R. (1982) Effects of divorce on parents and children. In *Non Traditional Families*. (Ed. M. Lamb). Erlbaum, Hillsale, NJ.

Hewson, P., Oberklaid, F. & Menahem, S. (1987) Infant colic, distress and crying. *Clinical Pediatrics*, 26, 69–76.

Howes, C. (1990) Can the age of entry into child care and the quality of child care predict adjustment in kindergarten? *Developmental Psychology*, 26, 292–303.

Hunt, J., Cooper, B. & Tooley, W. (1988) Very low birth weight infants at 8 and 11 years of age role of neo natal illness and family status. *Pediatrics*, 82, 596–603.

Kellmer Pringle, M. (1980) *A Fairer Future for Children*. Macmillan Press, London.

Klaus, M.H. & Kennel, J.H. (1976) *Maternal Infant Bonding*. C.V. Mosby, St Louis.

Klein, H. (1991) Couvade syndrome. Male counterpart to pregnancy. *Int. Jnl. of Psychiatry in Medicine*, **21** (1), 57–69.

Lamb, M.E. (1981) *The Father's Role in Child Development*. John Wiley, New York.

Lamb, M.E. (1987) *The Father's Role – Cross Cultural Perspectives*. LEA, New York.

Lemmer, C. (1987) Becoming a father. A review of nursing research on expectant fatherhood. *Maternal Child Nursing Jnl*, **16** (3), 261–75.

Levy Shiff, R. & Mogilner, M. (1989) Mothers and fathers' interactions with their pre term infants during the initial period at home. *Journal of Reproductive and Infant Psychology*, 7, 25–39.

Maguire, J. (1991) Sons and daughters. In *Motherhood*. (Ed A. Phoenix, A. Woollett and E. Lloyd). Sage, London.

Mayall, B. (1986) *Keeping Children Healthy*. Allen and Unwin, London.

McCormick, M. (1989) Long-term follow up of NICU graduates. *JAMA*, 261, 1767–72.

McCormick, M., Brooks Gunn, J. Workman Daniels, K., Turner, J. & Peckham, G. (1992) The health and developmental status of very low birth weight children at school age. *JAMA*, **267** (16), 2204–80.

McHaffie, H. (1991) A study of support for families with very low birth weight babies. *Nursing Research Unit Report*. Dept. of Nursing Studies, University of Edinburgh.

Newson, J. & Newson, E. (1968) *Four years old in an urban community*. Penguin, Harmondsworth.

Nicolson, P. (1990) A brief report of women's expectations of men's behaviour in the transition to parenthood. Contradictions and conflicts for counselling psychology practice. Special issue: sexual and marital counselling. Perspectives on theory, research and practice. *Counselling Psychology Quarterly*, **3** (4), 353–61.

Niven, C.A. (1992) *Psychological Care for Families Before, During and After Birth*. Butterworth Heineman, Oxford.

Parke, R. & Salby, R. (1983) The development of aggression. In *Handbook of Child Psychology Vol 4: Socialization, Personality and Social Development*. (Ed. P.H. Mussen). Wiley, New York.

Parke, R.D. & Swain, D.B. (1980). The family in early infancy – social and inter-actional and attitudinal analyses. In *The Father–Infant Relationship – Observational Studies in a Family Context*. Praeger, New York.

Perrin, E., West, P. & Culley, B. (1989) Is my child normal yet? *Advances*. **6** (3), 14–17.

Phoenix, A., Woollett, A. & Lloyd, E. (1991) *Motherhood Meanings: Practices and Ideologies*. Sage Publications, London.

Ragozin, A.S., Basham, R.B., Crnic, K.A., Greenberg, M.T. & Robinson, N.M. (1982) Effects of maternal age on parenting role. *Developmental Psychology*. 18, 627–34.

Reading, A. (1982) The management of fear related to vaginal examinations. *Jnl. of Psychosomatic Obstetrics and Gynaecology*, **1** (3/4), 99–102.

Reading, A. (1983) *Psychological Aspects of Pregnancy*. Longman, London.

Richards, M. (1983) Parent–child relationships: some general considerations. In *Parent Baby Attachments in Premature Infants*, (Eds. J. Davis, M. Richards & N. Robertson), Croom Helm, London.

Robson, K. & Moss, H. (1970) Patterns and determinants of maternal attachment. *Jnl. of Pediatrics*, 77, 976.

Rosenblatt, D. (1984) *The Effects of Obstetric Medication on Newborn Behaviour.* Unpublished PhD thesis.

Rutter, M. (1982) *Maternal Deprivation Reassessed*. Penguin, London.

Scarr, S. & Dunn, J. (1987) *Mothercare Other Care*. Pelican Books, Harmondsworth.

Schaffer, H.R. (1976) *The Growth of Sociability*. Penguin, Harmondsworth.

Schaffer, H.R. (1986) Child psychology: the future. *Jnl. of Child Psychology and Psychiatry*, 27, 761–9.

Shaffer, D.r. (1988) *Social and Personality Development* 2nd Edn. Brooks/Cole, Pacific Grove CA.

Shaffer, D.R. (1993) *Developmental Psychology – Childhood and Adolescence*. Brooks Cole, California.

Shapiro, J. (1987) The expectant father. *Psychology Today*, **21** (1), 36–42.

Stainton, M. (1985) The fetus: a growing member of the family. Family relations. *Jnl. of Applied Family and Child Studies*, **34** (3), 321–6.

Tizard, B. (1986) The care of young children: implications of recent research. *Thomas Coram Research Unit Paper 1.*

Tizard, B. & Hughes, M. (1984) *Young Children Learning*. Fontana, London.

Whiting, B. & Whiting, J. (1975) *Children of six cultures*. Harvard University Press, Cambridge, Mass.

Woollett, A., Lyon, L. & White, D. (1983) The reactions of east London women to medical intervention in childbirth. *Jnl. of Reproductive and Infant Psychology*, 1, 37.

Zajonc, R.B. & Markus, G. (1975) Birth order and intellectual development.*Psychological Review*, 82, 74–88.

Zeannah, C.H., Keener, M.A., Anders, T.F. & Vieira Baker, C.C. (1987) Adolescent mothers' perceptions of their infants before and after birth. *American Journal of Orthopsychiatry*, 57, 351–60.

Chapter 11

Stillbirth and Neonatal Death

Most babies are born healthy with few problems. However, prematurity and stillbirth can still occur; incidents of neonatal death are all too familiar. It is difficult for staff and parents to be adequately prepared (Reinharz, 1988). While counselling skills can often minimize much of the pain and suffering, they cannot take away the actual loss. A way forward starts with the ability to approach bad news and to understand the needs of those affected at the time of trauma. Support should consider a variety of factors, including the psychology of the pregnancy, various bereavement and mourning issues, high risk indicators of pathological grieving and future conception (Moscarello, 1989).

Premature babies

Neonatology is an evolving branch of medicine dedicated specifically to the care and treatment of premature babies (Richards & Roberton, 1983; Merenstein & Gardner, 1993). It has moved ahead rapidly in developed countries in the last few decades and small babies can now be treated with great success (Kelnar & Harvey, 1987).

With the advent of neonatology, many babies who would have died ten years ago are the subject of intensive input and may well survive. However, the experience of intensive care, its traumas and hurdles, its anxiety filled days and often the need to pace life day by day can be stressful for parents, siblings and staff.

Perrin, *et al.* (1989) examined the notions held by parents of the fragility of their child in the absence of objective evidence, comparing premature and full term babies. Parents of premature babies who remained healthy, perceived their children to be more vulnerable than parents of healthy full term babies. The greatest sense of vulnerability was, not surprisingly, expressed for children with ongoing health and/or developmental problems. The authors concluded that prematurity led to a greater sense of infant vulnerability than neonatal problems.

From the parents' point of view, a premature baby raises a multitude of difficulties, especially since the outcome for any individual baby is never certain. Their birth experience is, by definition, too early and is often shrouded in the trappings of emergency, panic and heightened medical intervention. Irrespective of infant outcome, the experience itself is often highly stressful, and the long-term ramifications have been noted (Benfield, *et al.*, 1978; Minde, *et al.*, 1978; Klaus & Kennell, 1983).

However, parental emotional response is often not directly related to severity of infant condition (Benfield, *et al.*, 1978). Staff input is focused on the baby, but the mother and father (indeed, the wider family) also need care and attention and should be seen as 'front line'. High maternal anxiety coupled with information seeking may be taxing on overstretched staff (these variables were in fact the ones found to be predictive of a superior relationship with the baby on discharge (Mason, 1963)). Different couples may show different coping styles. Individuals may vary in their approach, given the fact that care can extend over long periods of time. Adjustments are made according to the progress of the baby, the staff attitudes, the time of day and the emotional and physical state of the parent. Some styles may be hampered by cramped public environments, where parents who feel certain emotions are reluctant to show them. Other parents may pick up a social norm and take their cue from other parents whose stay pre dated theirs. Studies note the following specific coping styles.

Intense commitment (Newman, 1980)
Some parents (when allowed) can become intensely committed to the baby, being constantly present at their bedside and interactive. They may want to take over nursing roles. This can be viewed as positive (especially in a busy unit or one which can cope with such a challenge) or it can be viewed as negative (where staff find the strain of training the parent and trusting the parent too difficult and taxing).

Distance (Newman, 1980)
Some parents may find the units too overwhelming and therefore may retreat. Their visiting can become sparse or when present they may be passive and not interact. This may be a way of coping with the possibility of an impending death. It may also be a way of pacing a barrage of emotions in a practical way, or it may simply reflect exhaustion or exclusion.

Family models (Minde, et al. 1978)
Some parents turn to their family models of behaviour to mimic crisis styles. Some families show variation between the members which must be respected.

'Good patient'
Some parents feel vulnerable and believe that their baby is at the 'mercy' of the staff. They may thus endeavour to be 'good' patients. 'Good' can be

interpreted as someone who does not ask too many questions, does not get in the way, is compliant and smiles sweetly all the time. However, this is not necessarily good for the parents in terms of their own psychological adjustment. Emotions need venting, staff procedure and protocols need explaining and even challenging and questions are crucial.

Parents have to cope with a high level of conflicting emotional reactions. The experience of a premature baby is more difficult, given that the prognosis is invariably shrouded in uncertainty, and every new development is emotionally draining. In this situation, the problems they face include the following:

Fear for the life of the baby
This can be in absolute terms (will she or he live or die?); or in relative terms (will she or he be okay?).

Environmental obstacles
Parents suddenly find themselves in a high technology environment, surrounded by buzzing machinery and intimidating contraptions.

Dependence on technology
Parents will find that the life of their baby is dependent on technological intervention, which can start to control their own lives. They may either be intimidated by the complexity of the machinery, or they can get to know how various machines function and stay rooted to their monitors, or they can attempt to become proficient operators and master the technology for themselves.

Dependence on specialists/experts
As care is taken over by experts in uniforms (Stacey, 1992; Phoenix, et al., 1991) who understand the machinery which keeps the baby alive, if they are unable to operate the technology themselves, parents are often awed or subdued into distance and passivity. When the time comes to take over from these experts their confidence may be difficult to build up.

Sensory effects
The environment of the special or intensive baby units not only affects the sensory channels of the parents (via noise, unfamiliar sights, high temperatures) but may also affect the small infant. Smeriglio (1981) stressed the need for sensory stimulation for such babies. Varied clothing, toys and sounds may go a long way to helping with this.

Loss and grief
There are two levels of loss. The obvious one refers to the death of the baby. However, the temporary loss of the 'other' imagined baby, the one they expected to be born on time, who smiles and has pink cheeks, has

somehow to be mourned. The image of the new, underweight, under-developed baby has to be accommodated. Some parents find this difficult as the baby looks fragile, even ugly to some. Staff can make this worse by referring (anecdotally) to such babies as 'froglets', 'chickens' or 'little scraps of humanity'.

Challenging decisions
Some parents may have to face challenging decisions at the time when they are least capable of making these. These decisions may have long lasting implications, yet there is often scant time to reflect, gather supporting opinions or anticipate courses of action. These vary from life and death decisions to some minor choices – but they can all be taxing and draining on parents.

Disappointment
Parents have to navigate their way through special care stays whilst balancing hope with keen disappointment. They may feel let down by the professionals treating their child, or by their baby or themselves. Blame and guilt may also feed into the disappointment and set up conflicting emotions when they are holding on to straws of hope and pacing themselves through the difficult days in special care units. The course of a stay on a unit usually fluctuates instead of progressing in an orderly linear process. Thus, parental mood swings may be apparent so that one day there may be hope and happiness, which will be bitterly dashed the next.

Abrupt transition from being pregnant to being a mother
Some women find the transition of attention from themselves to their babies quite distressing. During pregnancy, the mother was the centre of attention, as they were during labour which, invariably, had high input due to the prematurity of the birth itself. Suddenly, the mother is moved backstage as all eyes focus on the baby. She may have had a caesarean section, she may have stitches and will also have the same physical and emotional feelings of any mother. Everything may have happened abruptly and she may find this difficult and need more time and patience, when these can be severely lacking or not readily available.

Need to protect
Parents not only need some protection and nurturing at such times, but they may also want to protect each other, their new baby and other siblings. Such protection can be expressed by intense involvement on the part of parents. Staff sometimes withhold information in the belief that they are shielding parents from pain, as well as by helping them and pacing the situation.

Ongoing uncertainty
In many cases, prematurity leaves a little seed of doubt which may nag

at the back of a parent's mind during the first few years of their baby's life.

Reduced feedback
Such tiny babies may fail to respond to parental caretaking efforts and parents may find it difficult to feel close to them.

Table 11.1 summarizes some of the major potential stress elements for parents of premature babies and pointers in the research literature on how these interact with parental coping.

Table 11.1   Potential stress elements and factors which affect levels of coping for parents of premature babies

Elements	Studies
Medical staff behaviour attitudes and stress	Merenstein & Gardner (1993) Griffin (1990) Spinks & Michaelson (1989)
Medical condition and progress of the baby	Merenstein & Gardner (1993)
The process of separation and facilitation of contact	Gennaro (1991)
Family involvement and access	Ballard (1984) Newman & McSweeney Rostov (1991) Shea-McAleavey & Jamusz (1991) McHaffie (1991)
Environmental stressors	Perehudoff (1990) Mann, *et al.* (1986) Wolke (1987)
Training, teaching and handling	Goldson (1992) Niven (1992)
Staff tolerance and accommodation of psychological trauma	Merenstein & Gardner (1993)
Provision of emotional support	Macnab (1985)
Formation of attachments	Plunkett (1986)
Structured care and discharge planning	Jones (1991)
Follow up	Kenner & Lott (1990)

Bereavement and death

Bereavement and death can take many forms, either through stillbirth (expected or unexpected), neonatal death or infant death. The death of a baby is always traumatic, whether this occurs as a stillbirth or in the neonatal period. Some deaths are anticipated and some are a complete shock. Such cases need special handling by all concerned and this involves acknowledgement, time, space, and the ability to grieve and create memories. Parents need explanations and they need to pace their understanding. This may lead to counselling sessions over extended periods; open access is not only important but should be programmed and planned in advance rather than left up to the parents.

Such explanations must, of necessity, extend to the whole family including siblings and grandparents if appropriate and their individual needs ought to be accommodated. Parents may have ongoing worries, especially concerning subsequent pregnancies (Forrest, 1983) and a wide range of fears and uncertainties (Klaus & Kennell, 1983).

Fertility treatments and resultant multiple births have a special role to play in cases of bereavement (Stacey, 1992), where a situation may be created in which a parent has to mourn the death of one baby, whilst going through with the day to day trauma of a second, ill baby. These two experiences each need their own time in which to be addressed and the parents should be allowed (indeed encouraged) to separate them.

Theut, *et al.* (1990) examined the longer term impact of stillbirth and neonatal death on couples after the birth of a subsequent baby. They followed up 25 couples, who comprised of 16 with a previous miscarriage, 7 with a previous stillbirth and 2 with a previous neonatal death. Subjects who had experienced late perinatal loss were shown to manifest higher levels of unresolved grief over a year after the subsequent birth of a baby, in comparison to subjects who had had an early miscarriage.

Losses can be associated with a wide range of issues (Conway & Valentin, 1987) including: loss of child, experience of pregnancy, birth, breastfeeding, parenting, control, relationships and a concept of self. Six factors mediated the grieving process in this study:

- Multiple losses.
- Existing relationships.
- Perceptions of being the victim or the cause of a loss.
- Gender.
- Recognition of the loss.
- Cultural factors.

The impact of the loss never disappeared (despite the fact that acute emotions could be tempered over time). Often such long-term grief receives little attention and has been found to contribute to marital discord, sibling anger, sleep disturbance, illness and family dysfunction (Best & Van Devere, 1986).

Raphael (1977) points out that bereavement must be viewed in the context of the family and goes on to describe different family patterns which may affect the impact and reactions surrounding a bereavement. The different patterns include families who are:

- Treating death as a taboo.
- Seeking out someone to blame.
- Avoiding close relationships of any kind.
- Attempting to ensure that things go on as before.
- Functioning with openness and sharing of real feelings.

Facing death for adults may be easier if they can foresee the death and plan accordingly. Farewells are important. When death is immediate, information needs and explanations will differ. Some parents go through 'anticipatory' grieving. This is a process whereby grieving is carried out during the extended illness of the baby. This may mean that when the baby, especially an ill baby, finally does die, much of the grieving has already been experienced. Some studies show that parents can begin to distance themselves and despite the fact that this is perfectly reasonable, much staff anger is recorded. Adults and children have a need for information and to have their questions answered. Sometimes questions are asked to which there is no answer. Fictitious or vague answers are not helpful.

Sudden infant death

The sudden death of a seemingly healthy infant gives great cause for alarm. Communication can play a key role in the handling and emotional reaction of parents to the death of an infant in such circumstances. Input should include (Mandell & McClain, 1988):

- Sensitive information provision.
- Autopsy explanations.
- Guidance for surviving children.
- Sensitivity to the effects on any subsequent pregnancy.

Wortman (1990) cautions that intense distress and depression is not an inevitable consequence of such a loss and that failure to experience such distress does not necessarily lead to subsequent difficulties. Preventative methods need to be provided at an early stage, ideally at parentcraft classes. Currently notions of sleeping position, infection and situational factors are under study. Emerging data needs to be fed into parenting protocols early on.

Miscarriage

Miscarriage is discussed at length in Chapter 4. However, many of the emotions and reactions are similar to neonatal death. Jackman, *et al.* (1991) studied 27 women who had experienced an early miscarriage. Dissatisfaction with aspects of medical care were commonly reported. It was rare for any dialogue or discussion to take place about whether to view the fetal remains or how to dispose of them. Although many negative emotions occurred immediately surrounding the miscarriage, most women said these became less acute with time. Yet levels of psychological distress were still present in 44 per cent of the subjects in the year following the miscarriage. An important factor in this study was that women who experienced problems with the ability to discuss the miscarriage and aspects of its medical management at a follow up medical appointment exhibited higher levels of psychological distress.

Cognitions surrounding miscarriages may give clues to later emotional adjustment. Many women have specific ideas about blame and cause. Madden (1988) studied 65 women to examine such cognitions, some of which were predictive of depressive moods on follow up. The presence of an existing older child was protective against depression. Day & Hooks, (1987) found with 102 women, that family resource variables were stronger predictors of crisis and recovery than community resources, supporting the notions that family cohesion and support are helpful.

Information and support are key elements. Although two thirds of parents are satisfied with the levels of these factors immediately after the incident in studies (e.g. Helstrom & Victor, 1987) this decreases to just over half who are satisfied, with the passage of a few weeks.

The parents' own explanations for fetal loss may affect their levels of coping and adjustment. Dunn, *et al.* (1991) examined both maternal and paternal explanations for fetal loss and found the following themes:

- Blaming the mother.
- Physical problems with the fetus.
- Physical problems with the mother.
- Fate
- No explanation.

Of the five explanations, none included any blame for the father.

The process of understanding can be twofold, with parents taking in the doctor's explanations, but formulating their own hypotheses. They may hold these simultaneously, or endorse one to a greater extent than the other. When good communications and helpful explanations were given by doctors (Dunn, *et al.*, 1991), these were not only satisfying but were recalled by parents after two years.

Support in times of trauma

High psychiatric morbidity has often been reported at the time of neonatal death or soon thereafter (White, *et al.*, 1983). In this study, some parents reported excessive problems well after the first year follow up. The levels of necessary support may be difficult to give for staff working on a demanding and stressful ward. Staff need to understand that birth when fused with death can be extraordinarily confusing (Bourne & Lewis, 1984).

The amount of counselling available may vary from unit to unit. Counselling intervention has been shown as effective for long-term adjustment (Black, 1974, 1978). Parkes (1980), in a review of grief counselling, has concluded that such services can reduce the risk of psychiatric and psychosomatic problems after bereavements. Forrest, *et al.* (1982) carried out a study on 50 families who had experienced a neonatal death. Twenty-five received counselling and the remainder received routine hospital care. Follow up (at 6 months) revealed a significant reduction in disturbance for the counselled group. By 14 months, the groups had equalized and by this time 80 per cent were reporting no symptoms and only 20 per cent still had problems. It seems from this study that counselling can reduce the intensity and duration of suffering and problems, although it is not a prerequisite. Future studies need to examine the nature of counselling input, optimum practice and the characteristics of clients who will benefit and those who will not.

Counselling is not the only form of support. There are a variety of very straightforward interventions which can ameliorate suffering. Psychological theory postulates that mourning is a process of finding a place for unpleasant memories. This is not the same as denial or dismissal, as it does not shut them out but instead allows them an explanation and place. Therein lies the advice to ensure that the parent can create memories. This process hinges on the availability of such memories to conjure up the image prior to coming to terms with its loss. For adult losses there are lifetime memories, but for babies memories will be obviously difficult. Their lives will have been fleeting and may have been filled with such high levels of intervention that memories are actually abhorrent. The key advice is to allow the parent the freedom to follow their instincts, to ensure that no barriers are placed in their way, and to facilitate the permission to obtain and retain memories. This can be done in multiple ways. Parents may want to hold their baby, to simply see their baby, to retain a photograph of their baby, to keep a small lock of hair, a piece of clothing or the name label. If parents do not wish to do this it is important that these items are kept in case they later change their mind.

Some staff avoid creating memories for parents (such as physically showing them the baby) if the child has had some form of handicap. The literature suggests that parents who do not see their baby have distressing memories associated with high fantasy. These are worse than the distress reported by those who do see their baby. Forrest *et al.* (1982) reported that parents of deformed babies tended to focus on the normal aspects of the infant and no subjects in their study showed distress or were horrified. From this study, staff can learn to help parents focus on positive aspects, such as little hands or tiny toes, as parents may take their cue from staff when they themselves are uncertain.

The bereaved child and the dying child

A body of literature is emerging on dying and bereavement with relation to bereaved children. When the death of a parent, sibling or close relative leaves a bereaved child, the age of the child will often have implications for the input they will need, the optimum coping mechanisms they will require and the way the bereavement is handled. Although it is unrealistic to place rigid age divisions, children differ markedly as their development progresses.

Babies

It is difficult to know the extent to which a young baby grasps the meaning and impact of a bereavement. There are probably emotional feelings which may well comprise the precursors to mourning and grief. Given that dialogue is not possible with such a young child, the level of interaction should be matched to the child's needs. If the death that the baby experiences is that of the mother, then there is a dramatic effect on the mothering relationship which will become disrupted and difficult to replace. Although the tasks of mothering can be replaced by many people, it is important to bear in mind that the child's needs extend beyond gratification and feeding. The practical advice must be to allow for a key individual to take over the mothering of the infant. Ideally such an individual should be someone who can have sustained input over considerable time so that the child does not have to experience a loss of mothering on more than one occasion. With young babies it is difficult to understand their responses and reactions, and interpret them accordingly. They may show distress but this may be as a result of a reaction to their needs or to a lost individual. As it is hard to differentiate on the data that is known, the needs of the child should be made paramount in any consideration of care, in order to minimize the hurt and distress they will experience.

The longer term effects of bereavement on very young children are unknown. Studies which have attempted to examine them often have many methodological flaws which render them useless. Retrospective studies reveal little concrete data, but are most useful in steering subsequent research. Prospective studies suffer from flaws where it is impossible to tease out the incidental effects of a loss (such as changed socio-economic circumstances, changed psychological mood and state of a care-giver, changed responses to needs) and the absence of the parent. The overwhelming message from the literature focuses on quality of subsequent mothering as an important key factor in life adjustment. When young babies are faced with a loss, this ought to be a primary goal in care planning and resource input.

Older children

For older children the levels of meaning will vary. This will depend on family factors, age, developmental and cognitive abilities of the child, individual circumstances and subsequent life circumstances. Again, the loss may be typified by a reaction of pining and despair. The hardest part for the child to deal with is the fact that the person they loved will not return. Again, irrespective of the age of the child, it seems that the level of care offered in its place is crucial in determining the psychological and life adjustment of the bereaved child.

Family adaptation to the loss determines the level of discussion, understanding, explanation and help that a child will receive at the time of bereavement. This will also directly affect children's knowledge about the illness, their understanding of the patterns of emotional adjustment and responses from other family members, as well as themselves, how they respond to crisis situations, their ability to accommodate and adjust to new roles, and how to resolve the loss.

Lansdown & Benjamin (1985) and Lansdown (1990) note that young children can hold a meaningful discourse on death and have a quite sophisticated understanding of the notions involved in death and loss. Very often the limiting factors for children relate not to their ability to understand but to the willingness of adults to explain. Studies showing children do not have an understanding of certain aspects of death or bereavement are limited as they do not explain whether children are incapable of understanding, or whether they have similarly been denied the relevant information.

One area of parental loss that has given way to systematic insight does not apply to death, but to divorce, where there is still a loss, and hence any learning from this literature may be useful in the absence of direct source material. Overall, the studies have attempted to equate later disorders or behavioural problems to earlier loss. Studies have shown anti-social behaviour (Newman & Denman, 1971; Douglas, 1970). It is difficult to draw cast-iron conclusions from these studies as they do not give pro-spective data and thus one cannot conclude that all children suffering from loss will have subsequent problems. Furthermore, it is unclear which factors contribute to the problems if the relationship is real. This is a key component as any preventive work must be focused on the right remedy.

Psychological effects of bereavement

Children

Children who lose a sibling or a parent at or during childbirth will have specific psychological needs. All too often these do not receive sufficient attention, as health care workers usually focus on the bereaved parents. A brief overview should serve to alert workers to the range and depth of childhood reactions. Van Eerdewegh, *et al.* (1982) in a study of bereaved children found an increase in general symptomatology. This included mood, bouts of sadness, crying and irritability, many reports of sleep difficulties, reductions in appetite, withdrawn social behaviour, temper episodes and bedwetting. In a similar prospective study by Raphael (1977), parental reports plus child assessments revealed high levels of behavioural symptoms in the period directly after the loss, lasting for weeks and sometimes months. A fifth of the sample experienced at least two symptoms, which included withdrawal, bouts of aggression (where previously this had not been noted), clinging to adults and severe separation fussing, sleep and appetite disturbances and alterations in habits.

Other research has gone further to relate reactions to bereavements and losses to more physical problems. If there is a link between medical conditions and psychological distress, these studies should be noted with care. For example, Morillo & Gardener (1980) found links with thyrotoxicosis and bereavement, and Herioch *et al.* (1978) found links with juvenile rheumatoid arthritis and loss.

After bereavement some children suffer from adjustment disorders which need specific attention and are neither simple nor transient. Future psychological problems have also been tracked. Felner, *et al.* (1981) recorded school problems in bereaved children and difficulties in adaptation. School refusal and disinterest was also recorded by Black (1974) and Van Eerdewegh, *et al.* (1982). Generally staff need an awareness of possible minor and major problems in later life, ranging from transient school refusal to more severe problems such as psychiatric disorders, depression, disrupted or difficult relationship patterns, increased sensitivity to losses and increased trauma at anniversary times (similar to adults) and sometimes individual life crises occurring at the age-anniversary point of the experienced loss.

At the point of the bereavement any adjustment disorders should be noted as they may affect decisions made for a child which, in turn, may ameliorate or eradicate the possibility of future problems. In general, the factors which seem to contribute to the course of bereavement reaction include the quality and level of pre-existing relationships, the individual circumstances of the death, the availability and quality of support both immediately after the death and in the longer term as well as the presence of additional stresses. Birtchnell (1971) noted a protective effect of older siblings and hence family breakup ought to be resisted or only considered when alternatives are non-existent.

There is a growing body of knowledge describing children's concepts of death which can aid understanding of how one should talk to children about death. As the child grows older, their ideas about death will begin to tally with adults. Each individual child should be treated according to their individual developmental insight and progress. Perceptions of death are closely allied to perceptions of illness. Great care should be taken to understand what children know and do not know, what they believe, what they expect and how they explain certain phenomena to themselves.

Reilly, *et al.* (1983) examined children's concepts of death. They examined notions of permanence and the extent to which the child understood this idea. They found dramatic changes across age groups, with only half the 5 year olds stating that they would die, just under three quarters of 6 year olds and over 80 per cent of 7 year olds. Thus in the short space of three years, a marked change occurs for the majority of children in grasping the fact of their own mortality. Another study by Kane (1979) looked at specific notions associated with death and measured the extent to which children of different age groups had grasped such ideas. These factors included the following, and knowledge of them increased with age.

- Realization
- Separation
- Immobility
- Irrevocability
- Causality
- Dysfunctionality
- Universality
- Insensitivity
- Appearance
- Personification

Such studies are often helpful in pointing out the way in which dealing with death for children can be focused. However, they are limited in that they do not tell us about individual children and their needs. Counselling covers informing and subsequent questioning whenever questions surface. Honesty is always the best policy and a child's understanding should not be underestimated.

Adults

There are no theories of bereavement which are prescriptive, i.e. which can generalize, predicting stages and outcome of mourning. The theories that exist are descriptive and as such have the power to describe common experiences and elements but do not accommodate the wide range of individual variation and experience. Workers should use the body of understanding to help guide them through the unknown, to help anticipate and assist the bereaved and to help with a level of understanding when confusion reigns. They should not, however, use the theories as dogmatic menus, as they will then fail to react to the individual and may not provide optimum help. Such theories describe a range of immediate emotions which generally cover:

Shock
An initial numbness which may be transitory or extended.

Denial
Shock may be followed by a reaction of denial, which serves to delay or dismiss full comprehension of the importance of the situation.

Anger
Reactions of anger are not uncommon. Anger should not be taken personally. A death may free the parent to make deeply felt criticism and should be listened to rather than simply compartmentalized as 'bereavement anger'. Anger is often directed at health care professionals. On the one hand this should not be personalized – on the other hand, it may be the only time when inadequacies in the system are highlighted.

Depression
Many studies describe a subsequent phase of depression which some people can experience. This may be short lived or prolonged. It may express itself in terms of withdrawal, low mood, depressed affect, crying or emotional outbursts, anger or recriminations. It may be debilitating and consuming and may hinder the individual from participating in surrounding life. This may be particularly difficult for a new mother and father who have other children and will be marked when there are multiple births and the parents have to oscillate their emotions between the bereavement and hope for the surviving infant.

Reconstitution
This variety of moods invariably culminates in a reconstitution type phase, when the individual slowly reaches the ability to integrate the bereavement and pick up the threads of a meaningful life. This feeds into the coping phase often described in the literature and can be facilitated by workers.

Essentially, bereavement is not a denial of the strong and negative emotions, of the life of the baby or its death. Rather, it is the process whereby a place is found for uncomfortable, distressing and unpleasant memories. Rather than forgetting, there is a need to remember and accommodate. Thus, as stated earlier in this chapter, workers are encouraged to assist parents in the creation of memories.

Pathological grieving is said to occur when an individual somehow becomes stuck. They may grieve for extended periods of time, are unable to assume their life roles and responsibilities again. Psychological help can take the form of easing them through grieving processes, helping them confront some of the obstacles, or simply providing them with an opportunity to express their grief.

Some parents are unable to express their grief for many years. Such expression may only be possible on the safe arrival of a new baby and some births are often accompanied by the first experience of delayed grief for a previous death.

Help for bereavement comes in multiple forms. It is available in the interactions between staff and parents, in the care and attention to detail and emotions that is provided and in the facility to express and experience the emotions and reactions the parents may feel. There is rarely in-depth training on bereavement for staff. This is often compounded by the lack of debriefing after particularly difficult bereavements, the lack of guidance and the professional barriers which are erected to protect, but may be counterproductive for both the staff and the family.

Implications for practice

Although childbirth focuses on life and new beginnings, there is always the possibility of loss and bereavement. Staff need to understand that loss can relate to death but can also be emotionally linked with a wide range of grief situations in which a loss is partial or unrecognized. Theories provide a limited understanding and can only assist in generalized understanding. There are no prescriptive theories of bereavement which can dictate predictable emotions. In practice, workers need to be sensitized to grief laden situations, to examine their own practice and to understand the literature so they can be prepared for possible reactions which may be uncomfortable or challenging. Above all, they need to adjust their input, with sympathy and sensitivity to the individual. Only by doing this will they provide care in the true sense of the word.

References

Ballard, J. (1984) Sibling visits to a newborn intensive care unit. *Child Psychiatry Hum. Dev.* 14, 203.

Benfield, D., Leib, S. & Vollman, J. (1978) Grief responses of parents to neonatal death and patient participation in deciding care. *Pediatrics*, 62, 171–7.

Best, E. & Van Devere, C. (1986) The hidden family grief. An overview of grief in the family following perinatal death. *Int. Jnl. of Family Psychiatry*, 7 (4), 419–37.

Black, D. (1974) What happens to bereaved children. *Proceedings of Royal Soc. of Medicine,* 69, 38–40.

Black, D. (1978) The bereaved child. *Journal of Child Psychology and Psychiatry,* 19, 287–92.

Birtchnell, J. (1971) Early parent death in relation to size and constitution of sibship in psychiatric patients and general population controls. *Acta Psychiatrica Scandinavica,* 47, 250–70.

Bourne, S. & Lewis, E. (1984) Pregnancy after stillbirth or neonatal death. *Lancet,* July 7, 31–3.

Conway, P. & Valentine, D. (1987) Reproductive losses and grieving. *Jnl. of Social Work and Human Sexuality,* 6 (1), 43–64.

Day, R. & Hooks, D. (1987) Miscarriage. A special type of family crisis. *Jnl. Applied Family and Child Studies,* Jul 36 (3), 305–10.

Douglas, J.W.B. (1970) Broken families and child behaviour. *Jnl. Royal Coll. of Physicians of London,* 8, 203–10.

Dunn, D. Goldbach, K., Lasker, J. & Toedter, L. (1991) Explaining pregnancy loss – Parents' and physicians' attributions. *Omega Jnl. of Death and Dying,* 23 (1), 13–23.

Felner, R.D., Genter, M.A., Bocke, M.F. & Cowen, E.L. (1981) Parental death or divorce and the school adjustment of young children. *Am. Jnl. of Com. Psy.,* 9 (2), 181–91.

Forrest, G. (1983) Mourning perinatal death. In *Care of the High Risk Neonate:* (ed. M.H. Klaus and A.A. Fanaroff). W.B. Saunders and Co, Philadelphia.

Forrest, G., Claridge, R. & Bau, M.J. (1981) Practical management of perinatal death. *BMJ,* 282, 31–2.

Forest, G., Standish, E. & Baum, J. (1982) Support after perinatal death: a study of support and counselling after perinatal bereavement. *BMJ,* 285, 1475–9.

Gennaro, S. (1991) Facilitating parenting of the neonatal intensive care unit graduate. *Jnl. Perinat. Neonatal Nurs.,* 4 (4), 55.

Goldberg, S. (1978) Prematurity effects on parent infant interaction. *Jnl. Pediatr. Psychol.* 3, 137.

Goldson, E. (1992) The neonatal intensive care unit: premature infants and parents. *Infants Young Child,* 4, 31.

Griffin, T. (1990) Nurse barriers to parenting in the special care nursery. *Jnl. Perinatal Neonatal Nurs.,* 4 (2), 56.

Helstrom, L. & Victor, A. (1987) Information and emotional support for women after miscarriage. *Jnl. of Psychosomatic Obstet. and Gynec.,* 7 (2), 93–8.

Herioch, M., Batson, J. & Baum, J. (1978) Psychosocial factors in juvenile rheumatoid arthritis. *Arthritis and Rheumatism,* 21 (2), 229–37.

Jackman, C., McGeen, H. & Turner, M. (1991) The experience and psychological impact of early miscarriage. *Irish Journal of Psychology,* 12 (2), 108–20.

Jones, M. (1991) *Hospital Care of the Recovering NICU Infant.* Williams and Wilkins, Baltimore.

Kane, B. (1979) Children's concepts of death. *Jnl. of Genetic Psy.,* 134 (11), 53.

Kelnar, C.J. & Harvey, D. (1987) *The Sick Newborn Baby,* 2nd edn. Balliere Tindall, London.

Kenner, C. & Lott, J. (1990) Parent transition after discharge from the NICU. *Neonatal Network,* 9, 31.

Klaus, M. & Kennell, J. (1983) Care of the parents. In *Care of the High Risk Neonate* (Ed M.H. Klaus and A.A. Fanaroff). W.B. Saunders and Co., Philadelphia.

Lansdown, R. (1990) Paper presented at the Inst. of Child Health Conference, London.

Lansdown, R. & Benjamin, G. (1985) The development of the concept of death in children aged 5–9 years. *Child Care Health and Education*, 11, 13–20.

Macnab, A. (1985) Group support for parents of high risk neonates an inter-disciplinary approach. *Soc. Work Health Care*, 10, 63.

McHaffie, H. (1991) A study of support for families with very low birth weight babies. *Nursing Research Unit Report*. Dept. of Nursing Studies, University of Edinburgh.

Madden, M. (1988) Internal and external attributions following miscarriage. *Jnl. of Social and Clinical Psychology*, 7 (2–3), 113–21.

Mandell, F. & McClain, M. (1988) Supporting the SIDS family. *Pediatrician*, 15 (4), 179–82.

Mann, N., Haddow, R. & Stokes, L. (1986) Effects of night and day on pre term infants in a newborn nursery: randomised trial. *BMJ*, 293, 1265–7.

Mason, E. (1963) A method of predicting crisis outcome for mothers of premature babies. *Public Health Reports*, 78, 1031.

Merenstein, G. & Gardner, S. (1993) *Neonatal Intensive Care*. Mosby, St. Louis.

Minde, K., Trehub, S. & Corter, C. (1978) Mother– child relationships in the pre-mature nursery: an observational study. *Pediatrics*, 61, 373–9.

Morillo, E.W. & Gardner, L.I. (1980) Activation of latent Graves disease in children. *Clinical Paediatrics*, 19 (3), 16–63.

Moscarello, R. (1989) Perinatal bereavement support service. Three year review. *Journal of Palliative Care*, 5 (4), 12–18.

Newman, L. (1980) Parents' perception of their low birth weight infants. *Pediatrics*, 9, 182–190.

Newman, G. & Denman, S.B. (1971) Felony and paternal deprivation: a socio psychiatric view. *Int. Jnl. of Soc. Psy.*, 17 (1), 65–71.

Newman, C. & McSweeney, M. (1990) A descriptive study of sibling visitation in the NICU. *Neonatal Network*, 9, 27.

Niven, C.A. (1992) *Psychological Care for Families Before, During and After Birth*. Butterworth Heinemann, Oxford.

Parkes, C.M. (1980) Bereavement counselling: does it work? *BMJ*, 231, 3–6.

Perehudoff, B. (1990) Parents' perceptions on environment stressors in the special care nursery. *Neonatal Network* 9, 39.

Perrin, E., West, P. & Culley, B. (1989) Is my child normal yet? *Advances*, 6 (3), 14–17.

Phoenix, A., Woollett, A. & Lloyd, E. (1991) *Motherhood Meanings, Practices and Ideologies*. Sage, London.

Plunkett, J. (1986) Patterns of attachment among pre term infants of varying biological risk. *J. Am. Acad. Child Psychiatry*, 25, 794.

Raphael, B. (1977) *The Anatomy of Bereavement: A Handbook for the Caring Profession*. Unwin Hyman, Boston.

Reilly, T.P. (1983) Children's conception of death and personal mortality. *Jnl. of Paed. Psy.*, 8, 21–31.

Reinharz, S. (1988) What's missing in miscarriage? *Journal of Community Psychology*, 16 (1), 84–103.

Richards, M. & Roberton, N. (1983) Parent child relationships: some general considerations. In *Parent Baby Attachment in Premature Infants* (Ed. J. Davis, M. Richards, N. Roberton). Croom Helm, Kent.

Rostov, P. (1991) The family's perspective. In *Hospital care of the recovering NICU infant*. (Ed. M. Jones). Williams & Wilkins, Baltimore.

Shea-McAleavey, C. & Jamusz, H. (1991) Sibling visiting: a plan for change. *Dimens. Crit. Care Nurs.*, 10, 218.

Smeriglio, V. (1981) *Newborns and Parents – Parent Infant Contact and Newborn Sensory Stimulation*. Lawrence Erlbaum, New Jersey.

Spinks, P. & Michaelson, J. (1989) A comparison of the ward environment in a special care baby unit. *Jnl. of Reproductive and Infant Psychology*, 7, 47–50.

Stacey, M. (1992) *Changing Human Reproduction*. Sage, London.

Theut, S., Zaslow, M., Rabinovich, B. & Bartko, J. (1990) Resolution of parental bereavement after a perinatal loss. *Jnl. of Am. Acad. of Child and Adol. Psychiatry*, **29** (4), 521–5.

Van Eerdewegh, M.M., Bieri, M.D., Parilla, R.H. & Clayton, P.J. (1982) The bereaved child. *B.J. Psychiatry*, 14, 23–9.

White, M., Reynolds, B. & Evans, T. (1983) Handling of death in special care nurseries and parental grief. *BMJ*, 289, 167.

Wolke, D. (1987) Environmental and developmental neonatology. *Journal of Reproductive and Infant Psychology*, 5, 17–42.

Wortman, C. (1990) Successful mastering of bereavement and widowhood. In *Successful Aging* (Ed. P. Battes & D. Battes), Cambridge University Press, New York.

Chapter 12

Sexual Function and Becoming a Parent

Sexual interest, activity and appraisal are often documented as changing or fluctuating during pregnancy and the post partum period (Alder & Bancroft, 1988). Robson, *et al.* (1981) documented that pre-pregnancy sexual levels are usually not resumed until as long as one year post partum.

Many couples referred to psychosexual counselling have problems which are associated with parenting and relationships. Marital satisfaction is reported to decline during parenting and child bearing phases (Alder, 1989). However, few studies control for the passage of time, and often longitudinal studies show a consistency in pre- and post-pregnancy ratings (Feldman & Nash, 1984; Cowan & Cowan, 1988). Sexual interest and activity during pregnancy have been reported to change in some studies (Masters & Johnson, 1966), but not in others (Reamy & White, 1987; Falicov, 1973). An overall decline in sexual activity is commonly reported (Tolor & Di Grazia, 1976).

Post partum sexual function has not been studied in great depth (Alder, 1989). There is wide cultural variation, with sexual taboos post partum lasting for differing periods of time. This is often linked with lactation. Most studies concentrate on the female partner and there is little consistent documentation on sexual attitudes and desires between partners, yet alone their reaction to changes in sexual activity which may occur over the course of pregnancy and early childhood.

Sexual concerns and pregnancy

During late pregnancy there are often concerns surrounding sexual intercourse, either as a result of medical advice (Alder, 1989), fear of affecting the baby (Masters & Johnson, 1966) or fears of triggering labour. These may not be unfounded, given the high concentration of prostaglandins noted in semen. However, the presence or absence of sexual activity in the week prior to delivery has not been associated with pregnancy complications (Zlatnik & Burmeister, 1982) or prematurity (Solberg, *et al.*, 1973).

Post partum sexual concerns are often ignored by staff. Post partum sexual problems may emerge from the following factors (Debrovner & Shubin, 1985):

- Fear of infection.
- Fear of injury.
- Fear of discomfort during sexual activity.
- Fears about pregnancy.
- Emotional factors.
- Lowered libido if post partum depression is a complication.
- Exhaustion.
- Anger.
- Resentment.
- Caesarean section.
- Body image variations.
- Fears and/or worries surrounding lactation (breast sensitivity, leaking, altered body image).

It is important to remember there is a wide range of individual and couple variation and any study which presents averages may hide individual variation – much of which may have predated the pregnancy. Masters & Johnson (1966) conclude that the majority of couples have resumed sexual intercourse by two months post partum whilst other studies (Kenny, 1973) note an increase in sexual desire post partum. Further studies (e.g. Falicov, 1973; Jacobsen, *et al.*, 1967) report interrupted return to sexual intercourse accounted for by:

- Episiotomy and tenderness.
  This is a much overlooked problem, with rates as high as 40 per cent recording problems (Reading, 1982).
- Exhaustion
- Time constraints
- Lack of desire

Bachman (1986) discussed the occurrence and causes of vaginal or lower pelvic pain during intercourse resulting from obstetrical trauma. Pain could emanate from vaginal or caesarean deliveries. When partners are questioned there appears to be a change in frequency but not in quality of sexual relations (i.e. it may not occur as often, but enjoyment is greater). Table 12.1 shows the results of the available surveys.

Alder & Bancroft (1988) examined the relationship between breast feeding and sexuality. They hypothesized that mothers who breast fed their babies would have differing hormone levels to those who partially or fully formula fed their infants. Although they did find some differences, it is unclear whether these can be accounted for by hormonal changes or by factors which accounted for breast feeding (for example,

Table 12.1   Results of studies examining resumption of sexual intercourse after pregnancy

Study	n	Resumption of sexual intercourse
Masters & Johnson (1966)	71	Majority resumed by 6–8 weeks
Tolor & Di Grazia (1976)	216	69 per cent twice weekly at six weeks post partum 35 per cent more than four times a week at six weeks post partum
Jacobsen *et al.* (1967)	–	90 per cent resumed sexual intercourse by three months (10 per cent not having done so)
Falicov (1973)	19	Two thirds resumed by eight weeks post partum
Robson *et al.* (1981)	–	33 per cent resumed by six weeks post partum Majority by 12 weeks post partum
Grudzinkas & Atkinson (1984)	–	50 per cent resumed by six weeks post partum

breast feeding mothers were more likely to come from higher social classes) or factors associated with the logistics of breast/formula feeding. Alder & Bancroft found that the breast feeders delayed resuming sexual intercourse for longer, experienced greater levels of pain during intercourse and reported reduced sexual interest compared with their pre-pregnancy levels than the non-breast feeders. However, by six months these differences were undiscernible. No relationship was found between mood change and sexuality, but no consideration was made of some of the practical details associated with breast feeding, such as disturbed sleep, inability to share feeding with a partner, or cumulative exhaustion.

Marriage and the family

There is a lack of a critical tradition when examining the psychology of marriage. Most of the literature emerges in the course of examining marital breakdown and thus examines deviance from the presumed norm (Hart, 1976; Brannen & Collard, 1982). Yet the state of divorce is so common that these notions become unhelpful. The newer bodies of literature are beginning to take on board an examination of the factors which contribute to successful or meaningful marriages. Yet such studies may often be partial and non academic, in that they present presumptions of 'good' and 'bad' marriages and often show a social predisposition in favour of marriage. Although it is often easier to dichotomize marriages into 'failures' and 'successes', this is simplistic. Some marriages which continue do not necessarily represent excellent relationships. In addition, most dialogue on marriage focuses on the relationship role between the partners without due and adequate consideration of the family structure, especially the children.

Marital trends show interesting variation. For example, in the UK in the 1990s, divorce rates are increasing but remarriage rates are also on the up. However, a closer scrutiny of the trends also shows that divorce rate within remarriage is increasing. The effect of marriage on birth rate is unclear. Cohabiting in the UK is an increasing trend. As early as 1979, statistics showed that 20 per cent of couples married for the first time had previously cohabited. The role of cohabitation is one that can also be analysed within the family literature. Very often it is seen as a fundamental part of courtship rather than an 'experiment' in living together, often fuelled by the opportunities society creates for people to live together.

The process of marriage can be viewed in terms of role differentiation, life planning, carer (Rapoport & Rapoport, 1971) and family ramifications. Power issues are commonly debated in the literature and the role of the woman has received much attention (Oakley, 1974). Much psychological input has been focused on marital problems and marital therapy. Psychosexual problems often result in marital problems, or indeed are manifestations of marital problems. The three major approaches to marital therapy are:

(1) A systems approach

This approach (Minuchin, 1974) focuses on the family as an entity which is greater than the sum of its individual parts. The emphasis of such therapy is on the current behaviour of the family and the process of interaction which maintains its balance (or homeostasis). The therapy involves observation of family functioning, analysis of proximity and distance between family members, examination of boundaries and territory and examination of the rules (stated or implicit) which govern interactions. The intervention is aimed at identifying enmeshment, where there is overinvolvement at the expense of individuality which can blur boundaries. It also attempts to identify disengagement, where boundaries are loose. The main aim of the intervention is therefore to modify the existing structure into a healthier balance.

Other family problems can emerge when communication is malfunctioning or faulty. Therapy in such circumstances is aimed at shifting the balance of power. This is achieved by observation and interpretation of functioning, or at times by presenting couples with paradoxical interventions which may succeed in altering behaviour or perceptions.

(2) A behaviour approach

This theory has emerged from the literature on social learning. It examines learning patterns and associations and uses intervention to interrupt or reorder such links. For example, couples may often provide negative feedback to each other, may be involved in coercive behavioural chains or may maintain certain behaviours because of their direct (or indirect) rewards.

The success of this approach may be improved by integration of cognitive theory. Thus the theory does not simply focus on behavioural aspects of the couple, but examines the thoughts, meaning, intentions and cognitive interpretations of the individual partners. Adjustments to such cognitive styles may effect change.

(3) Psychodynamic approach

This theory is based on an understanding of the stages of development from child to adult. Problems with such stages may result in a client being 'stuck' in one stage, or being unable to integrate into adult life. When clients are unable to integrate, this may be reflected in their relationship patterns. They may seek out a partner who represents their unrealized self or, on the other hand, they may project parts of their unacceptable self onto their partners. In such therapy it is not uncommon for only one partner to be the focus of therapy.

How widespread are psychosexual problems?

Studies which attempt to examine the full range and nature of sexual problems often have systematic flaws. They invariably report clinic based populations (i.e. those already seeking out help) and it is therefore difficult and even misleading to generalize these figures to the whole population. Furthermore, psychosexual problems are often not absolute. For example, premature ejaculation for one couple may not be premature for another. Lack of desire for sex in a member of one couple may pose enormous problems, but may not be seen as problematic in another. It is with this caveat that a general outline of the range of reported sexual difficulties will be described, with brief mention of the current interventions which are available, together with their effects and evaluation.

The starting point for understanding psychosexual problems must come from a comprehensive understanding of 'normal sexuality'. There are wide margins of agreed and accepted behaviour and normal in this context is better used in the statistical sense (i.e. close to the norm) than in a judgemental sense.

There are a variety of factors which affect sexual expression. These can be summarized as:

Social norms

Sexual behaviour is often private, yet it is regulated to a great extent by social and cultural norms, expectations and accepted patterns. Deviations occur but are often censured (either informally or formally within a legal system).

Sexual partners
In western society, monogamy is generally accepted as a norm, with wide cultural variation. This can, however, often result in 'serial monogamy' (i.e. couples change partners – at times with great frequency – but such changes are consecutive rather than simultaneous). Anthropological studies show that many societies practise polygamous marriages (one male, many females) and fewer (0.5 per cent) are polyandrous (one female and many males).

Expectations
Sexual expression cannot be separated from individual expectations.

External factors
Certain constraints may directly affect sexual relationships such as war, or availability of partners, or sexual freedom.

Age at marriage
Age at marriage has varied over time, dipping into the lower twenties and then climbing again. The reasons for this variation are largely culturally and economically bound.

Sexual experience
Sexual experience is usually measured by age of first intercourse. Teenage pregnancy is noted across the world and thus must be a certain indicator of early sexual exposure. As noted in Chapter 3, first experiences are invariably unprotected. Males report earlier first experiences than females. However in some cultures, younger girls have their first sexual experience with older men.

Contraception
Contraceptive behaviour and availability has a dramatic effect on sexual experience and expression. The advent of the contraceptive pill provides a marked example. This allowed for sexual expression without the constraints of pregnancy threat. Availability, cost, social acceptability and safety are all triggers for contraceptive choice. Methods can be divided along different parameters. There are those under female control (e.g. the pill and IUD) and those under male control (e.g. condoms). There are those which are utilized within the sexual encounter (e.g. condoms, cap) and those utilized outside of the encounter (e.g. the pill, IUD, vasectomy). There are many catalogued short and long term ramifications of a variety of contraceptive methods (see Chapter 3).

Understanding sexual problems

Sexual problems are often identified with great difficulty, sadness, trauma or distress. They can be categorized into two groups:

- *Excess* This includes problems where there is an excess, either in duration, frequency, intensity or appropriateness.
- *Deficiency* This refers to behaviours which do not materialize or occur at all or in the desired manner (frequency, duration, intensity or situation appropriate).

It is vital that clear and precise histories are taken, with an exact description of the nature of the problem, the situations in which it occurs, the length of time it has been present and situations where no such problem exists. Most problems are couple based. Some therapists will only treat couples. However, there are problems which present clearly defined as male or female. These are:

Problems associated with men

Premature ejaculation
This is hardly ever biological, except in cases where the man has had good control which suddenly ceases: occasionally this may point to prostate difficulties. However, if ejaculation is always premature, then situational factors need to be examined. Premature ejaculation begs the question 'how early is premature?'. Studies in the USA show that the average thrusting time can be as short as two minutes. The reasons underlying premature ejaculation are usually associated with the man never gaining control – often a skill which can be learned via masturbation. When there is no opportunity to gain control – i.e. where there is consistent anxiety or punishment in early experience – control is frequently not gained. Men may resort to strategies which involve distraction. This in fact often confounds the problem whereby the subject does not attend to his own sensations and shuts out or misinterprets feedback.

Failure of erection
Generally, the longer a man can retain an erection, the more resistant it becomes. There has been an age effect noted where the time to erection becomes longer and the amount of stimulation needed becomes greater with increasing age. Impotence rates are difficult to ascertain with certainty. Rates are reported at about 70 per cent at the age of 70. Evidence suggests that if sexual behaviour is maintained, the ability is maintained. There does seem to be an organic component with age, but the reasons are unclear. The increase of impotence over the years is often accompanied with an increase in premature ejaculation. For some men the problem lies

with the fact that they can generate an erection but then lose it. However, if they are able to generate an erection at any point, then the causes tend not to be organic. In young men the majority problem is psychogenic. The reasons for this are not certain. Organic factors may be implicated, which include genital or abdominal operations. If the individual has no erection at all, then consideration must be given for a referral to urology or to an investigation into the effects of other allied factors such as:

- Drugs
- Chronic alcoholism
- Diabetes
- Anti hypertensive medication
- Barbiturate consumption
- Major tranquillizer consumption.

In general, the younger the man, the better the outlook and prognosis.

Failure to ejaculate
Any failure to ejaculate must be clearly defined. There are conditions where it is retarded or absent, whilst some men fail to ejaculate yet have the sensation and experience of orgasm. In these cases it is most likely that the ejaculation is retrograde (i.e. backwards to their own bladder). This can often result after surgery, particularly after prostate or urethral surgery. There seems to be little that can be done for such individuals. They are usually identified not for sexual problems but because they fail to conceive. If conception is a problem, live sperm can be retrieved from the urine and inseminated into the partner. Pregnancies have been known to occur as a result of such intervention.

Other men have no orgasm and no ejaculation. Psychological explanations for the man or the couple are often linked to fear of impregnation, cultural or personality concerns. This group can respond well to standard interventions.

Problems associated with women

Pain on intercourse
This is commonly referred to as vaginismus and results in a failure to achieve penetration. A 'tough hymen' is rarely the cause of this (if it is the cause, the problem can be eased fairly quickly with intervention). The woman will usually report sharp pain on thrusting and great difficulty in achieving entry to the vagina. Medical history may often reveal no use of internal sanitary protection and a woman who has rarely touched herself or inserted her own fingers to explore her vagina.

The problem is caused by the contractions of an annular ring muscle around the vaginal wall. It can sometimes occur as secondary to an episiotomy, which provokes such pain on intercourse so as to cause the woman to clench her muscles at the thought of the pain recurring.

Anorgasmia
It is speculated that anorgasmia occurs in as many as one third of women. Primary anorgasima refers to women who have never been orgasmic. Interventions are usually carried out in progressive stages, with initial utilization of masturbation techniques. Secondary anorgasmia occurs in women who have previously been orgasmic but have now ceased to be so. The key here is to examine relationship problems and difficulties. A woman who is orgasmic on masturbation and not on intercourse will respond well to psychological interventions. Generally, the problem is associated with a sexual partner who either ejaculates too quickly or fails to stimulate her. There may also be problems with the woman not 'letting herself go' and these can sometimes be linked to a number of early learning experiences.

Pain
Some women report a pain on intercourse which feels like being rubbed with sandpaper. This description invariably suggests a situation where there is a lack of lubrication. Solutions to inadequate lubrication include the use of synthetic lubricants, variations in sexual behaviour to allow for lubrication or an investigation into other causes such as infection (e.g. candida/thrush).

Sharp pains after thrusting
Other women report sharp pains after thrusting which invariably indicate that the woman is not excited during intercourse and the vaginal channel is not fully lengthened. The pain experienced results from impact on the cervix. Help can come in the form of intervention to either vary sexual position or ensure lubrication is adequate. Occasionally problems may be associated with a retroverted (forward facing) uterus.

Dull ache
Women who report a dull ache after sexual activity usually note that this remains for anything up to 12 hours after intercourse. It is invariably a result of insufficient resolution of the blood vessels. When orgasm occurs, the muscles contract and pump blood out. When there is no orgasm, the blood takes time to resolve and therefore feelings of discomfort can result.

Bad episiotomies
There has been wide reporting (Reading, 1982) of the ramifications of poor episiotomies and widespread pain and problems which these can cause. The best cure for this problem is prevention of episiotomies in the first place. Practitioners should think very carefully before carrying out unnecessary or marginally necessary procedure and should take extreme

time and effort to ensure high quality suturing and post-episiotomy care. The long-term silent suffering from episiotomy pain is avoidable with good midwifery and obstetric care.

Lack of desire

The most major problem which most practitioners have to deal with is the lack of sexual desire. This book is not the place for an extensive dialogue on the causes and interventions surrounding this problem. The major techniques under employ are those of Masters & Johnson. Good texts include Hawton (1985), Bancroft (1989), Valins (1989) and Dickson (1985).

Relationship issues surrounding childbirth

The desire for a pregnancy, the pregnancy itself and the arrival of a new baby can have dramatic effects on a relationship. These are not necessarily always either good or bad, but may challenge currently vibrant relationships with change, accommodation and adjustment. Scott Heyes (1984) reports that childbirth affect nuturance and interdependence factors within relationships. This fascinating study reveals the particular problems for women who simultaneously experience increase in emotional and physical burdens and their own need of nuturance. Such nuturance was provided by over three-quarters of partners but was rarely perceived as sufficient. It was noted that despite change, to accommodate need, frustration and unmet needs often persisted. One can speculate that such demands (both of change and of unrequited need) may place strain on any relationship, which may be expressed in terms of disharmony, depression or break up.

As stated earlier in this chapter, sexual intercourse patterns may change during pregnancy and post partum, and this in turn may affect relationships. Niven (1992) conceptualizes this in terms of 'male deprivation' rather than a comprehensive look which also includes the female and the needs of the couple as a whole.

Implications for practice

Psychosexual issues are rarely included in childbirth and pregnancy debates. This oversight contributes to a form of denial of where the baby has come from and the relationship into which the baby and the parents return. There is something asexual about maternity care and the very conspiracy of silence serves to overshadow any discussion of sexuality and sexual issues. This must represent a lost opportunity for care and may result in a poor understanding of the totality of needs for any woman. There should be no revelation that sex and pregnancy are linked, but it is astounding that midwifery and obstetric training rarely includes psychosexual issues. Midwives and obstetricians are ideally placed for a discussion and dialogue on a host of sex-related topics, ranging from pregnancy to contraception, sexually transmitted diseases and psychosexual problems.

References

Alder, E. (1989) Sexual behaviour in pregnancy after childbirth and during breast feeding. *Bailliere's Clinical Obstetrics and Gynaecology*, **3** (4).

Alder, E. & Bancroft, J. (1988) The relationship between breast feeding, persistence, sexuality and mood in post partum women. *Psychological Medicine*, 18, 389–96.

Bachman, G. (1986) Dyspareunia due to obstetrical trauma. *Medical Aspects of Human Sexuality*, **20** (3), 21–5.

Bancroft, J. (1989) *Human Sexuality and its Problems.* Churchill Livingstone, London.

Brannen, J. & Collard, J.L. (1982) *Marriages in Trouble.* Tavistock, London.

Cowan, P. & Cowan, C. (1988) Changes in marriage during the transition to parenthood – must we blame the baby? In *Transition to Parenthood*, (Ed. G. Michaels & W. Goldberg). Cambridge University Press, Cambridge.

Debrovner, C. & Shubin, R. (1985) Pregnancy and post partum sexual concerns. *Medical Aspects of Human Sexuality*, **19** (5), 84–90.

Dickson, A. (1985) *A Woman In Your Own Right.* Quartet, London.

Falicov, C. (1973) Sexual adjustment during first pregnancy and post partum. *Am. Jnl. of Obstet. & Gynec.*, 118, 991–1000.

Feldman, S. & Nash, S. (1984) The transition from expectancy to parenthood: impact of the first born child on men and women. *Sex Roles*, 11, 84–96.

Grudzinkas, J. & Atkinson, L. (1984) Sexual function during the puerperium. *Archives of Sexual Behavior*, 13, 85–91.

Hart, N. (1976) *When Marriage Ends: A Study in Status Passage.* Tavistock, London.

Hawton, K.K. (1985) *Sex Therapy: A Practical Guide.* Oxford University Press, Oxford.

Jacobsen, L., Kaij, L. & Nilsson, A. (1967) The course and outcome of the post partum period from a gynaecological and general somatic standpoint. *Acta Obstetrica et Gynecologica Scandanavica*, 46, 183–203.

Kenny, J. (1973) Sexuality of pregnant and breastfeeding women. *Archives of Sexual Behavior*, 2, 215–29.

Masters, W. & Johnson, V. (1966) *Human Sexual Response*, Little Brown, Boston.

Minuchin, D. (1974) *Families and family therapy.* Harvard University Press, Cambridge, Massachusetts.

Niven, C. (1992) *Psychological Care for Families Before, During and After Birth.* Butterworth Heinemann, Oxford.

Oakley, A. (1974) *The Sociology of Housework.* Martin Robertson, London.

Rapoport, R. & Rapoport, R.N. (1971) *Dual Career Families.* Penguin, London.

Reading, A. (1982) How women view post episiotomy pain. *BMJ*, 284, 28.

Reamy, K. & White, S. (1987) Sexuality in the puerperium: a review. *Archives of Sexual Behavior*, 16, 165–86.

Robson, K., Brant, H. & Kumar, R. (1981) Maternal sexuality during first pregnancy and after childbirth. *B. Jnl. of Obstet. & Gynec.*, 88, 882–9.

Scott-Heyes, G. (1984) Childbearing as a mutual experience. Unpublished Dip. Phil thesis, New University, Ulster.

Solberg, D., Butler, J. & Wagner, N. (1973) Sexual behavior in pregnancy. *New Eng. Jnl of Med.*, 288.

Tolor, A. & Di Grazia, P. (1976) Sexual attitudes and behavior patterns during and following pregnancy. *Archives of Sexual Behavior*, 5, 539–51.

Valins, L. (1989) *Vaginismus*. Ashgrove Press, Bath.

Zlatnik, F. & Burmeister, L. (1982) Reported sexual behavior in late pregnancy: selected associations. *Jnl. of Reproductive Medicine*, 10, 627–32.

Chapter 13

Child Development

'It's a long trip from the beginning of cortical behaviour to adolescent rebellion and moral judgement.'

(Scarr & Dunn, 1987)

The course of early child development is affected by many variables. These can include genetic factors, environmental influences (before, during and after birth), parenting and stimulation factors, and basic human needs such as nutrition, exercise and protection.

The complexity of infant function is rarely appreciated fully. Often this reflects a lack of sophistication in measuring infant responses, rather than the absence of such responses. As the area of child development becomes more advanced, so does understanding of children's progress.

There are numerous influences on child development which have been studied in detail (Lansdown, 1988; Shaffer, 1985). A few will be outlined to give some insight into the way psychological understanding can shed light on infant development. Many of these factors are interdependent, but may include separate studies of temperament, sex differences, behavioural differences, the impact of early experiences, the contribution of the family, school and social factors.

Growth covers many elements. These include motor development; cognitive development in terms of understanding, attention, language, memory, perception and intelligence; personal development, which involves personal relationships, social and emotional development; personality development, moral development and the emergency of a concept of 'self'. Much of this can be observed via mechanisms such as play, art, language or social interactions. A variety of theories exist which attempt to encapsulate and explain child development (such as Piaget, Bruner and Freud – see for example, Bremner (1988) or Smith & Cowie (1988).

The newborn has the capacity to learn, perceive, react and interact socially. The infant can imitate gestures from a very early age. By the time a baby is born, it has nearly its full complement of neurons. This has provoked investigators into looking very closely at early experience in terms of its effect on development as a whole. Sameroff & Chandler (1975) point out that 10 per cent of the US population has handicaps or defects that are present either at or soon after birth.

Antenatal experience and its impact on development

Work has been carried out on both animal and human subjects, which tries to trace links between antenatal events and later development. The animal literature, although interesting, provides mainly questions to be asked rather than answers which are directly applicable to humans. Much research on animal development simply cannot be generalized to human behaviour (for example, early work on thalidomide, which has been dramatically linked to physical development interference in humans, had no such effect on animals). Studies on the effects of discrete substances or events on subsequent development are fraught with difficulties. They are usually retrospective and therefore only include those subjects who have had effects, rather than population based samples. There are also often problems with definitions, measurement and recall. Numerous studies have examined various events to possible outcomes including the following factors.

Aspirin

Some work has examined the link between congenital malformations and aspirin intake during pregnancy. Teratogenic potential of aspirin is thought to be enhanced when administered with benzoic acid, which is commonly found in food colouring (Kimmel, *et al.* 1971).

Radiation

Heavy doses of radiation have been shown to be linked with abnormalities. There is, however, no knowledge of chronic radiation effects.

Lead

Lead poisoning has been shown to cause abnormalities. Again, there is little understanding of the ramifications of smaller doses of lead and where the cut off points or periods lie.

Mercury

Mercury is another substance which has been linked to negative outcomes in high quantities, but little is known of the effects of traces or small doses of mercury.

Disease

There is a great level of documentation of the effects of a variety of diseases on subsequent child development. The most thoroughly investigated teratogen is that of rubella, which has now been described and refined in terms of contact time (Sever, 1970; Kopp, 1983). It is unclear why some babies are unaffected. Effects relate mostly to sensory deficit (visual and auditory) aphasia, agnosia cataracts and heart defects. Other diseases, such as herpes, toxoplasma gondii, cytomegalovirus, syphilis and Human Immunodeficiency Virus have been related to microcephaly, retardation, general impairment, visual problems and immune deficiency. Where presence of these conditions is detected, avoidance or containment protocols are sometimes available (e.g. caesarian section in the presence of herpes simplex). When treatment is available (e.g. syphilis), screening is considered, with all its allied concerns and difficulties (see Chapter 12).

Man-made substances

Some man-made substances have been linked with developmental impairment. These include anti-convulsants (Riley & Vorhees, 1986), anticoagulants, testosterone and anaesthesic gases, sex hormones, lithium and even vitamins (Shaffer, 1988). They have been studied in terms of developmental effects, still birth, retardation, miscarriage and epilepsy. One substance which has been much studied is thalidomide, which has resulted in a very high level of limb defects, lifelong suffering and recently a case of a second generation effect. Diethylstilboestrol (DES) was a drug given to women who repeatedly miscarried. Only many years later was a connection found between DES ingestion and subsequent fertility and reproductive problems (Kelley Buchanan, 1988).

With any medication, it is important to differentiate the impact of the primary condition for which the medication is being taken and the effect of the medication itself. Furthermore, decision making about altering or desisting from the medication must weigh up the costs and benefits for both the mother and the baby.

Habit-forming substances

There is a wealth of literature on the effects on child development of alcohol, so-called recreational drugs and tobacco products (Butler & Golding, 1986). Streissguth, *et al.* (1989) examined the links between antenatal alcohol consumption and IQ of the child at 4 years of age. They concluded that a daily consumption of 44 ml during pregnancy related to an average decrement in IQ of 5 points. Fetal alcohol syndrome has dramatic implications. These effects can be seen as acute or chronic although it is unclear whether the syndrome is directly associated with ethanol transfer, or linked to the life stresses prompting the alcohol use in the first place. Whatever the mechanisms, learning disability and a range of distinctive features are often noted. A number of problems have been associated with hallucinogen and narcotic use (Shaffer, 1993), including sudden infant death, abnormalities, miscarriage and stillbirth. The study cautions for consideration of allied factors in these mothers, which may include malnutrition, illness or multiple teratogen exposure.

Nutrition

The lack of an adequate diet can initially reduce fertility and subsequently affect the development of the fetus. Nutritional problems can be caused because of poverty and inadequate availability of food, or because of poor placental functioning, which effectively restricts the amount of nutrition to the developing fetus. Cognitive impairment has also been documented, where protracted and severe malnutrition was present (McLaren, *et al.*, 1973). Yet such malnutrition usually indicates a variety of other problems, which may account for or at least contribute towards the problems themselves. These factors include the wider socio-economic problems occurring in the presence of malnutrition such as poverty, disease, family breakdown, low emotional support, war, ravages of disease, and other excessive environmental conditions. Malnutrition may also affect variables such as miscarriage and stillbirth. It is unclear whether the effects of malnutrition are irreversible.

Psychosocial factors

These cover a vast array of topics, some of which are covered in Chapters 5–7. The very presence of antenatal care and supportive systems has been associated with lower perinatal mortality.

Birth and delivery factors and their effect on development

Freud places a great emphasis on the passage of birth for later development. There is no empirical evidence to back such claims, but there is no evidence to refute them either. There are many variables which may contribute to factors during this period. They may emanate from the baby, from the mother, from the system, or from secondary sources such as medication given, time of day, availability of expertise and resources. Developmental problems as a result of birth and delivery factors may cover the following factors.

Anoxia at birth

Although severe anoxia is documented in terms of developmental inter-ruption, there is very little evidence which charts the severity of anoxia in terms of severity of handicap. Most studies are retrospective, following up children who have already been identified as experiencing problems. This means that all children who may suffer from episodes of oxygen restriction at birth have not been charted. The study methodologies utilized so far also make it difficult to ascertain whether it is anoxia which is the primary source of problems, or whether another unknown factor is linked to anoxia and this, in turn, contributes to developmental delay or interruption. There is no guidance about what period of anoxia is potentially harmful, although it is clearly known that at a certain level of deprivation, an infant is unlikely to survive.

Drugs given during childbirth

The use of anaesthesia during childbirth is increasing. Chamberlain (1975) showed that 70 per cent of birthing mothers used pethidine during childbirth. Regional and hospital figures vary. Some mothers are given multiple anaesthesia (such as entonox and pethidine) and it is difficult, if not impossible, to separate out or catalogue the individual effects if any exist. Pethidine, the most commonly used drug, has been studied exten-sively. Richards (1983) found that mothers who had pethidine had chil-dren with poorer reflexes; this in turn limited mother–infant interactions. Rosenblatt (1979) looked at infants with high pethidine absorption and found this group had a lowered Apgar score and the half life of the drug was in the region of 18 hours. It was also found that such babies were more likely to fuss at six weeks and were less easy to settle.

Behaviour at and around birth

There is much literature examining events at or around birth and their short- and long-term consequences on the child. These tend to focus on the early interactions of the mother and baby (and the corresponding deleterious effects of early separation of mother and infant: Klaus & Kennell, 1976). Other factors examine maternal handling of the infant (Sander, 1969) or infant temperament and behaviour. The infant may also contribute greatly to the individual situation. It is necessary to examine the complexity of the post partum period with an appreciation of the many complex and inseparable factors which may affect it.

Development can be studied according to various strands, such as motor development, cognitive development, perceptual development, social development or language development. However, the reality is that child development is a complicated interaction of all these threads which provides a diversity of progress for almost every child. Therefore, although it is helpful to consider developmental themes and stages, the range and variation is often dramatic. This text will only consider the young infant.

Social/environmental factors

The traditional debates on development have usually dichotomized progress as a result of either genetic or environmental causes. More current psychological theories attempt to integrate these positions. Firstly, there is no reason why genetic factors should be fixed. It is more helpful to respect the dynamic nature of the interaction between environmental and genetic factors and to perceive the infant as a vibrant, self shaping force.

Psychiatric disorders in the mother have often been examined in terms of susceptibility in the child (Andrews, *et al.*, 1990). Studies have consistently found links which may relate to the provision of parenting environments which are either interrupted or dispersed with chronic or intermittent disorder. Such situations can adversely affect the developmental environment and have been found to be associated with a greater rate of psychiatric disorders in children (Keller, *et al.*, 1986).

Schaffer (1977) describes in great detail the complex role played by the infant in social interactions. Such roles depend, to a large extent, on the infant's individual capabilities. Although infants are entirely dependent for their care, there is a need nonetheless to appreciate how sophisticated and developed their abilities can be, even when only a week old.

In order to interact socially, an infant must have an ability to perceive, orientate and maintain attention to social stimuli. The infant must be alert, responsive and exert some motor control to maximize input from social surroundings. Many studies on infant state have formed the basis for understanding early infant functioning (Brazelton, 1973), as they can affect the quantity and quality of function response. States can be affected by hunger, temperature, noise, light, movement and sound.

Newborn abilities

Newborn babies have a wide range of skills, including the ability to see, hear, smell, taste and respond to touch, pain and stimulation (Scarr & Dunn, 1987). Newborns also exhibit complex social behaviours. They smile to other humans, react differentially to their parents or primary caregiver, and they show preference to human faces over abstract shapes.

Many theories of infant development attempt to explain underlying abilities and the evolution of acquired cognitive skill. These theories can be divided into four categories:

- *Biological theories* These describe growth and maturation from the standpoint of pre-wired species.
- *Learning theories* Studies explain how development proceeds according to social learning, trial and error, punishment and praise paradigms.
- *Cognitive theories* These were developed by Kohlberg (1969) and Piaget (1952) and attempt to examine underlying cognitive networks and how they evolved.
- *Psychodynamic theories* These theories attempt to explain infant and child development in terms of needs, relationships, pleasure and emotions.

Despite total dependance, the newborn arrives with considerable skills. Some reactions have been monitored in utero such as turning reactions to sound and variation in movement pattern. Very young infants can show preferential turning towards and away from stimuli, be they auditory, olfactory or visual (McGurk, 1974). It seems that many of the infant abilities are only revealed with evolving sophistication in our ability to test or examine their behaviour.

From the age of 2 weeks, an infant will fixate, or scan moving images of subjects' faces, in preference to stationary images (Carpenter, 1974). Slater, *et al.* (1985) showed with a variety of experiments that newborns exhibited a high degree of visual organization with clear preference for moving stimuli. They even show longer fixation for faces rated as attractive by adult raters. Infants can modify the shape of their hands to correlate with the object they reach, although this ability is said to be dependent on visual or tactile experience of the objects (Pieraut Le Bonniec, 1985). Infants can also discriminate patterns of fine detail and show a preference for high density contrast or motion (Fantz, 1961, 1963).

Infants respond to auditory cues and show preference, quite early on, for known voices (Mills & Melhuish, 1974). Although it is unclear whether there is 'intention' behind such acts, it is clear that parents can infer intention and this sets up a process of attribution of meaning and corresponding emotional development.

Sophisticated methodologies have allowed researchers to catalogue the extent to which infants perceive and react to patterns. Such methods include measuring habituation, scanning patterns, attention fixation or behavioural reactions to various visual stimuli. Studies using the methodologies have highlighted that very young babies (within 48 hours of birth) can discriminate visual patterns. They appear to seek out patterns actively, showing preference for movement, contrast and human like features. By the end of the first year, babies can utilize such information and adjust their behaviour accordingly. Depth perception evolves fairly early and experiments which manipulate looming objects have shown that infants can react to depth and distance. Some studies have examined differential anticipatory hand shaping and have inferred that young infants can adjust their hand size according to stimulus object sizes. Most researchers emphasize the importance of sensory experience and learning in the evolving process of cognitive skill acquisition.

Although there is a wide range of work on visual perception, there are also indications of sophisticated evolving abilities in the domain of auditory perception. Young babies can recognize voices and show preferential turning to maternal voice. Acuity and the ability to distinguish slight variations in vowel sounds has been measured in very young infants. As children grow, their abilities to distinguish various sound patterns grow in sophistication. Shaffer (1993) postulates that infants have integrated senses from birth, evidenced by their negative reactions to sensory incongruities.

There are numerous environmental factors which may affect such evolving abilities. These include the effects of deprivations, the influence of cultural and environmental factors on form recognition as well as gender differences.

Early social interactions

Although early theory suggested that socialization was a process which was imposed on a seemingly blank or inactive child, more up to date psychological theory (Schaffer, 1985) has set out in detail a mutuality model, which represents the child as an active partner in social development. This sets up an interdependent social system in which the close and wider social environment are enjoined in a web effect, which allows simultaneously for a diversity of approach and an interrelationship between parental input and the contributions of the child.

Detailed studies of paired maternal/infant behaviour in very young infants have shown intricate and synchronized behavioural interactions. This meshing has been observed in feeding patterns, 'burst' (typified by a stage of activity followed by a pause), dialogue patterns, turn taking in communication with early vocalizations, visual and gestural contributions (Schaffer, 1977).

Language development is reliant upon conversational activity with proficient language users – be they parents or non parents, siblings or others. Babies can respond to speech from very early on, yet specific language skills take time to evolve. During this period of progress, there is a great variety of language and communication which predates speech. There are not absolute theories which explain language acquisition. Current theories focus on learning theories which emphasize the role of imitation and reinforcement. On the other hand, there are those theories which claim an innate language wiring. Interactionist theories explain language acquisition by an interplay between innate abilities and environmental learning.

Social relationships have been studied in terms of parents, siblings and peer groups. Any study of social integration and growth is also contingent upon an understanding of the infant's self perception. As the infant grows and matures, personality and moral development will form an integrated part of their self expression.

Temperament

The study of temperament has been an attempt to incorporate the lay views on disposition and the extent to which they may influence behaviour, development or interact with the quantity or quality of care received. Temperament seems to vary with time, situation and to evolve with age. Chess & Thomas (1987) have provided a descriptive framework for temperament that includes notions of different categories of child, as set out in Table 13.1.

Table 13.1   Chess & Thomas: framework for examination of infant temperament

Temperament cluster	Subjects '(percentage)
Easy child	40
Slow to warm up	15
Difficult	10
Uncategorized	35

Temperament also has implications for situational variables and blending. Problems were more likely to occur (Chess & Thomas, 1987) when difficult children, for example, were in a family context of conflict.

Parenting

There is extensive literature available on parenting, but on close examination it often refers to mothering only. Fathers are only just becoming involved in studies, reflecting changes in research rather than sudden change in paternal roles. Such maternal bias can be seen throughout the literature. For example McGuire (1991) states:

'Overall many parental characteristics may be relevant to prenatal child health, but a key area to focus on is a mother's attitude, both to herself as a potential parent and to the developing child'.

Such sentiments show scant appreciation of the effect the father may have (on both the child and the mother) and endorses a societal view that mothers should take both the responsibility and the blame for child rearing.

Developmental problems

There is a wide range of possible problems experienced by young and growing children. Congenital disorders are apparent at birth, yet they may only become noticeable at older age. Such disorders may arise from genetic or other factors. Handicaps, in a variety of forms, may pose a series of barriers and impairment in everyday life. The term 'handicap' has been replaced with 'special educational need' or 'challenges' in order to formulate the issues in terms of service, requirement and reaction, rather than stigma and negativity (see Chapter 14).

Psychological problems are exceedingly common in young children (Rutter, 1976). Indeed, most children show some psychological problems at some time during their lives, which either take the form of emotional or behavioural difficulties. These are often transient and seen as part of 'normal development'. Some problems are common within a given age group, but become cause for concern if they are present in another age group. All concerns must be viewed in terms of evolving development and with an understanding of age and society norms. If a problem persists or causes major concern, it is then that intervention is sought, as this reflects adult coping as an issue as well as child behaviour.

Children, especially young children, must be viewed within their environmental circumstance. Understanding comes from an analysis of assessment of the problems, in conjunction with an understanding of the levels of resulting limitations.

What is normal?

The concept of normality is complex, given that some behaviours are considered normal for some children and abnormal for others; normal in some circumstances and abnormal in others. Much of this variation relates to expectation, social and cultural norms and tolerance. Normality can change over time and is deeply influenced by current fashion, experiences, religious and legal factors, cultural norms and taboos.

What is fitting?

The next analysis to be made is whether the problem(s) fit the norm for the age and developmental stage of the child. Some behaviours are seen as problematic, not because of the behaviour per se, but because the child is too old to exhibit such behaviour.

Duration

Transient behaviour difficulties are much less of a worry than those which are maintained over extended time.

Situation

Life circumstances should always be examined when children's behaviour varies from the general or their own norm. Under stress, children may often revert to a behaviour pattern they have previously used. Situations that trigger such changes are usually those which are demanding, stressful, challenging and which create change or uncertainty. Some children associate different situations with different stresses, exhibiting symptoms within a confined situation but symptom free when outside of that situation.

Nature of the behaviour

The quality of the behavioural symptoms need to be examined. Generalized symptoms in multiple areas are more indicative of problems than isolated symptoms. The intensity and frequency of occurrence of the behaviours may also contribute to a classification of problems. Variations within the individual are often indicative of problems, if a child suddenly changes from their own norm.

Limitations caused by such behavioural problems can be considered according to the criteria of suffering, social restriction, interference with development and effects on others (Rutter, 1975).

Table 13.2 sets out the classification and description of different childhood disorders.

In summary, assessment for the presence of psychological disorders in children essentially entails an examination of the nature of the problem and the level of impairment it will cause.

Nature of the problem

The following criteria should be examined:

(1) The age and sex appropriateness of the behaviour.
(2) The level and degree of persistence of the problem.
(3) The life circumstance within which it occurs.
(4) The socio-cultural setting of the child.
(5) The extent of the disturbance.
(6) The type of symptoms which are being manifested.
(7) The severity of the symptoms and the frequency with which they occur.
(8) The extent to which this behaviour marks a change in the child's lifestyle and the nature of this change (was it sudden, dramatic or slow? What were the surrounding events such as the arrival of a new baby, commencement of school, mother going out to work, parental strain?).
(9) The situational triggers of the behaviour. This relates to an identification of which situations the behaviour occurs in and whether it is different (or absent) in other situations.

Table 13.2 Synopsis of childhood disorders

Syndrome	Description	Gender
Emotional Disorders		Sex distribution is said to be roughly equal. Some conditions are more frequent in girls in later adolescence.
Anxiety	May relate to fears and phobias specific or generalized. Emerges early and sometimes again at puberty as a result of stressful situational experience, observation, family learning, or insecurity.	
Depression	Unusual pre adolescence. Qualitatively different from adult experience. Often more transient and situation specific. Resembles adult experience more as child grows older. Physical symptoms less than in adults (such as early morning waking, weight loss, and reduced physical activity). Family history and environmental triggers may play a key role.	
Suicide	Rare in the pre-adolescent, increasing in adolescents.	
Obsessive Compulsive States	Typified by the ritual or constant use of compulsive actions or thought patterns. These are invariable, irrational and unreasonable and the child may well have insight into this and attempt to resist them. Often they are a coping mechanism specially in anxiety laden situations or times.	
Hypochondriasis	Complaints of physical illness, unjustified in symptoms or an exaggeration of symptoms, invariably internal aches and pains (headaches, tummy aches). May set up patterns of attention and stress avoidance together with the special rules of 'illness behaviour' which serve to reinforce the complaints and endorse learned patterns.	
Mutism	An uncommon condition but one where the child who is well able to speak, chooses to remain silent. Often linked to specific situations.	

Table 13.2 Continued

Syndrome	Description	Gender
Psychosomatic problems	These invariably result from extreme experiences of anxiety where the emotional problem is converted into physical symptoms and can result in severe symptoms such as paralysis or blindness. Other conditions such as asthma are thought to have possible psychological components.	
Hyperkinetic Syndrome	Abnormal motor function with marked overactivity. Markedly severe with early onset. Difficulties with maintaining attention and concentrating for any period of time. Highly distractable and uninhibited with many impulsive tendencies. Educational and learning problems are often profound and prognosis for severe problems is generally poor.	Affects boys greater than girls in a ratio of 4.5:1 (especially in the under 5s).
Childhood Autism	Present from early in infancy. Marked by delay and obstruction in language development, understanding, and functional use of language. Typified by an array of ritualized behaviours and marked by an impediment to evolve social relationships. Can be severe or mild. Mental retardation commonly associated. Usually a poor prognosis, but can be variable.	More common in boys than girls
Schizophrenia	Rarely seen until later adolescence. Marked by an insidious onset with bouts of perplexity, thought disorder or disturbance, altered interactions and relationships, emerging delusions, persecutory thoughts and onset of hallucinations. Not really considered prior to at least 7–8 years of age. Poor prognosis, and usually indicative of longer term adult problems.	Equal sex distribution
Enuresis	Comprises primary and secondary problems. Primary when the child has never learnt bladder control, and secondary when the child loses bladder control after an incident (such as the arrival of a new baby or a traumatic	

Table 13.2 Continued

Syndrome	Description	Gender
	event) Frequency surprisingly high (up to 20 per cent of 7 year olds in some thorough studies).	More common in boys than girls
Encopresis	This refers to problems of bowel control. It may include faeces retaining (constipation) which then results in abnormal bowel movements, masses and physical discomfort. On the other hand the child may have normal motions but may place them in random places or inappropriate places. Again, this can be primary or secondary. Primary for a child who has never attained bowel control and secondary for a child who has achieved bowel control but selectively loses it. Usually associated emotional distress and social reaction. Decreases as a function of age.	More common in boys than girls
Tics	These refer to quick movements, invariably involuntary and purposeless, in the absence of neurological deficits. They can be associated with situations (often stress perceived or stress inducing) and cause much social discomfort. Usually only come to clinic attention after about a year duration. Many recede spontaneously. Less likely to do so if associated with mental retardation or other conditions.	More common in boys than girls
Anorexia Nervosa	An eating disorder, associated with severe weight loss and sometimes associated with bulimia. Rarely present in very young children. Tends to be noted in adolescence. Numerous explanations and treatments including problems with facing adulthood, maturity or growing sexuality, behavioural control and family problems. Potentially life threatening disorder, sometimes associated with emotional disturbance in adulthood.	More common in girls than boys

Table 13.2   Continued

Syndrome	Description	Gender
Obesity	Nutritional disease with far reaching physical and psychosocial ramifications. The earlier on the onset occurs, the more likely the child will have problems as an adult. Uncertainty about aetiology and prognosis.	
Developmental disorders	Typified by specific delay in achieving developmental milestones. Notably associated with speech delays or disorders and corresponding reading retardation. Often runs in families.	More common in boys than girls.
Truancy	Non attendance at school is seen in Western societies as a problem. It is often divided into two groups, those who are not at school and not at home. The other group is at home either because they are kept at home (reflecting family or parental problems ramifying to the child) or reflecting a reluctance for the child to attend – often termed school refusal. This can be accounted for by numerous explanations. Social or travel phobias may make school attendance intolerable. Fear of school itself may prompt refusal, as would separation anxiety. It may also be a symptom of a more global social withdrawal.	
Conduct disorders	Typified by behaviours which meet with social disapproval. Commonly divided into: **Delinquent acts:** theft, truancy, arson, wilful damage (to property and person) **Non-delinquent acts:** fighting, bullying, lying, aggression. Generally poor prognosis. Often family background of disharmony, discord and/or inconsistent limits and discipline, multiple members. Often associated with reading difficulties, learning problems and educational delay. Also linked with personality problems in adult life.	More common in boys than girls

Level of impairment

The following points should be considered:

(1) The amount of emotional suffering caused should be examined, to the child him/herself and to the wider family and social group.
(2) The social restriction resulting from the problem should be examined.
(3) The extent to which the problem interferes with development must be assessed.
(4) Clearly the physical effect the problem has on the child and on others must be determined.

Interventions

Interventions with children can be short- or long-term. A variety of outcome studies have been reported (Quay & Werry, 1979). These cover individual interventions, family, or group work. Theoretical models on which interventions are based on numerous (Quay & Werry, 1979) and include behavioural, family, psychodynamic, cognitive and learning theories.

Aetiological factors

Numerous studies have been carried out to examine aetiology and prevalence. Whole population studies are superior to clinic audits, as the latter are not representative.

Some studies have examined factors associated with the various rates of disorder. These include the environment and the social circumstance in which the child grows up, marital relationships, parental psychiatric disorder, socioeconomic status and school factors. Although these factors do seem to be associated with level of disorder, it is unclear in what way they contribute and how they may be avoided.

Assessment tools

A variety of techniques have been employed in examining the nature and extent of childhood problems. These range from interview to a variety of forms of testing and observation.

All forms of assessment must be carried out with great care and attention so as to ensure that assessment tools are helpful, interviews are productive and no harm is caused. Traditionally, psychological assessment tools have been judged according to their standards of validity, the extent to which they are predictive, have content and construct validity.

Furthermore, they must be able to be repeated and administered accurately.

Implications for practice

A major goal of child health must be to encourage fulfilling childhood and to limit circumstances which may adversely jeopardize the child and the family. As such, there is an onus on health care workers to ensure, from the start, that fields of communication are open, that resources exist to assist parents in need and that routine provision is high on the agenda.

References

Andrews, B., Brown, G. & Creasey, L. (1990) Intergenerational links between psychiatric disorder in mothers and daughters. The role of parenting experiences. *J. Child Psychol. Psychiat.*, **31** (7), 115–29.

Brazelton, T. (1973) *Neonatal Behavioural Assessment Scale.* Heinemann Medical Books, London.

Bremner, J.G. (1988) *Infancy.* Blackwell Scientific Publications, Oxford.

Butler, N. & Golding, J. (1986) *From Birth to Five.* Pergamon, Oxford.

Carpenter, G. (1974) Visual regard of moving and stationary faces in early infancy. *Merrill Palmer Quarterly of Behavior and Development*, 20, 181–94.

Chalmers, I. & Richards, M. (1977) *Benefits and Hazards of the New Obstetrics.* Spastics International Medical Publications, London and Philadelphia.

Chamberlain, G. (1975) *Obstetrics.* Blackwell Scientific Publications, Oxford.

Chess, S. & Thomas, A. (1987) *Origins, Evolution and Behavior Disorders.* Harvard University Press, New York.

Dunlea, A. (1984) The relation between concept formation and semantic roles: some evidence from the blind. In *The Origins and Growth of Communications*, (Ed. L. Feagans, C. Garvey & R. Golinkoff). Ablex Publishing Corp, Norwood, New Jersey.

Fantz, R.L. (1961) The origin of form perception. *Sci. American*, 204, 66–72.

Fantz, R.L. (1963) Pattern vision in newborn infants. *Science*, 140, 296–7.

Keller, M., Beardslee, W., Dorer, D., Lauori, P., Samuelson, H. & Klerman, G. (1986) Impact of severity and chronicity of parental affective illness on adaptive functioning and psychopathology in children. *Archives of General Psychiatry*, 43, 930–37.

Kelley Buchanan, C. (1988) *Peace of Mind During Pregnancy.* Facts on File, New York.

Kimmel, C., Wilson, J. & Schumacher, H. (1971) Studies on metabolism and identification of the causative agent in aspirin teratogenesis in the rat. *Teratology*, 4, 15–24.

Klaus, M. & Kennell, J. (1976) *Maternal Infant Bonding.* Mosby, New York.

Kohlberg, L. (1969) Stage and sequence: The cognitive developmental approach to socialization. In *Handbook of Socialization, Theory and Research.* (Ed. D.A. Goslin), Skotie, Rand McNally.

Kopp, C. (1983) Risk factors in development. In *Handbook of Child Psychology Vol 2* (Ed. M. Haith & J. Campos). J. Wiley, New York.

Lansdown, R. (1988) *Child Development*. Heinemann Professional Publishing, Oxford.

McGuire, J. (1991) Sons and daughters. In *Motherhood* (Ed. A. Phoenix, A. Woollett and E. Lloyd). Sage, London.

McGurk, H. (1974) Visual perceptions in young infants. In *New Perspectives in Child Development* (Ed. Foss). Penguin, London.

McLaren, D., Yatkin, U., Kanawati, A., Sabbagh, S. & Kadi, Z. (1973) The subsequent mental and physical development of rehabilitated marasmic infants. *Jnl. of Mental Deficiency Rsrch*, 17, 273–81.

Mills, M. & Melhuish, E. (1974) Recognition of mothers' voices in infancy. *Nature*, 252, 123.

Piaget, J. (1952) *The Origins of Intelligence in Children*. International Universities Press, New York.

Pieraut Le Bonniec, G. (1985) Hand eye coordination and infants construction of convexity and concavity. *British Journal of Developmental Psychology*, 3, 273–80.

Quay, H. & Werry, J. (1979) *Psychopathological Disorders of Childhood*. John Wiley, Chichester.

Richards, M. (1983) *Parent Child Relationships: Some General Considerations in Parent Baby Attachment in Premature Infants* (Eds J. Davis, M. Richards, N. Robertson). Croom Helm, Kent.

Riley, E. & Vorhees, C. (1986) *Handbook of Behavioral Teratology*. Plenum, New York.

Rosenblatt, D. (1979) Unpublished PhD thesis.

Rutter, M. (1976) *Helping Troubled Children*. Penguin, London.

Sameroff, A. & Chandler, M. (1975) Reproductive risk and the continuum of caretaking casualty. In *Review of children development research Vol 4* (Ed. D. Horowitz, M. Hetherington, S. Scarr Salapatek & G. Slegel). University of Chicago Press, Chicago.

Scarr, S. & Dunn, J. (1987) *Mothercare Othercare*. Penguin Books, Harmondsworth.

Schaffer, H.R. (1977) *Interactions in Infancy*. Academic Press, London.

Shaffer, D.R. (1985) *Developmental Psychology*, Wadsworth.

Shaffer, D.R. (1993) *Developmental Psychology: Childhood and Adolescence*, 3rd edn. Brooks Cole, California.

Sever, J. (1970) Viruses and embryos. In *Congenital Malformations* (Ed. F. Fraser & V. McKinsick). Excerpta Medica, Amsterdam.

Slater, A., Morison, V., Town, C. & Rose, D. (1985) Movement perception and identity constancy in the new born baby. *British Jnl. of Developmental Psychology*, 3, 211–20.

Smith, P. & Cowie, H. (1988) *Understanding Children's Development*. Blackwell Scientific Publications, Oxford.

Streissguth, A., Barr, H., Sampson, P., Darby, B & Martin, D. (1989) IQ at age 4 in relation to maternal alcohol use and smoking during pregnancy. *Developmental Psychology*, 25, 3–11.

Chapter 14

Mental and Physical Problems

The taboo subject of the possibility of a handicapped child is rarely raised in antenatal classes. Yet the fear of handicap is often pervasive for all pregnant women. Much antenatal testing is set up to detect various forms of handicap. Few doctors or midwives have training in disability, yet when a baby is born with problems (physical or emotional), there is much help (practical and emotional) that can be offered to the parents – who invariably will provide the bulk of care and input, especially so in the early years of the child's life.

A child with a handicap is a child first and foremost who, secondly, has a handicap which affects some, but rarely all, of the aspects of their behaviour. Personality characteristics may be due to background factors, regardless of handicap. Invariably there will be a range of individual differences, whatever the condition. Handicaps themselves are not always single and not always simple in their effects. Often the presence or definition of a 'handicap' are subject to influences such as current knowledge, and societal views and attitudes. The boundaries and cut off points which define handicap are murky and may fluctuate with time as new information and new demands evolve. In their 1979 research, Wynn & Wynn estimated that there were a total of 130 000 severely handicapped children in the UK, with another 30 000 handicapped children being born each year. The origins of some handicaps are understood, but many are not. They may arise during pregnancy, at birth or postnatally. In general the earlier in development that the handicap originates, the more severe it is (Lewis, 1987).

Multiple handicaps

It is not uncommon for a child to have more than one handicap. For example, some children who are challenged by cerebral palsy may also have mental handicaps. Some children with handicaps may also have sensory disturbances or epilepsy. Rutter (1970) found that one in four of the children with handicaps had more than one challenge, of those 90 per cent who were found to be intellectually retarded had more than one problem and 29 per cent of those physically handicapped had a secondary problem.

Secondary handicap

Any handicap is likely to create limitations which further restricts the child's behaviour, either directly or indirectly. For example, a child with limb control problems may subsequently be limited in the extent they can indulge in exploration and learning. Behaviour problems are often seen as secondary to mental handicap, for example as a result of boredom or handling difficulties (Shakespeare, 1975).

Cultural context

All impairments should be viewed in terms of the society in which the handicapped child will live. Society will convey norms and values, provide a willingness or reluctance to help or reject and is ultimately responsible for the institutions and services which can aid or impede the problems.

Any condition in any individual can become a handicap if it causes a problem to the person or people they in turn live with. A disability is often categorized into mental or physical, which can be congenital or acquired. The reaction to a handicap in a child will vary according to multiple factors, as shown in Table 14.1.

The reaction of the staff to a handicapped infant can often be as intense as that of the parents (Davis & Fallowfield, 1991). Parents can be devastated when faced with the news that there is a problem with their child, whether this is given during pregnancy, at the birth or later. They will have to mourn the loss of their imagined child and adjust to the reality of a different child to the one they had been expecting (Davis & Cunningham, 1985). Although such reactions are often likened to a grief reaction, they differ in that whilst the grief may be ongoing, the emotional adjustment will have to be made in the presence of the baby, rather than in the absence or void often signified by the death of a baby. The caring needs of the baby are also demanding and the parent may be given little time to mentally accommodate the new situation.

Information plays a key role in adjustment and coping (Wilkinson, 1989). Parents require much information and sometimes never fully understand their child's condition. Information recall is often hampered by extreme emotional state when the news is broken. Care givers are usually available to give information in the early days, at the very time when parents are unable to digest fully the enormity of the news. Information and the availability of dialogue should be paced with their

Table 14.1   Factors affecting reaction to handicap

(1) Social	Circumstances including social class, family size, family support, age of child at the onset of problems and the demands their condition will engender.
(2) Emotional	Factors which encompass both the emotional temperament of the individual and their family and the emotional ramifications of the handicapping conditions.
(3) Preparedness	'Preparedness' is ongoing – it relies on information facilities and support.
(4) Economic	Factors such as income, housing and financial burden.
(5) Experience	Whether handicap has been previously experienced in the family, the extent to which the parents have a notion of care giving and the extent to which other care givers are able to assist the parents.
(6) Societal demands	This is the backdrop against which limitations may be noticed and which set the agenda of demands.
(7) Family	Attitudes, expectations and support from the family and for the family may be key factors in coping and adjustment. These in turn may directly affect the functioning of the individual child.

growing ability to concentrate, understand, formulate questions and address practical issues (Leventhal & Nerenz, 1983). Professional behaviour has been linked directly to parental adaptation (Woolley, *et al.*, 1989). Plans for the provision of information should include:

- *Explanations*, to assist in understanding with ongoing dialogue.
- *Details of help which is available*, including avenues of provision from formal and informal sources.
- *Expectations* of the parents may need to be discussed and realistic boundaries provided.
- The *impact* of the handicap on the child and the family will change over time and flexibility is needed to accommodate and adjust to their needs as and when they occur.
- *Future planning* should be an ongoing process, not the subject of a single discussion. Families should have a meaningful ongoing dialogue with carers to plan for short- and long-term input.
- *Action* is always preferable to complacency. Prevention, intervention and postvention all have a part to play.
- *Social functioning* can be directly affected. The child and the family may have severe restraints on even the simplest social activities such as visits, holidays or guests. Respite and assistance should be available to ameliorate this.

Table 14.2   Emotions and their related response to handicap

Emotion	Response
Grief	Bereavement reactions at the loss of the expected 'normal' baby.
Fear	Avoidance of the child, the issues, discussions or staff.
Revulsion	Distancing or rejection.
Confusion	Information seeking, placing blame.
Threat	Lowered self esteem. Fear of future handicap.
Shame	Isolation, avoidance, withdrawal.
Challenge	Over-reaction, pursuance of treatments, commitment to interventions.
Anger	Blame, self hate, relationship stress.
Positive emotions	Not all experiences are negative, and the whole process can be interspersed with joy, reward and love.

A wide range of emotions are experienced with related responses. These are outlined in Table 14.2.

Psychological effects of a handicap

There are many psychological ramifications for children with a handicap. These include:

Self concept
Early sensory motor restrictions may affect the ability to generate a meaningful self concept. Frustration at not being able to achieve every day or demanding tasks may additionally slow the process. Body image may be an integral part of a self concept and handicap may pose challenges for an individual who sees any differences between their ideal and actual self image.

Communication problems
These can be a primary effect of the handicap or can occur as a secondary factor because the child is spoken to less often. Communication challenges can occur at many levels, including language acquisition, com-

munication abilities, conversation difficulties, non verbal problems, interruptions and the usage and interpretation of cues.

Experience limitations
Experience is intricately laced into growth and development. Any limitation on experience may feed into allied development.

Realization of the handicap
For any individual child, realization and self awareness may come suddenly or slowly. Adjustment and accommodation may be affected by how they are told of their condition and how insight is gathered. If the handicapping condition is acquired later in life, there may be consistent differences from conditions which are congenital. In these sorts of situations, the child will have to alter a previously held self concept and range of abilities. If the gap is insurmountably wide, maladjustment may result. Reactions may include denial, anxiety, depression, withdrawal, fantasy and egocentricity (Ringness, 1961).

Marginality
Group affiliation factors. It has been found that those totally affected adjust better than marginally affected individuals.

Privacy
Privacy is a challenge for people who may be reliant on others for their tasks of daily living. They may have little occasion for privacy and may experience little control over their privacy and personal space.

Breaking the news
How a child is told that they have a handicap may dramatically affect their long-term reaction. Openness and frankness is the best policy. Overall satisfaction with disclosure is poor. Levels can, however, be enhanced by highly professional behaviour. Cunningham, *et al.* (1984) reported high satisfaction for parents who were informed that their child had Down's syndrome by paediatricians working with a model based approach.

Families of the handicapped

Children with problems are usually not isolated but function within a family, with whom they are intricately bound up from the moment of realization that they have a handicap. Even so, Hewett (1970) reports that a fifth of children questioned felt very isolated. Families will face a multitude of crises, such as decision making about the place of upbringing, overprotection, dissatisfaction with services, discipline problems, difficulties going out with the child, limited contact with other children and traumas at providing adequate stimulation over extended periods for a demanding child.

Studies such as Hewett (1970) and Rutter (1970) found effects on parental relationship such as strain, quarrelling, disharmony and higher divorce and separation rates. Siblings may also feel the effects from the demands made upon them by the other child, his/her needs, role in the family, consumption of family resources and attention. Indirectly, there may be effects with reluctance on the part of the sibling to bring friends to the home and some experience of jealousy, as well as love and caring.

Cognitive, motor and educational deficits are often concomitants of handicap, which can be hounded by problems of adequate and accurate assessment, difficulties resulting from absence from school and the interference of drug and drug effects on performance and learning.

Parents have been harnessed into the formal educational care of their children with varying levels of success (Davis & Cunningham, 1985). Studies have shown that parents can be more effective than therapists for a range of reasons. Parents may simply have greater opportunity and occasion for intervention. They may also be highly motivated and have greater influence and control. On the other hand, the strain and level of adaptation of the family can also be reflected in the educational attainments of the child and thus preventive strategies should ensure that families receive adequate and appropriate input and support. Davis & Cunningham reported great parental satisfaction with educational training and high levels of appreciation for support. Training and professional input not only impart skills which affect the child, but can also alter levels of the parents' commitment and confidence.

Davis & Fallowfield (1991) notes that needless distress can be caused to parents by professional behaviour, such as ill informed or hurtful remarks, brusque manner, patronizing approach, failure to listen and communication generally.

Coping with physical handicap and sensory handicap (visual or auditory impairment)

Physical handicaps in a young baby present a range of challenges. Often they differ from mental handicap in that they are visible (such as a cleft palate or cerebral palsy).

Visual and auditory impairment are present at birth or may become apparent during early babyhood (Lewis, 1987). Expectations about development and concomitant supplementary input will be reviewed.

Visual handicap

Visual problems are rarely total, and many visually challenged children do have some level of sight. Blindness has been defined for legal reasons and for educational needs. There is a wide range of children with different visual abilities and different needs. Progress is often linked to the form and nature of the visual impairment as well as its timing. In general, children who have had vision at some time (of any form) have different needs and abilities when compared to those with no vision and no previous vision. Some children may have visual impairment in addition to other problems and it is difficult to tease out which contributes to developmental patterns and how these interact. The child who has visual problems will need to gather information about the environment through touch and sound. Lewis (1987) summarizes the developmental implications as follows:

- A child with no sight will be slower to reach out.
- Mobility may be affected or delayed.
- Blindisms may develop – these are behaviours such as eye poking or body rocking and are explained in terms of autostimulation.
- Mobility is affected often by the lack of environmental incentives to movement and the environmental cues and aids for accurate navigation. Mobility does develop and is often linked with sound cues.
- Posture may be affected, as there is no input from observing others. Posture adaptation can be taught when the child is older.
- Perception and perceptual development in blind children has been studied. The commonly held belief that such children have greater acuity in non affected senses or a 'sixth sense' is untrue. What does seem to occur is that blind children utilize their non affected senses to perceive their world and gather environmental cues.
- Cognitive development may be directly or indirectly affected by visual problems. The problems themselves may limit the type and amount of information the child can integrate and assimilate. This may result in a very different understanding of objects and their relationships.
- Social development may be affected, although blind children have shown differential smiling to parental voices as early as four weeks old. However, an idea of permanence may be more difficult for a child relying on auditory cues, as visual cues are much more helpful in organizing experience. This may result in a great dependence on family by the child. Interactions can be affected by different or absence of non verbal cues, which often supplement social interactions. Lack of eye contact, facial response and a restricted environmental understanding may affect feedback loops and communication channels. Social interactions are often dependent on these; active effort and education may be required to adjust or compensate.
- Communication development may be affected by visual impairment. The ability to speak, however, will greatly facilitate other aspects of development, as the child can begin expression and enquiry. The obstacles to language development stem mainly from the fact that

people from whom the child will be assimilating language and words do not experience the environment in the same way as the child itself.

- Language development follows similar patterns to sighted children but may differ in content, with different word usage (Dunlea, 1984), different levels of asking for assistance and different rates of word increases (Burlingham, 1979; Willis, 1978). Continued development may show marked differences, especially in integrating pronouns and diversifying and generalizing concepts.
- Echolalia is often reported, which is the tendency to repeat all phrases heard. Urwin (1981) suggests that this serves to maintain dialogue channels.
- Reading development is a key to other areas of input. Braille reading, utilizing raised dots, is much harder than visual reading and thus may be acquired at a later age and result in a slower reading pace.

Hearing impairment

As with visual impairment, hearing loss is rarely total and usually refers to a wide range of abilities, varying in degree as well as in nature. Hearing impairment is difficult to measure in young babies. Developmental findings show:

- Motor development is similar in terms of gross motor milestones, but fine motor adjustments, particularly those utilizing balance, may differ in focus (Wiegersma & Van der Velde, 1983).
- Language development is a key skill. There are opinions which endorse the utilization of signing and those which encourage oral communication. The pros and cons are well articulated in texts such as Lewis (1987). The current challenge is to understand the processes of language acquisition when oral communication is not available. This will then give some insight into the complexity of the language ultimately acquired and of the possible intervention aids. If a deaf child has any residual hearing, the ability to use oral communication is greatly facilitated.
- Word acquisition has been studied and it appears that deaf children in some studies utilize many more social words than naming words. This can be explained in terms of priorities for interaction and seen as highly adaptive. Profoundly deaf children have significant barriers in acquiring language skills.
- Cognitive abilities in deaf children are difficult to measure, given that many tests are language bound. Deficiencies may reflect language barriers or language biases in responses, rather than true cognitive barriers. Measurements of cognitive performance on non verbal scales or tests that are not language dependent show a very similar range.

Lewis (1987) concludes that 'cognitive development can occur and does occur in the presence of poor spoken language skills'.

● Object concepts do seem to develop and it appears that sound is not an essential component, although it obviously aids the understanding of objects. What may differ is the route of development rather than the ultimate outcome.

● Thinking is often linked to language. There are diverging schools of thought which postulate that language and thought are or are not intricately dependent. Although it was initially thought that hearing impairment may resolve this, it is clear that even if language is not available in the generally recognized form, hearing impaired children may still have access to some form of language (such as signs) and this cannot resolve the issue.

● Reading and writing may be particularly difficult for deaf children. Lewis (1987) recommends that workers should concentrate on the level of comprehension and understanding for the deaf child who is reading, rather than simplistic judgments of how intelligible reading aloud is.

● Social interactions and relationships can be affected by hearing impairment. Many social problems are linked to communication. It is not surprising that allied behavioural difficulties are noted which reflect emotional frustration or confusion (Gregory, 1976).

Implications for practice

Handicap must be considered as one of the possible factors in pregnancy and childbirth. There needs to be clear exposure, learning and understanding for all staff so that parents in situations who face any challenging aspect associated with their baby can acquire insightful care. There is an extensive body of understanding which is constantly evolving. Such knowledge should feed into ongoing maternity services.

References

Burlingham, D. (1979) To be blind in a sighted world. *Psychoanalytic Study of the Child*, 34, 5–30.

Cunningham, C., Morgan, P. & McGucken, R. (1984) Down's Syndrome: is dissatisfaction with disclosure of diagnosis inevitable? *Developmental Medicine and Child Neurology*, 26, 33–9.

Davis, H. & Cunningham, C. (1985) Mental Handicap: People in Context. In *Personal Construct Theory and Mental Health*. (Ed. E. Batton). Croom Helm, London.

Davis, H. & Fallowfield, L. (1991) *Counselling and Communication in Health Care*. Wiley & Sons, Chichester.

Dunlea, A. (1984) The relation between concept formation and semantic roles: some evidence from the blind. In *The Origins and Growth of Communication* (Ed. L. Feagans, C. Garvey & R. Golinkoff), Ablex Pub., Norwood, New Jersey.

Gregory, S. (1976) *The Deaf Child and his Family.* George Allen & Unwin, London.

Hewett, S. (1970) *The Family and the Handicapped Child: A Study of Cerebral Palsied Children in their Homes.* George Allen and Unwin, London.

Leventhal, H. & Nerenz, D. (1983) A model for stress research and some implications for the control of stress disorders. In *Stress Reduction and Prevention* (ed. D. Meichenbaum & M.E. Jaremko), 5–38. Plenum Press, New York.

Lewis, V. (1987) *Development and Handicap.* Blackwell Scientific Publications, Oxford.

Ringness (1961) Self concept of children of low, high and average intelligence. *Am. Jnl. of Met. Deficiency,* 65, 453–61.

Rutter, M. (1970) *Helping Troubled Children.* Penguin, Harmondsworth.

Shakespeare, R. (1975) *The Psychology of Handicap.* Methuen, London.

Urwin, C. (1981) Early language development in blind children. The British Psychological Society Division of Educational and Child Psychology, Occasional Papers, 5, 78–93.

Wiegersma, P. & Van derr Velde, A. (1983) Motor development of deaf children. *Jnl. of Child Psychology and Psychiatry,* 24, 103–11.

Wilkinson, S. (1989) Psychological aspects of physical disability. In *Health Psychology* (Ed. A. Broome), Chapman & Hall, London.

Wills, D. (1978) Early speech development in blind children. *Psychoanalytic Study of the Child,* 34, 85–117.

Woolley, H., Stein, A., Forrest, G. & Baum, J. (1989) Imparting the diagnosis of life threatening illness in children. *BMJ,* 298, 1623–6.

Wynn, M. & Wynn, A. (1979) *Prevention of Handicap and the Health of Women.* Routledge and Kegan Paul, London.

Index